Advanced Neuroimaging: From Theory to Clinical Practice

Advanced Neuroimaging: From Theory to Clinical Practice

Editor: Miles Scott

AMERICAN
MEDICAL PUBLISHERS
www.americanmedicalpublishers.com

AMERICAN
MEDICAL PUBLISHERS
www.americanmedicalpublishers.com

Cataloging-in-publication Data

Advanced neuroimaging : from theory to clinical practice / edited by Miles Scott.
p. cm.
Includes bibliographical references and index.
ISBN 978-1-63927-855-8
1. Nervous system--Imaging. 2. Brain--Imaging. 3. Brain--Magnetic resonance imaging.
4. Brain--Tomography. 5. Neurology. I. Scott, Miles.
RC349.D52 A38 2023
616.804 754--dc23

American Medical Publishers,
41 Flatbush Avenue,
1st Floor, New York,
NY 11217, USA

ISBN 978-1-63927-855-8 (Hardback)

Contents

Preface

This book has been a concerted effort by a group of academicians, researchers and scientists, who have contributed their research works for the realization of the book. This book has materialized in the wake of emerging advancements and innovations in this field. Therefore, the need of the hour was to compile all the required researches and disseminate the knowledge to a broad spectrum of people comprising of students, researchers and specialists of the field.

Neuroimaging uses quantitative (computational) techniques to study the form and function of the central nervous system in a non-invasive manner. It is used extensively in studies concerning brain disorders and psychiatric diseases. Clinical neuroimaging is used for identifying tumors, strokes, brain injuries, and neurodegenerative diseases. Conventional neuroimaging techniques include computed tomography (CT) and magnetic resonance imaging (MRI). There are two major categories of neuroimaging, namely, structural imaging that focuses on quantifying brain structure and functional imaging, which is used to study the functions of CNS. Medical practitioners also make use of advanced neuroimaging techniques to obtain functional information with respect to the pathophysiology of different CNS disorders. Advanced neuroimaging techniques include diffuse optical imaging (DOT), event-related optical signal (EROS), functional magnetic resonance imaging (fMRI), magnetoencephalography (MEG), positron emission tomography (PET), single-photon emission computed tomography (SPECT), etc. This book discusses the theoretical and clinical aspects of neuroimaging. It will also provide interesting topics for research in neuroimaging, which interested readers can take up. This book is a complete source of knowledge on the present status of this important field.

At the end of the preface, I would like to thank the authors for their brilliant chapters and the publisher for guiding us all-through the making of the book till its final stage. Also, I would like to thank my family for providing the support and encouragement throughout my academic career and research projects.

Editor

1

Functional MRI of Awake Behaving Macaques Using Standard Equipment

Reza Farivar and Wim Vanduffel

1. Introduction

Functional magnetic resonance imaging (fMRI) is perhaps the most important development in the measurement of human brain function in recent neuroscience history. The technique allows for noninvasive whole-volume measurements of brain function in humans and repeatable non-invasive measurement of activity over the whole brain, providing a correlate of neural activity without use of tracers or electrodes. Well-developed commercial MRI systems with built-in support for functional imaging are widely available, as are a plethora of tools, both free and commercial, for the analysis of human functional brain images. The combination of non-invasiveness and the broad availability of equipment and tools to perform fMRI have made this technique popular and broadly adopted.

While human fMRI can go a long way to answering fundamental questions about organization of function in the brain, much of the information we obtain from fMRI is correlative—for example, while activity in an area may correlate with a task, it is impossible to assume that the activity *causes* the observed behaviour. In order to draw causal links between brain function and behavioural performance, it is necessary to directly alter the brain either prior to or during fMRI. While some coarse techniques exist to manipulate human brain function, such as transcranial magnetic stimulation, non-invasive methods comparable to localized chemical deactivations (Liu, Yttri et al. 2010) and local electrical microstimulation (Tolias, Sultan et al. 2005; Ekstrom, Roelfsema et al. 2008; Moeller, Freiwald et al. 2008; Ekstrom, Roelfsema et al. 2009) in the monkey do not exist for human imaging, and direct microstimulation or temporary deactivation by cortical infusion in a normal human subject is ethically unthinkable.

Studying brain function in humans alone is also limiting in that very little is known about the structure of the human brain—at least when compared to what we know about the macaque brain, for example. Axonal tracing requires local injection of a tracer molecule followed by death and histological analysis, all of which is ethically infeasible in humans. In monkeys, this data has provided for a rich map of connectivity that can not only aid us in interpreting single-cell and fMRI results, but also formalize relationships between brain regions that can then be tested directly with temporary deactivation. For example, recently Schmid, Mrowka et al. (2010) used fMRI in awake-behaving macaques to demonstrate the neural basis for blind-sight —the residual visual capacity following loss of primary visual cortex (see (Leopold 2012 for a review). The anatomical basis for blind-sight has long been hypothesized to be the branching connections of the lateral geniculate nucleus of the thalamus (LGN) to other visual areas—in other words, while the V1 input to the cortical visual hierarchy is lost following ablation of V1, other visual areas receive indirect input via the thalamus. This hypothesis had not been directly tested, until Schmid et al. (2010)—that study was made possible by the fact that the projections of the LGN to the cortex are well known in the monkey.

Functional MRI in awake-behaving macaques thus affords us the possibility of studying primate brain function in a well-defined model (i.e., well-defined structure and connectivity) and to perturb the cortex using causal manipulations such as temporary deactivation, electrical microstimulation, or optogenetic manipulation (Boyden, Zhang et al. 2005; Gerits, Farivar et al. 2012). However, a number of challenges must be overcome to carry out a successful awakebehaving macaque fMRI study. Some aspects are general to animal neurophysiology studies— need for restraint, training, behavioural monitoring, etc.—while other aspects are unique to performing studies in the MRI scanner. These include the need to refrain from use of metallic material near the head, even if non-magnetic due to potential eddy current artifacts (Bernstein, King, et al. 2004), as well as issues pertaining to radio frequency (RF) noise, animal movement during scanning, motivation to perform specific behavioral tasks, environmental constraints for these tasks, etc. In this chapter, we begin with a comparison of human and monkey fMRI to highlight some of the differences and continue to discuss some of our solutions to the challenges of functional MRI with awake-behaving macaques. We close by discussing some unique possibilities afforded by fMRI in awake-behaving macaques.

1.1. Primate imaging and human comparison

A typical fMRI session with a human subject may follow this pattern: the participant is debriefed on both the experiment and aspects of the MR imaging, particularly noise issues and the importance of remaining still in the scanner. The participant's questions are answered and the experimenter, with the help of another individual typically, sets up the subject in a commercially available, clinical-grade head coil, places cushions around the subject's head and sometimes restrains the subject further by using a bite bar. The subject's behaviour may be monitored during the scanning as the subject tries to cooperate with the instructions given, and after each run, the experimenter talks with the subject to make sure all is well. During the scan, the subject does his utmost not to move and to pay attention to the task or stimuli, as requested by the experimenter.

A typical scan with an awake monkey may go a little differently: the experimenter restrains the monkey from his cage—good pole and collar training can go a long way to reduce this first step in a long line of frustrating steps. The animal is placed in an MR-compatible chair, and his head is subsequently restrained using an implanted headpost that is then attached to the chair. Custom-made RF coils are then placed around the animal's head and tested on a vector network analyzer to ensure adequate performance. The animal is water restricted to increase its motivation to participate, but the level of motivation will vary depending on various factors, such as time of day being scanned, frequency of being scanned, amount of prior training in a simulator box, etc. During the scan, the animal receives juice reward for performing the required task, whether central fixation or more complicated tasks requiring response by way of eye movements or hand manipulations. While a well-trained monkey will perform this task well above 90% of the time, the animal will make many fast movements during a given scan. During some runs, for unclear reasons, the animal may choose not to behave according to training, and often after a short break, good behaviour returns to standard.

In short, a great deal changes between scanning humans and monkeys, and they begin with the fact that one has a cooperative human subject, and an innately uncooperative monkey who may do what you ask (most of the time) in return for juice. The monkey makes many more movements during a scan despite the fact that his head is rigidly fixed to the chair, and this has a strong negative influence on image and data quality, regardless of whether he performs his trained task.

1.2. Issues of particular relevance to imaging awake non-human primates

In this section, we will briefly discuss some of the demands of functional imaging in awake animals, and then discuss some of our solutions in meeting those demands.

First, we need a stable preparation. By stability we mean two different things—that the animal moves as little as possible, and that its performance during a scan is consistent. The movement of the animal requires means of head restraint that balance animal comfort with robust restraint against movements. Importantly, the means of head restraint must be fully MRcompatible, precluding use of metals anywhere near the brain. The head restraint method depends on a stable platform, typically the primate chair, which also needs to be non-magnetic and mechanically stable. The aspect of stability pertaining to the performance of the animal requires extensive training outside of the magnet which can last months to a year, depending on the specifics of the task, with conditions as comparable to the MRI conditions as possible— i.e. with simulated MRI noise at the same level as that of the MRI, same distance to screen, etc. The training regimen should also aim to create a stable pattern of performance for a reasonable amount of time (typically 2-6 hours). In other words, the animal should be occupied with a specific task throughout an entire scan, otherwise in absence of a task at hand, it may resort to fast movements which are detrimental to the quality of the images.

Second, we need high performance receive coils to pick up the small signal changes acquired during functional imaging scans. The coil design and layout are limited by the first requirement outlined above, namely that the coils must work around the head restraint employed. Importantly, given the drop in the signal-to-noise ratio (SNR) as a function of the distance between the coil and the subject (Mispelter, Lupu et al. 2006) the coils must be placed as close to the animal's head (brain) as possible. There is the added challenge of the monkey's jaw muscles that add considerable distance between the coils placed at the sides and the brain.

Third, we need to image at high spatial and temporal resolutions. Both require fast imaging methods which can be realized with high-speed and high-powered gradient systems and parallel imaging using phased array receive RF coils (Roemer, Edelstein et al. 1990; Kimmlingen, Eberlein et al. 2004). While standard gradients (i.e., G ≈ 45mT/m and SR ≈ 200mT/m/s) on most 3-Tesla scanners can be sufficient to image volumes as small as 1.5x1.5x1.5mm, faster (>400mT/m/s) and stronger (>70mT/m) gradients allow us to encode voxels as small as 0.5x0.5x0.5mm (Janssens, Keil et al. 2012; Kimmlingen, Eberlein et al. 2004). Multi-channel Phased array RF coils allow us to speed up the acquisition of a single image even further by acquiring multiple image fragments simultaneously (Roemer, Edelstein et al. 1990; Kimmlingen, Eberlein et al. 2004). These increases in speed and performance are important both to minimize image acquisition artifacts and to mitigate the effects of subject movement.

Finally, given that functionally-relevant signal fluctuations are a small (<5%) of the overall signal and their fidelity may be further compromised by the increase in spatial and temporal resolution, we will need to find ways to enhance the strength of our functional signals. While some of this may be achieved through specific experimental designs, MR contrast agents—specifically MION (mono-iron oxide nanoparticles; Mandeville, Marota et al. 1998; Vanduffel, Fize et al. 2001, Leitte et al 2002)—can boost the functional signal drastically, by 3-4 fold at 3-Tesla.

1.3. Access to specialized equipment

A major appeal of our approach is that it does not require large-scale specialized equipment, such as a dedicated animal MRI. Our techniques can be easily incorporated in any standard clinical scanner, preferably 3-Tesla system with multiple receive channels. While dedicated animal-only MRI systems certainly have their own merit, the cost of such systems, above the costs of clinical-grade scanners that are available at many research facilities, prohibits their purchase by all but the wealthiest institutions.

2. Our approach

Below we outline the basic setup used for primate imaging in our group. We begin with a discussion of animal restraint because other aspects of the setup are restricted by this component.

2.1. Animal restraint

A now-common method of head restraint for neurophysiology studies involves attaching a metal post directly to the skull with titanium screws which tend to fuse to bone tissue (Betelak, Margiotti et al. 2001; Adams, Economides et al. 2007). Metallic objects close to the head would preclude any attempt to image the brain due to strong susceptibility artifacts (Matsuura, Inoue et al. 2005), and thus this method has been modified to make it appropriate for use in the MRI environment (Logothetis, Guggenberger et al. 1999; Vanduffel, Fize et al. 2001). In place of titanium screws, especially made ceramic screws (zirconia) are used that result in very little noticeable susceptibility artifacts (Logothetis, Guggenberger et al. 1999; Scherberger, Fineman et al. 2003). The screws form a contact with the skull and the headpost is not directly held in place with these screws but instead it is embedded in acrylic that also embeds the ceramic screws. We have found that when used as a base material around the screws, a highly pure poly(methyl methacrylate) formulation (C & B METABOND) can result in a much more rigid and stable headpost preparation. In this way, a rigid connection is established between the headpost and skull (Betelak, Margiotti et al. 2001).

The head is then held in place using the headpost which is attached to the chair. The chair and the headpost holder are all made of non-metalic material, usually acrylic sheets and ultem components where rigidity and high tolerance against cracking is necessary—acrylic, while very rigid, cracks under force. Ultem components retain rigidity while being more resistant to cracking and breaking under pressure. It is important to note that several alternative methods of invasive head restraint have been proposed and used (e.g. Pigarev, Nothdurft et al. 1997; Keliris, Shmuel et al. 2007).

The design of the chair must take into account the placement of the RF coils, eye illumination, juice reward, as well as any other experimental attachments necessary. These items must be rigidly attached such that they interact very little with one another and are not disturbed by animal movements. As we will discuss further below, the rigidity of the RF coils is key to stable measurements, and the chair design must take this into consideration (AppliedPrototype 2011).

In our experience, an approach that balances animal comfort with strong restraint is key. Many researchers may find that too much restraint, such as additional restraint on limbs, may make the animal uncomfortable and result in reduced cooperation and thus performance. A welcomed contribution to this area is the development of non-invasive head-restraint methods, such as that recently developed by Srihasam and colleagues (Srihasam, Sullivan et al. 2010). This method does not require implanting of headposts while promising an adequate restrain on the head for animals without additional head apparatuses, such as recording wells.

2.2. Coil designs

Magnetic resonance signals are weak—the ratio of nuclei in the low energy state to high energy state, which is directly proportional to the strength of the measured resonance signal, is on the order of 0.0031% even at very high field strengths (e.g., 9.4T; De Graaf 2007, p. 7). This means that accurate and robust measurement of resonance signals requires sensitive RF coils. Coil sensitivity is affected by a number of factors, such as choice of conductor, size of the coil, and most importantly, distance of the coil to the brain. With reduced coil size (i.e, ~4cm diameter instead of >10cm diameter for human head coils) and close proximity to the brain (a tight-fitting coil rather than a one-size-fits-all helmet as used for humans), one can optimize coil sensitivity, but this comes at the cost of reduced field of view (FOV; e.g., Logothetis, Merkle et al. 2002). This reduced FOV is compensated by using an array of coils such that each coil becomes sensitive to one part of the brain, and the combination of all the coils together image the entire brain (Roemer, Edelstein et al. 1990). An added benefit of so-called multi-channel phased arrays is that image acquisition time can also be accelerated by a method analogous to image-tiling (Pruessmann, Weiger et al. 1999; Sodickson, Griswold et al. 1999). While this does reduce the image SNR by up to 33% (Dietrich, Raya et al. 2007), it benefits us by allowing for faster imaging which (a) reduces image deformations, (b) allows us greater temporal resolution, and (c) grants us a greater degrees of freedom in our statistical analysis. In short, with parallel imaging we can make more measurements in less time with a small sacrifice in image SNR (de Zwart, van Gelderen et al. 2006).

We now almost exclusively use phased-array coils in our studies because of the advantages listed above. Phase-array coils for human applications typically make use of a helmet design for a complete sampling of the head (e.g., Wiggins, Triantafyllou et al. 2006), but in our experience helmet designs for monkeys pose difficulties due to obstruction by the headpost. In place of a helmet, a two-paddle design has many advantages, such as being easy to place over the head of many different monkeys and allowing them to be placed tightly around the head, thus maximizing the sensitivity of the coils. We now routinely use both 4-channel (two paddles with two channels each; e.g. Khachaturian 2010) and 8-channel coils (two paddles with 4 channels each), with the latter allowing for up to 3-fold acceleration as well. The receive channels are paired with a local transmit coil placed just above the head.

Because fMRI measurements can be heavily affected by temporal noise in addition to image SNR, it is imperative that the RF coils are rigidly placed so as to minimize movement or vibration (Roemer, Edelstein et al. 1990; Mispelter, Lupu et al. 2006). This applies to both the transmit coils and the receive channels. Vibration of the transmit coil can produce variations in the transmit field, adding temporal noise to our measurements (Mispelter, Lupu et al. 2006). Vibrations of the receive channels also adds temporal noise because movement of the receive coils away from the brain has the effect of changing the intensity of the signal detected by the coil, thus bringing about large changes in image intensity (Mispelter, Lupu et al. 2006). The receive channels are designed for use at a specific distance to the brain (Mispelter, Lupu et al. 2006), and changes in this distance will negatively affect the sensitivity of the coil which will result in both a decrease in signal and an increase in noise.

2.3. Sequence setup

The ideal functional imaging sequence would grant us high resolution, geometrically veridical images with high SNR at very short intervals. There is unfortunately a delicate balancing act as parameters that increase our resolution also decrease our SNR and prolong our imaging time while decreasing image veridicality. It is impossible to prescribe imaging parameters as this will vary depending on the setup at hand, the types of coils used (single loop or phased arrays), the performance of the gradients, the desired resolution, and finally, the type of signal measured. Discussion of these parameters is beyond the scope of this chapter, but a few general guidelines are helpful in animal imaging.

Given the size of the monkey brain as compared to the human brain (80 compared to 1250cm^3; Gonen, Liu et al. 2008), voxel sizes used in humans (typically 2-3mm isotropic) would tend to be far too large for use in primate imaging as they would obstruct many small details of importance in the functional maps. While one may strive towards voxel sizes of 1mm or less, slightly above that is acceptable for imaging macaque brains. The size of the voxel is dictated by the size of the imaging matrix, which in turn dictates how many voxels are to be measured in a given slice. Naturally, the larger the matrix size, the longer it will take to complete an image. The time to acquire one 2-D image depends on a number of factors, including matrix size, echo time, bandwidth, partial Fourier encoding, parallel imaging, amongst others (Bernstein, King et al. 2004). Thus it is not feasible to provide a formula to calculate acquisition time of one slice as it depends on a number of factors, many of which are also dependent on available hardware specifications. In general, however, increasing the matrix size increases echo time (TE) and the slice acquisition time—the increasing TE causes increased image blurring and image deformation and increasing slice acquisition time decreases temporal resolution (Bernstein, King et al. 2004). While for BOLD imaging at 3T the optimal TE is around 30 msecs (Fera, Yongbi et al. 2004), with MION contrast agents, one can decrease the TE to below 20 msecs (Leite, Tsao et al. 2002; Leite and Mandeville 2006), allowing for faster slice acquisition, which decreases image deformations and permits higher temporal resolutions.

Because even a well-restrained animal will move during acquisitions, the effect of movements on image acquisition must be carefully considered (Goense, Whittingstall et al. 2010). For example, as is typical of many fMRI studies, we routinely use interleaved acquisition whereby odd slices are acquired first prior to even slices. However, if an animal moves during single frame, then the odd and even slices are misaligned and standard 3d registration methods will be unable to correct for this. Worse, the misalignment can then propagate through the time series if slice-time correction is performed on the dataset (Sladky, Friston et al. 2011). Fortunately, a simple solution to this problem is to image in plane of head motion. For example, head restrained animals generally make very few lateral movements or rotations, but can use their bodies to push and pull their heads—thus the plane of motion is mainly sagittal. If one were to acquire horizontal or coronal slices, then such motion would pass through multiple slices and it would be impossible to visualize the motion and correct for them, since each slice is also acquired at a different time point. However, by acquiring sagittal slices, one can take optimal images of the movements and correct for them by applying 2-D slice-by-slice registration such as that offered by 2dImgReg of the AFNI toolset (Cox 1996). This correction can be done prior to slice-time correction so as to minimize the effects of head shifts in the sagittal plane on the rest of the dataset.

3. Preprocessing steps

A typical preprocessing stream for human functional data involves slice-time correction, 3D motion correction, and 3 Gaussian smoothing of the data prior to statistical analysis (Ashby 2011; Strother 2006). While the same steps may be used for processing of primate data, a few optimizations can be made.

As described above, by taking sagittal slices one can image the movements of the monkey head more adequately and correct for the 2-D movement using freely available tools from the AFNI toolkit (namely 2dImgReg). This software tool allows the specification of one image to serve as the "base" image—an image where no motion was present between the two interleaved passes. Individual slices from the series are then registered to their target slice in this base image using only 2-D image registration. The result generates x,y and pitch rotation for each slice. Slice-based correction can improve 3-D registration because the latter cannot deal with situations where motion occurs during the acquisition of a volume and this can introduce errors in the 3-D correction (Kim, Boes et al. 1999). Thus while we have only begun to use 2-D in-plane realignment to correct for rapid head motion of the monkey, its utility has been previously demonstrated in human fMRI (Kim, Boes et al. 1999), although it is not widely used in that field.

Because it is customary to include motion-realignment parameters in the general linear model as nuisance variables, the output of 2-D in-plane registration per slice poses a problem because we typically have 50+slices, and thus would have over a 150 parameters to include in our model. This impractical setup can be avoided by reducing the movement parameters using principal components analysis—since the motion in all the slices will likely be largely correlated, reducing them with principle components analysis will likely yield a good estimate of 2-D head motion that can then be used in the general linear model.

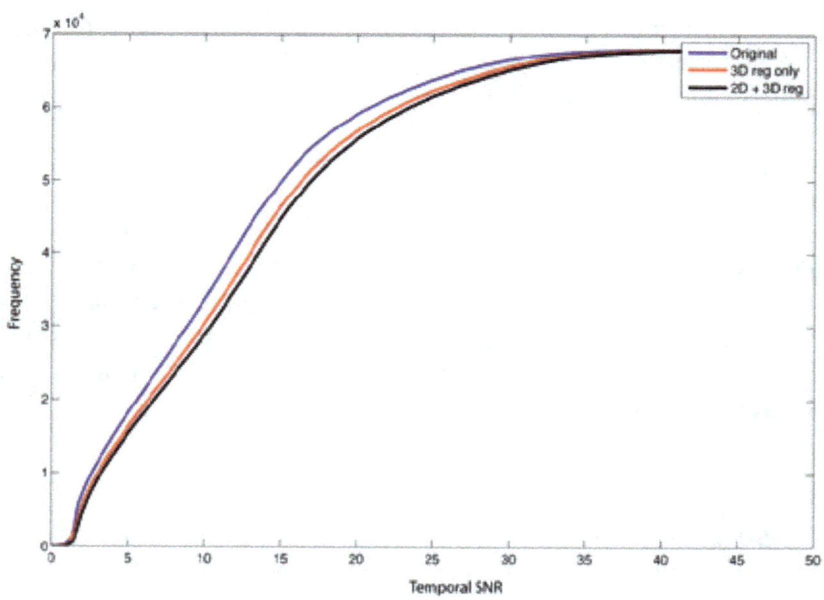

Figure 1. Cumulative histogram of voxel temporal SNR across different realignment strategies. The blue line depicts cumulative SNR without any motion correction. The red line depicts standard 3-D rigid motion correction, while the black line depicts the additional gain made by in-plane 2-D followed by 3-D rigid motion correction. 2-D in-plane registration can therefore improve temporal SNR, while the largest gain is made by 3-D rigid registration.

We can describe the potential sensitivity gain of such preprocessing steps by estimating temporal SNR, defined as time-course mean divided by time-course standard deviation

(Constantinides, Atalar et al. 1997). The cumulative histogram below (Figure 1) describes such a gain when using 2-D image realignment with sagittal slices followed by 3-D realignment, as opposed to the classic 3-D realignment typically performed. Over the entire volume of the brain (a crude measure), there is a gain of approximately 9% in temporal SNR by performing 3-D realignment, but this increases to an approximately 14% gain when it follows 2-D registration. Thus 2-D in-plane registration of sagittal slices followed by 3-D registration is a more appropriate strategy for image registration than classic 3-D realignment for motion correction.

Slice-time correction follows this 2-D motion correction because now the slices in the time series should be correctly aligned in space, permitting a meaningful correction to be performed in time. It is common to use sinc interpolation to correct for slice-time differences, but this method can propagate errors such as sudden changes in voxel values through the entire time series. It is thus advisable to use slower, more robust interpolators, such as Fourier or spline interpolators. Again, the AFNI tools offer a range of interpolators that can be used in place of sinc, as realized by the 3dTshift tool.

Three-dimensional movements, including lateral movements (if any) can then be corrected using any of a number of motion-correction tools—almost every package incorporates a motion correction algorithm, while a recent comparison (Oakes, Johnstone et al. 2005) suggests that those used by two of the more popular packages, namely SPM and AFNI, are quite comparable in performance, while the latter is substantially faster. Indeed, the AFNI tool 3dvolreg substantially outperforms SPM in 3-D motion realignment in speed and yields comparable results while not requiring the Matlab software package.

4. Functional-anatomical registration: Image deformation correction

Echo planar imaging (EPI), the method of choice for functional imaging, is prone to image deformations that can make the registration of the images to anatomical targets challenging (Farzaneh, Riederer et al. 1990; Andersson, Hutton et al. 2001). This is an issue that affects all EPI methods and animal imaging is no different. A number of solutions exist that either minimize deformations by acquiring segments of images more rapidly, or correct those deformations using informed or uninformed methods (i.e., using additional information about the imaging conditions obtained during the acquisition, or not).

First, a common method used to reduce deformation is to segment a single image into two or more pieces, and acquire each piece separately (Butts, Riederer et al. 1994). This method of segmented EPI is implemented prior to image reconstruction and involves acquiring interleaved lines of *k*-space in separate passes. The effect is that in each pass, very little time is spent acquiring the given lines, thus deformations are minimized. By acquiring multiple separate segments, the entire image is constructed out of minimally deformed acquisitions and the resulting image has high anatomical veridicality (Logothetis, Merkle et al. 2002; Goense, Whittingstall et al. 2010). The method, however, prolongs overall acquisition time substantially and is strongly vulnerable to even slight movements that would set the k-space lines out of alignment—thus it is very challenging to perform this with awake behaving animals. Using a more conventional single-shot method, one could also acquire an entire image with a smaller matrix—thus a lower resolution—which would reduce deformations but the decreased resolution has many other disadvantages including reduced anatomical veridicality (Bernstein, King et al. 2004).

Because of the challenges of effectively reducing deformations at the acquisition side, a number of efforts have been made to correct for deformations after acquisition. Here, two categories of approaches can be considered—the informed and uninformed methods. An informed method makes use of independent additional information about the deformations, such as a field map (Jezzard and Balaban 1995; Andersson, Hutton et al. 2001) to correct for them. The main idea behind the field map method is to acquire another un-deformed image at the same resolution and position as the deformation-afflicted images, and then calculate the degree of deformation between the ideal and acquired images. This deformation field map can then be used to correct deformations in all the functional images. The field-map method has proven generally satisfactory in human imaging, but for animal imaging it poses a serious challenge because it of the difficulty of making a stable field-map in an awake animal (see Jezzard 2012 for a review).

An interesting new development involves estimating deformations by measuring them in opposite directions (Holland, Kuperman et al. 2010). In echo-planar imaging, deformations are mostly in the phase-encoding direction (Jezzard and Balaban 1995). The method of Holland et al. (2010) involves acquiring two images in opposite phase-encoding directions. This means that each image will have deformation in the direction opposite to the other image (compression in one image will correspond to expansion in the other image). The balance between these two images would then be the un-deformed image, and the deformation map estimated from these two images can then be applied to the entire dataset. Furthermore, entire datasets or sessions can also be acquired in opposite phase-encoded directions to minimize imaging bias and combined so as to maximize overall image SNR— by combining minimally deformed voxels from forward and reverse phase-encoding directions.

4.1. 3-D Diffeomorphic demons correction

Image deformations can also be corrected by using the information available in the image itself in absence of secondary sources. In general, linear registration methods, such as affine registration methods that allow for translation, rotation, scale and shear, do not adequately correct for image deformations and one needs to make use of non-linear registration methods to achieve a good match between an EPI stack and an anatomical image. There are many non-linear methods that can be used to improve registration (for a review, see Zitova and Flusser 2003), but a danger of over-fitting is always present, as is the danger of creating new features —for example, if a gyrus in the functional image happens to fall closer to a sulcus after affine registration, some non-linear registration methods may force a dent in the gyrus to match the target image. We have found that non-linear registration using diffeomorphic demons (Vercauteren, Pennec et al. 2009) produces satisfactory and efficient results. The original demons algorithm (Thirion 1998) treats the registration problem as one of heat diffusion (an analogy to Maxwell's demons). In this formulation, the boundaries of the target image are considered permeable membranes that allow for the diffusion of the source (moving) image through the permeable interfaces by effectors (agents) in the membrane or image contour. The source (moving) image is warped on a deformable grid, which maintains spatial relations between image elements. When combined with diffeomorphism (Chef d'Hotel, Hermosillo et al. 2002; Vercauteren, Pennec et al. 2009), which treats two images as manifolds with a differentiable one-to-one displacement field between them, the diffeomorphic demons algorithm (Vercauteren, Pennec et al. 2009) provides for an efficient non-linear multimodal (i.e., EPI to T1-weighted) registration method. This registration method ensures that the spatial order of voxels is maintained during registration, so as to prevent excessive compression or expansion of features in the image. Figure 2 demonstrates the advantage of 3-D diffeomorphic registration of an EPI volume to an anatomical target, as opposed to a 12-parameter affine registration.

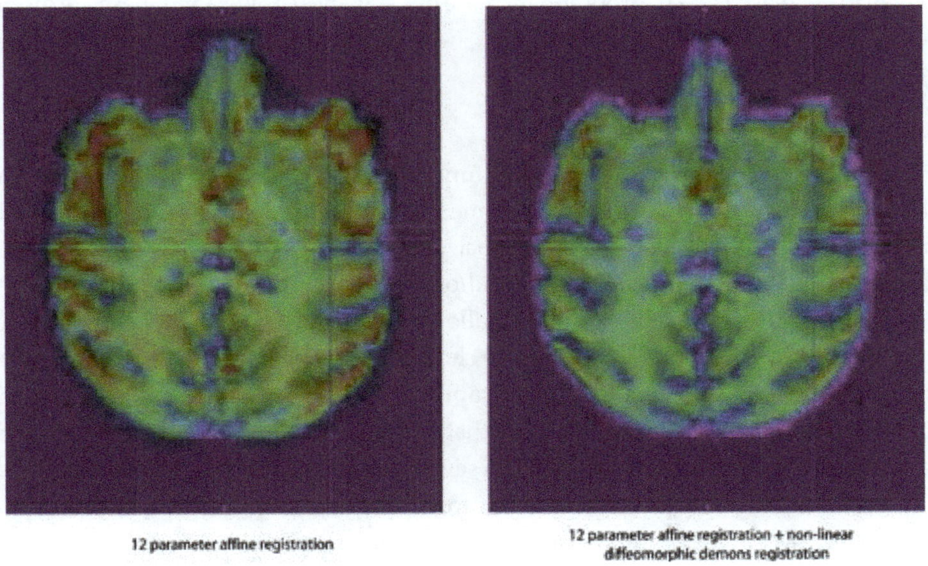

Figure 2. Comparison of 12-parameter affine registration (translation (x,y,z), rotation (pitch, roll, yaw), scale (ax,ay,az) and shear across x,y & z) with or without non-linear diffeomorphic registration for an EPI acquired with left-right phase encoding. The areas in red are regions that are poorly registered.

While EPI images in general have a very different contrast compared to MPRAGE anatomical images, images acquired with MION are even more different. This mismatch of the intensity distributions in the image can negatively affect the image registration. Hence it is useful to either use a mutual-information minimization strategy that avoids intensitybased matching, or modify the contrast profile of the T1-weighted anatomical such that it has a contrast comparable to the MION EPI images. In other words, we substitute a different image intensity look-up table such that the T1-weighted image looks more similar to a MION EPI image. The contrast profile or look-up table of an image may be modified through any of a number of image processing tools, including the Image Processing toolbox in Matlab or with the freely available Slicer package and its Histogram Matching module.

5. Statistical analysis

For the most part, statistical analysis of macaque functional images follows the same methods as those used in human imaging (Friston, Holmes et al. 1995). Specifically, the general linear model is used to make estimates of differential brain activity by convolving a known impulse response function, in our case the MION response function (Leite, Tsao et al. 2002; Leite and Mandeville 2006), with the onset of the stimulation events and adjusted for the duration of those events. The model response profile for all conditions are then fitted to the high-pass filtered data and the beta values estimated for two conditions are compared and tested for statistical significance with various corrections in place to reduce the possibility of Type I errors, such as Bonferroni correction, Gaussian Random Field (Worsley and Friston 1995), or false discovery rate (Benjamini and Hochberg 1995). However, a few additional steps can go a long way to decrease Type II errors and increase our statistical power, and these are discussed below.

5.1. Artifact rejection

The most overlooked but important aspect of functional image analysis is to simply look at the raw data and verify data quality. This may come as a daunting task, given the seemingly large amount of data. Yet a number of popular packages offer very simple methods of quickly assessing data quality with visual inspect and/or by quantitative methods. For example, the volume viewer in the FSL package (fslview) allows one to quickly load and animate through an entire functional volume time series while checking through in multiple orthogonal views for artefacts. The AFNI viewer allows one to rapidly click through voxels to visually check for unexpected signal changes. It is almost a fact that image fluctuations will occur when working with an awake and behaving animal, but the severity of the changes can be quickly assessed with these tools. Indeed, it is of great value to familiarize oneself with these tools to also evaluate the efficacy of the entire preprocessing stream.

A number of formal methods can be used to select and remove outliers from the dataset on the basis of additional data, such as behaviour of the animal, or based on movement estimates obtained from motion-correction tools (Goense, Whittingstall et al. 2010). In general it is preferable to exclude "bad" volumes from the analysis rather than correct for them, because the degree and effectiveness of any correction is hard to evaluate and indeed, some "corrections" may actually add more noise to the data than they remove. At least both AFNI's and SPM's GLM analysis tools (the latter via the ART repair toolkit; Mazaika, Hoeft et al. 2009) allows for exclusion of outliers. The ART repair tool readily allows for exclusion (or de-weighting) of the outlier volumes from the GLM analysis, with outliers selected on the basis of movement parameters and average signal intensity. In contrast, AFNI's GLM tool, 3dDeconvolve, allows for exclusion of volumes on any basis, allowing the experimenter to select volumes based on external measurements such as animal behaviour as well as on image realignment parameters, etc.

5.2. Behavioural and motion regressors

The exclusion of outliers can have drastic effects on reducing the noise in a dataset. Another approach is to reduce non-white noise by providing estimates of noise sources and incorporating this in the GLM analysis as regressors of no interest (Friston, Williams et al. 1996; Lund, Madsen et al. 2006). It is common and quite effective to include movement estimates obtained during motion correction in the GLM model. Additional regressors can be included, such as behaviours of no interest (e.g. saccades made during a fixation task) or external estimates of motion or jaw movement. A challenge with including regressors of no interest is that one does not know a priori how the regressors correspond to changes in voxel intensity values. For example, head movements will likely affect voxel values, but whether the direction of change or its magnitude or even its pattern would correspond to the movement estimates is not clear. In general, inclusion of additional estimates of noise sources does reduce variability in a dataset and is therefore recommended.

An approach that we are currently investigating is the inclusion of variability estimates obtained from non-brain tissue. In this approach, a brain mask is inverted to only select nonbrain voxels. Using principle components analysis, we then estimate a limited number of components that explain the majority of non-brain time-course variance. Finally, we include these estimates as regressors of no interest in the GLM analysis. In effect, we treat non-brain tissue as samples of noise, and estimate the main sources of this noise by reducing the data with principle components analysis. We assume that there are fewer noise sources than nonbrain voxels, and that the various noise sources result in correlated extraneous signals across multiple voxels. Based on these assumptions, we can then seek to estimate the noise sources by estimating principle components of the time-course of non-brain voxels, which will highlight noise components that may be distributed across a number of voxels. Noise signals may arise from eye, head, or jaw movement, or instabilities in the RF coil. The figure below (Figure 3) describes the amount of variance explained in the brain by non-brain components. Note that the components well capture the large fluctuations in the jaw muscles and the eyes, but also capture a significant amount of variability in the brain. This method is still under investigation, but it seems a quite promising method to reduce variability in time course data.

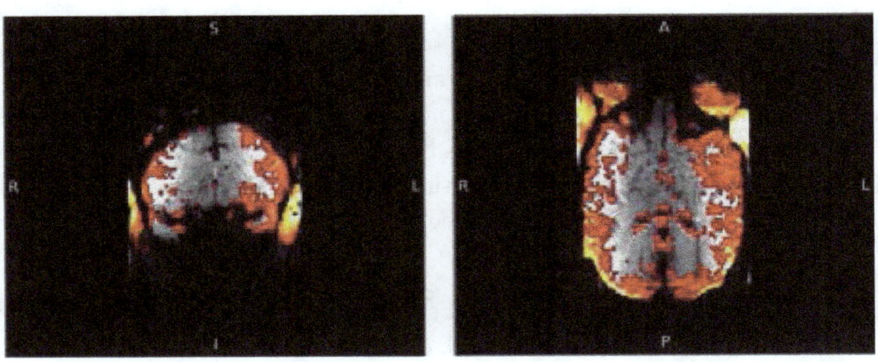

Figure 3. Variance explained by 20 non-brain principle components (corrected FWE < 0.05)

5.3. Experimental design strategies to minimize movement of an uncooperative animal subject

A major challenge of working with animals is that one has to motivate them to perform the task at hand. Typically this is done by restricting their fluid intake so that they are motivated to work for a liquid reward during the scans. However, even then it can be difficult or impossible to completely ensure the animal complies with the experimenter's wishes. The optimal solution involves motivating the animal so that it works for fluids, habituating it to the scanner environment by training it frequently in a simulated scanner environment, and minimizing the effect that its movements can have on the experiment itself. We routinely habituate our animals for months before the actual scans, and even then they are habituated in the scanner for a number of scans before their performance compares to that obtained outside of the scanner. The animal restraint, as discussed above, must be balanced against animal comfort given that the animal may be restrained for several hours at a time.

6. Combining methods with fMRI

While functional imaging in macaques bridges a crucial gap in comparing the function of human and non-human primate brains (Vanduffel, Fize et al. 2002; Orban, Fize et al. 2003; Orban, Claeys et al. 2005; Nelissen, Vanduffel et al. 2006; Kolster, Mandeville et al. 2009), a major advantage of working with an animal model is the ability to directly manipulate the brain to assess the causal interactions of brain networks. Our lab and others have now successfully implemented electrical microstimulation of the brain simultaneous with functional imaging to assess the role of FEF microstimulation on the cortical response to simple and complex visual stimuli (Ekstrom, Roelfsema et al. 2008; Ekstrom, Roelfsema et al. 2009), stimulation of face-selective patches in the macaque cortex (Moeller, Freiwald et al. 2008) and role of microstimulation in the propagation of information in the cortex more generally (Tolias, Sultan et al. 2005; Logothetis, Augath et al. 2010). The information obtained by this combination could not have been garnered using other methods, such as single-unit recordings, as this would require simultaneously measuring over large swaths of cortex—a task that is virtually impossible.

Another important development is the temporary deactivation of a brain area to assess its role in a more complex network. The application of muscimol, a GABA agonist, to temporarily shut down an area is now common and many labs have successfully applied this to measure the effect of deactivation on behaviour and single-unit responses. Our lab has now extended this to use with fMRI to allow us to measure both the brain response and its correlated behavioural change (Gerits, Wardak et al. 2009).

In addition to temporary deactivation, a number of groups have successfully combined local cortical lesions with fMRI. Pinsk, Moore, et al. (2005) were first to demonstrate feasibility of performing fMRI in awake-behaving macaques with straiate cortex lesions. Lesions to the striate cortex in humans lead to a phenomenon termed "blindsight" (see Leopold, 2012, for a recent review). Blindsight patients are essentially unaware of visual stimulation, yet they are able to respond to such stimuli without conscious awareness. Pinsk, Moore et al. (2005) were first to demonstrate that following striate cortex lesions, the extrastriate visual cortex continues to be responsive to visual stimuli as measured by fMRI. This finding was later corroborated by Schmid, Panagiotaropoulos et al. (2009) who showed that V2 and V3 in awake-behving macaques with focal striate lesions continue to be responsive to visual stimulation, albeit at 70% the pre-lesion rate, when measured with fMRI. They further demonstrated that retinotopy in V2 and V3 corresponding to the lesion in V1 did not change, suggesting that post-lesion activity in these areas was not driven by peri-lesion V1. This further highlighted the possibility that blindsight is mediated by sub-cortical inputs. Shmid et al (2010) provided the conclusive evidence that blindsight is mediated by sub-cortical inputs to extrastriate cortex—specifically the LGN. Using fMRI in awake-behving macaques with striate lesions, they first corroborated earlier findings of Pinsk et al (2005) and Schmid et al. (2009) and demonstrated that extrastriate cortex remains active following striate cortex, but at a lower level. They then temporarily deactivated the LGN with a GABA agonist while measuring the responses of the visual cortex of the macaques using fMRI. They found that deactivation of the LGN in striate-lesioned macaques completely abolished the residual response of the extrastriate cortex to visual inputs as well as residual behavioural function. This was the first direct evidence that projections from LGN to extrastriate cortex allow for blindsight to occur, and demonstrates the power of combining fMRI with causal manipulations to answering fundamental questions in systems neuroscience.

An exciting new development by our group is the integration of optogenetic methods (Boyden, Zhang et al. 2005) with fMRI in awake-behaving macaques (Gerits, Farivar et al. 2012). We have demonstrated that optogenetic stimulation of the frontal eye fields results in activation in a number of cortically-connected nodes, and for the first time, that optogenetic stimulation in primates can affect behavioural performance—in our case, saccade latency in a visually-guided task (Gerits, Farivar et al. 2012). These results are important for the further development and refinement of optogenetic methods to select sub-population of neurons in the cortex and evaluate their contribution to global brain activity as well as behaviour.

While fMRI provides images of population neural activity based on indirect measures, it is possible to combine it with simultaneous electrophysiological recordings (Logothetis, Pauls et al. 2001; Logothetis, Kayser et al. 2007; Oeltermann, Augath et al. 2007). This combination helps overcome an important challenge in interpreting the fMRI response and provide a confirmation and an additional metric of the underlying neural processes. However, a more practical approach is to use fMRI to guide subsequent electrophysiology outside of the MRI (e.g. Tsao, Freiwald et al. 2006; Freiwald and Tsao 2010). Of course, this does not allow for direct links to be made between BOLD signal fluctuations and underlying spiking activity, but it does allow for more refined examination of a patch of tissue identified by fMRI using single-cell recordings.

7. Impact and future directions

Functional MRI is useful for measuring activity over the whole brain, for identifying regions of importance for subsequent analysis, for assessing brain-wide effects of lesions, deactivations, or selected stimulations. Performing fMRI in awake-behaving macaques is not trivial and requires reconsideration of a number of factors, including restraint, training, coil design, image acquisition, data pre-processing, and additional refinements of the statistical analysis steps. Implementation of the solutions described above contributes to the feasibility of performing fMRI in awake-behving macaques, which opens the door to answering a large number of questions in systems neuroscience. The power of this utility is best realized when combined with temporary causal manipulations of cortical function, such as combining with electrical or optogenetic stimulation or with temporary and/or permanent deactivation, or in conjunction with single-cell recordings to understand in detail the contribution of single cell responses to behavioural outcomes.

Author details

Reza Farivar[1,2] and Wim Vanduffel[1,3]

1 Massachusetts General Hospital and Harvard Medical School, USA

2 McGill Vision Research Unit, McGill University, Canada

3 Katholieke Universiteit Leuven, Belgium

References

[1] Adams, D. L., J. R. Economides, et al. (2007). "A biocompatible titanium headpost for stabilizing behaving monkeys." J Neurophysiol 98(2): 993-1001.

[2] Andersson, J. L., C. Hutton, et al. (2001). "Modeling geometric deformations in EPI time series." Neuroimage 13(5): 903-919.

[3] Applied Prototype. (2011). "Vanduffel/HMS fMRI chair." from http://appliedprototype.com/AppliedPrototype/Vanduffel.html.

[4] Ashby, F. G. (2011). Statistical analysis of fMRI data. Cambridge, Mass., MIT Press.

[5] Benjamini, Y. and Y. Hochberg (1995). "Controlling the false discovery rate: A practical and powerful approach to multiple testing." Journal of the Royal Statistical Society, Series B (Methodological) 57: 289-300.

[6] Bernstein, M. A., K. F. King, et al. (2004). Handbook of MRI pulse sequences. Amsterdam ; Boston, Academic Press.

[7] Betelak, K. F., E. A. Margiotti, et al. (2001). "The use of titanium implants and prosthodontics techniques in the preparation of non-human primates for long-term neuronal recording studies." J Neurosci Methods 112(1): 9-20.

[8] Boyden, E. S., F. Zhang, et al. (2005). "Millisecond-timescale, genetically targeted optical control of neural activity." Nat Neurosci 8(9): 1263-1268.

[9] Butts, K., S. J. Riederer, et al. (1994). "Interleaved echo planar imaging on a standard MRI system." Magn Reson Med 31(1): 67-72.

[10] Chef d'Hotel, C., G. Hermosillo, et al. (2002). Flows of diffeomorphisms for multimodal image registration. IEEE International Symposium on Biomedical Imaging. Constantinides, C. D., E. Atalar, et al. (1997). "Signal-to-noise measurements in magnitude images from NMR phased arrays." Magn Reson Med 38(5): 852-857.

[11] Cox, R. W. (1996). "AFNI: software for analysis and visualization of functional magnetic resonance neuroimages." Comput Biomed Res 29(3): 162-173.

[12] De Graaf, R. A. (2007). In vivo NMR spectroscopy : principles and techniques. Chichester, West Sussex, England ; Hoboken, NJ, John Wiley & Sons.

[13] de Zwart, J. A., P. van Gelderen, et al. (2006). "Accelerated parallel imaging for functional imaging of the human brain." NMR Biomed 19(3): 342-351.

[14] Dietrich, O., J. G. Raya, et al. (2007). "Measurement of signal-to-noise ratios in MR images: influence of multichannel coils, parallel imaging, and reconstruction filters." J Magn Reson Imaging 26(2): 375-385.

[15] Ekstrom, L. B., P. R. Roelfsema, et al. (2008). "Bottom-up dependent gating of frontal signals in early visual cortex." Science 321(5887): 414-417.

[16] Ekstrom, L. B., P. R. Roelfsema, et al. (2009). "Modulation of the contrast response function by electrical microstimulation of the macaque frontal eye field." J Neurosci 29(34):10683-10694.

[17] Farzaneh, F., S. J. Riederer, et al. (1990). "Analysis of T2 limitations and off-resonance effects on spatial resolution and artifacts in echo-planar imaging." Magn Reson Med 14(1): 123-139.

[18] Fera, F., M. N. Yongbi, et al. (2004). "EPI-BOLD fMRI of human motor cortex at 1.5 T and 3.0 T: sensitivity dependence on echo time and acquisition bandwidth." J Magn Reson Imaging 19(1): 19-26.

[19] Freiwald, W. A. and D. Y. Tsao (2010). "Functional compartmentalization and viewpoint generalization within the macaque face-processing system." Science 330(6005): 845-851.

[20] Friston, K. J., A. P. Holmes, et al. (1995). "Statistical parametric maps in functional imaging: A general linear approach." Human Brain Mapping 2(4): 189-210.

[21] Friston, K. J., S. Williams, et al. (1996). "Movement-related effects in fMRI time-series." Magn Reson Med 35(3): 346-355.

[22] Gerits, A., C. Wardak, et al. (2009). Behavioral and brain-wide functional consequences of reversible LIP inactivation during visual search. Society for Neuroscience Annual Meeting, Chicago, IL, Online.

[23] Gerits, A., R. Farivar, et al. (2012). "Optogenetically Induced Behavioral and Functional Network Changes in Primates." Curr Biol.

[24] Goense, J. B., K. Whittingstall, et al. (2010). "Functional magnetic resonance imaging of awake behaving macaques." Methods 50(3): 178-188.

[25] Gonen, O., S. Liu, et al. (2008). "Proton MR spectroscopic imaging of rhesus macaque brain in vivo at 7T." Magn Reson Med 59(4): 692-699.

[26] Hackensack, NJ, Imperial College Press ; Distributed by World Scientific.

[27] Holland, D., J. M. Kuperman, et al. (2010). "Efficient correction of inhomogeneous static magnetic field-induced distortion in Echo Planar Imaging." Neuroimage 50(1): 175-183.

[28] Janssens, T., B. Keil, et al. (2012). "An implanted 8-channel array coil for high-resolution macaque MRI at 3T." Neuroimage 62(3): 1529-1536.

[29] Jezzard, P. (2012). "Correction of geometric distortion in fMRI data." Neuroimage 62(2): 648-651.

[30] Jezzard, P. and R. S. Balaban (1995). "Correction for geometric distortion in echo planar images from B0 field variations." Magn Reson Med 34(1): 65-73.

[31] Keliris, G. A., A. Shmuel, et al. (2007). "Robust controlled functional MRI in alert monkeys at high magnetic field: effects of jaw and body movements." Neuroimage 36(3): 550-570.

[32] Khachaturian, M. H. (2010). "A 4-channel 3 Tesla phased array receive coil for awake rhesus monkey fMRI and diffusion MRI experiments." J Biomed Sci Eng 3(11): 1085-1092.

[33] Kim, B., J. L. Boes, et al. (1999). "Motion correction in fMRI via registration of individual slices into an anatomical volume." Magn Reson Med 41(5): 964-972.

[34] Kimmlingen, R., E. Eberlein, et al. (2004). An easy to exchange high performance head gradient insert for a 3T whole body MRI system: First results. Procedings of International Society for Magnetic Resononacne Medicine. 11.

[35] Kolster, H., J. B. Mandeville, et al. (2009). "Visual field map clusters in macaque extrastriate visual cortex." J Neurosci 29(21): 7031-7039.

[36] Leite, F. P. and J. B. Mandeville (2006). "Characterization of event-related designs using BOLD and IRON fMRI." Neuroimage 29(3): 901-909.

[37] Leite, F. P., D. Tsao, et al. (2002). "Repeated fMRI using iron oxide contrast agent in awake, behaving macaques at 3 Tesla." Neuroimage 16(2): 283-294.

[38] Leopold, D. A. (2012). "Primary visual cortex: awareness and blindsight." Annu Rev Neurosci 35: 91-109.

[39] Liu, Y., E. A. Yttri, et al. (2010). "Intention and attention: different functional roles for LIPd and LIPv." Nat Neurosci 13(4): 495-500.

[40] Logothetis, N. K., C. Kayser, et al. (2007). "In vivo measurement of cortical impedance spectrum in monkeys: implications for signal propagation." Neuron 55(5): 809-823.

[41] Logothetis, N. K., H. Guggenberger, et al. (1999). "Functional imaging of the monkey brain." Nat Neurosci 2(6): 555-562.

[42] Logothetis, N. K., J. Pauls, et al. (2001). "Neurophysiological investigation of the basis of the fMRI signal." Nature 412(6843): 150-157.

[43] Logothetis, N. K., M. Augath, et al. (2010). "The effects of electrical microstimulation on cortical signal propagation." Nat Neurosci 13(10): 1283-1291.

[44] Logothetis, N., H. Merkle, et al. (2002). "Ultra high-resolution fMRI in monkeys with implanted RF coils." Neuron 35(2): 227-242.

[45] Lund, T. E., K. H. Madsen, et al. (2006). "Non-white noise in fMRI: does modelling have an impact?" Neuroimage 29(1): 54-66.

[46] Mandeville, J. B., J. J. Marota, et al. (1998). "Dynamic functional imaging of relative cerebral blood volume during rat forepaw stimulation." Magn Reson Med 39(4): 615-624.

[47] Matsuura, H., T. Inoue, et al. (2005). "Quantitative analysis of magnetic resonance imaging susceptibility artifacts caused by neurosurgical biomaterials: comparison of 0.5, 1.5, and 3.0 Tesla magnetic fields." Neurol Med Chir (Tokyo) 45(8): 395-398; discussion 398-399.

[48] Mazaika, P., F. Hoeft, et al. (2009). Methods and Software for fMRI Analysis for Clinical Subjects. Human Brain Mapping.

[49] Mispelter, J., M. Lupu, et al. (2006). NMR probeheads for biophysical and biomedical experiments : theoretical principles & practical guidelines. London

[50] Moeller, S., W. A. Freiwald, et al. (2008). "Patches with links: a unified system for processing faces in the macaque temporal lobe." Science 320(5881): 1355-1359.

[51] Nelissen, K., W. Vanduffel, et al. (2006). "Charting the lower superior temporal region, a new motion-sensitive region in monkey superior temporal sulcus." J Neurosci 26(22): 5929-5947.

[52] Oakes, T. R., T. Johnstone, et al. (2005). "Comparison of fMRI motion correction software tools." Neuroimage 28(3): 529-543.

[53] Oeltermann, A., M. A. Augath, et al. (2007). "Simultaneous recording of neuronal signals and functional NMR imaging." Magn Reson Imaging 25(6): 760-774

[54] Orban, G. A., D. Fize, et al. (2003). "Similarities and differences in motion processing between the human and macaque brain: evidence from fMRI." Neuropsychologia 41(13): 1757-1768.

[55] Orban, G. A., K. Claeys, et al. (2005). "Mapping the parietal cortex of human and non-human primates." Neuropsychologia.

[56] Pigarev, I. N., H. C. Nothdurft, et al. (1997). "A reversible system for chronic recordings in macaque monkeys." J Neurosci Methods 77(2): 157-162.

[57] Pinsk, M. A., T. Moore, et al. (2005). "Methods for functional magnetic resonance imaging in normal and lesioned behaving monkeys." J Neurosci Methods 143(2): 179-195.

[58] Pruessmann, K. P., M. Weiger, et al. (1999). "SENSE: sensitivity encoding for fast MRI." Magn Reson Med 42(5): 952-962.

[59] Roemer, P. B., W. A. Edelstein, et al. (1990). "The NMR phased array." Magn Reson Med 16(2): 192-225.

[60] Scherberger, H., I. Fineman, et al. (2003). "Magnetic resonance image-guided implantation of chronic recording electrodes in the macaque intraparietal sulcus." J Neurosci Methods 130(1): 1-8.

[61] Schmid, M. C., S. W. Mrowka, et al. (2010). "Blindsight depends on the lateral geniculate nucleus." Nature 466(7304): 373-377.

[62] Schmid, M. C., T. Panagiotaropoulos, et al. (2009). "Visually driven activation in macaque areas V2 and V3 without input from the primary visual cortex." PLoS One 4(5): e5527.

[63] Sladky, R., K. J. Friston, et al. (2011). "Slice-timing effects and their correction in functional MRI." Neuroimage.

[64] Sodickson, D. K., M. A. Griswold, et al. (1999). "Signal-to-noise ratio and signal-to-noise efficiency in SMASH imaging." Magn Reson Med 41(5): 1009-1022.

[65] Srihasam, K., K. Sullivan, et al. (2010). "Noninvasive functional MRI in alert monkeys."Neuroimage 51(1): 267-273.

[66] Strother, S. C. (2006). "Evaluating fMRI preprocessing pipelines." IEEE Eng Med Biol Mag 25(2): 27-41.

[67] Thirion, J. P. (1998). "Image matching as a diffusion process: an analogy with Maxwell's demons." Med Image Anal 2(3): 243-260.

[68] Tolias, A. S., F. Sultan, et al. (2005). "Mapping cortical activity elicited with electrical microstimulation using FMRI in the macaque." Neuron 48(6): 901-911.

[69] Tsao, D. Y., W. A. Freiwald, et al. (2006). "A cortical region consisting entirely of face-selective cells." Science 311(5761): 670-674.

[70] Vanduffel, W., D. Fize, et al. (2001). "Visual motion processing investigated using contrast agent-enhanced fMRI in awake behaving monkeys." Neuron 32(4): 565-577.

[71] Vanduffel, W., D. Fize, et al. (2002). "Extracting 3D from motion: differences in human and monkey intraparietal cortex." Science 298(5592): 413-415.

[72] Vercauteren, T., X. Pennec, et al. (2009). "Diffeomorphic demons: efficient non-parametric image registration." Neuroimage 45(1 Suppl): S61-72.

[73] Wiggins, G. C., C. Triantafyllou, et al. (2006). "32-channel 3 Tesla receive-only phased-array head coil with soccer-ball element geometry." Magn Reson Med 56(1): 216-223.

[74] Worsley, K. J. and K. J. Friston (1995). "Analysis of fMRI time-series revisited--again."Neuroimage 2(3): 173-181.

[75] Zitova, B. and J. Flusser (2003). "Image registration methods: a survey." Image and Vision Computing 21(11): 977-1000.

2

Simultaneous Measurement of fMRI and EEG – Principles and Applications

Yeji Han, Sung Suk Oh, Joong Koo Kang and HyunWook Park

1. Introduction

Functional MRI (fMRI) and electroencephalogram (EEG) are the most widely used neuroimaging techniques which assist neuroscientists in investigating human brain function. FMRI measures the induced magnetic field change, usually the change in the blood oxygenation level dependent (BOLD) contrast, which reflects physiological changes of neuronal activity (Ogawa et al., 2000). EEG measures the summed electrical activities of neurons by detecting the electric potential difference at the scalp. As the sources of the signal measured by fMRI and EEG are different, the spatial and temporal information of the two techniques are also different. For example, EEG has millisecond resolution which is much higher than fMRI's temporal resolution, characterized by the lag of the hemodynamic response of 6-7 seconds (Friston et al., 1998). Low temporal resolution of fMRI is inevitable not only because the BOLD contrast is developed over seconds by accumulated changes of the magnetic field, resulting from neuronal activities and vascular changes (Rosenkranz & Lemieux, 2010), but also because several seconds are required to perform each MRI measurement. Instead, fMRI has excellent spatial resolution which is much higher than EEG. Moreover, the spatial as well as the temporal resolution of fMRI is expected to further increase as the field strength of MRI system is still increasing (Ogawa et al., 2000; Regatte et al., 2007). Thus, EEG and fMRI are complementary for brain research in regard to the types of information they can provide, and it is important to utilize both EEG and fMRI signals to get a more comprehensive view of brain activities.

To combine the information provided by fMRI and EEG, one can consider performing data fusion after separately acquiring data using each modality, as it is done for many other multimodality approaches such as combining MRI with positron emission tomography (PET) or combining MRI with computed tomography (CT). Combining PET or CT images with MR images is rather straight-forward because only a correct image registration process is required for a successful fusion of multimodality data. Combining EEG and fMRI data is more complicated; the two types of data are different as fMRI data is presented in the image domain whereas EEG represents information using waveforms in the time domain. Thus, it is recommended to simultaneously acquire fMRI and EEG data so that the data can be more easily interpreted afterwards. In fact, when fMRI and EEG are simultaneously measured, a more accurate interpretation of the data is possible because the timing information is commonly available for both of the measurements, making it more concise to figure out which parts of the fMRI and EEG signals originated from the identical brain activity.

While simultaneous recording of the two modalities can provide high spatio-temporal information for brain research, there are several issues that have to be considered to successfully perform a simultaneous fMRI-EEG measurement, such as patient safety, fMRI image quality, and EEG quality. Patient safety and image quality can be usually coped by using a properly designed MR-compatible EEG instrument. However, degradation of EEG quality cannot be prevented during the acquisition process and several post-processing techniques have to be employed to remove artefacts in the acquired EEG data.

In this chapter, a practical approach for simultaneous fMRI and EEG measurement will be discussed in detail. In section 2, an actual measurement technique and required hardware/ software will be presented. Then, common artefacts of EEG signal and removal techniques will be discussed in section 3. In section 4, a practical example of simultaneous fMRI-EEG experiment will be demonstrated.

2. Simultaneous measurement of EEG and fMRI

The first report on a combined use of fMRI and EEG was presented in 1993 (Ives et al., 1993), which showed that signals of brain activities could be obtained with both high spatial and high temporal resolution. In the following years, more experiments have been conducted to confirm the possibility of recording EEG inside an MR scanner (Huang-Hellinger et al., 1995; Lemieux et al., 1997). Nowadays, it has become more common to measure fMRI and EEG simultaneously and many practical applications have been introduced for epilepsy, sleep, and other brain functions.

When an experiment with a simultaneous measurement of fMRI and EEG is conducted, the first step is to prepare a proper EEG instrument. The EEG instrument is composed of electrodes which detect the EEG signal and a recording system which amplifies and digitizes the detected EEG signal. To record EEG signal within an MRI system, electrodes are attached to the patient head and placed inside an MR scanner while the recording system (the amplifier and the digitizer) is placed inside or outside the MR scanner according to different needs. Thus, it should be guaranteed that the electrodes are made with MRcompatible materials because anything placed inside an MR scanner should not contain ferrous material due to safety as well as potential susceptibility artifacts in the MR image. If an experiment requires the amplifier and digitizer placed inside the MR scanner, it should be ensured that they are manufactured with MR-compatible materials and can operate properly in the high magnetic field.

For EEG quality, the number of electrodes located at the subject's brain scalp is a critical factor because it determines the overall spatial resolution (Reilly, 2005) and the numbers of electrodes in commercially available EEG instrument ranges from 32 to 256. Another factor which influences the EEG quality is the arrangement of electrodes and electrode wires connected to the amplifier/digitizer. To prevent possible signal artefact induced by the magnetic field change, they have to be set on the subject's head without any loops. To minimize the problems related to the electrodes and the electrode wires, an electrode cap is generally used (Bonmassar et al., 2002; Srivastava et al., 2005). In addition, immobilization of the subject's head, the electrodes, and the electrode wires are also important factors for the EEG quality, as well as for the fMRI quality, because the change of the loop area created by the electrode wires in the static field also induces artefacts. To reduce movements of the electrodes and the electrode wires, various techniques are being employed, such as weighing down the electrode wires using sandbags (Benar et al., 2003), padding (Hoffmann et al., 2000), and placing a tight bandage over the subject's head (Benar et al., 2003). Additionally, a vacuum cushion is widely used to reduce the subject's head motion (Benar et al, 2003).

For a simultaneous fMRI-EEG experiment, most of the published literature have conducted experiments using either BrainAmp (BrainProducts GmbH, Munich, Germany) or EMR32 (Schwarzer GmbH, Munich, Germany) because both of them allow the use of an amplifier, which is non-magnetic, shielded, battery-operated, and designed for use in the MRI scanning environment. The EEG signals are amplified, converted to digital signals, and transmitted from the MR scanning environment to a computer located in the control room via optical fibers. Figure 1 shows a typical example of the commercially available MRcompatible EEG instruments, which include electrode caps (32 and 64 channels), a vacuum cushion, and a sandbag.

Using a properly prepared EEG instrument, EEG, electrocardiogram (ECG), and electrooculogram (EOG) signals are recorded, usually with a sampling rate of 5 KHz to capture the rapid change of artefacts caused by switching the magnetic field gradients during fMRI acquisition (Allen et al., 2000). After the EEG signal is measured, artefacts have to be removed as explained in the following sections. Attenuation of the artefacts caused by the gradient fields is employed by initially filtering with a cut-off frequency, typically smaller than 70Hz. The resulting signals are then down-sampled to 200 Hz. Since 200Hz is the sampling rate used for the conventional EEG measurement, down-sampling can reduce the processing time without degrading the EEG quality (Allen et al., 2000).

When EEG and ECG signals are measured, the EEG signals can be represented with different montages by using different references (Fisch, 1999). One of the most widely used montages is the referential montage, which defines a reference electrode at an inactive position, such as the midline position between two hemispheres of the brain. The reference may also be defined at such positions, where the distances from the left channel and the corresponding right channel are equal, eg. earlobes. Thus, the referential montage represents the EEG signal compared to the background EEG signal. The bipolar montage refers to the potential difference between two adjacent electrodes, with longitudinally or transversely directed chains (Fisch,

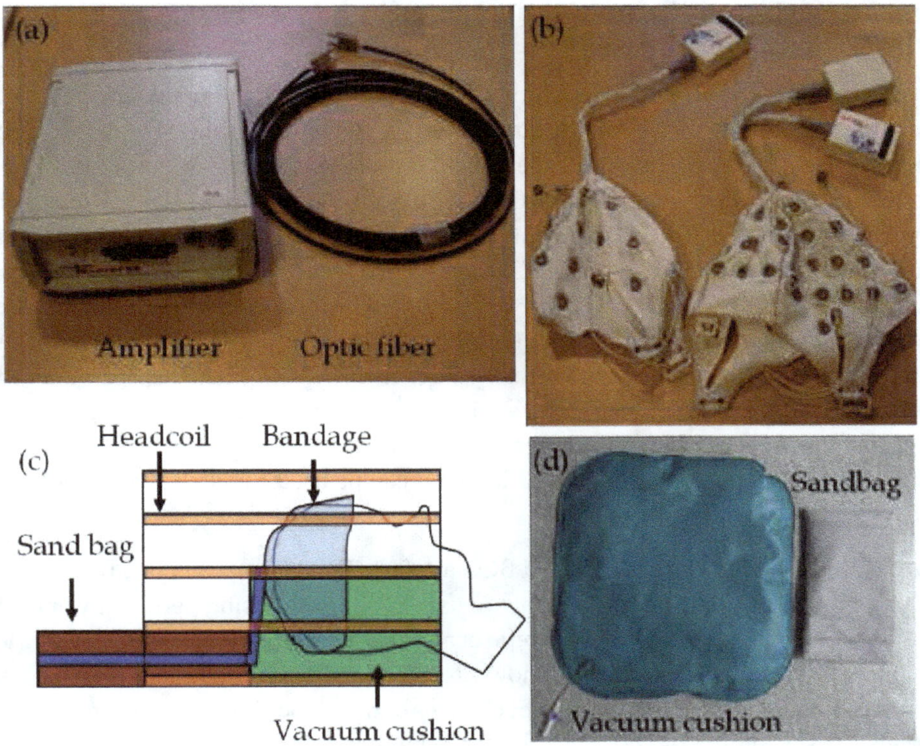

Figure 1. The EEG Instrument. (a) amplifier and optic fiber, (b) electrode caps, (c) illustration of EEG measurement inside an MRI system with an RF headcoil, and (d) aiding materials for movement reduction.

1999). This montage is known to be useful for localization. The third type of montage is the average reference montage, where the common reference is obtained by averaging all EEG signals. Lastly, the Laplacian montage averages several neighboring electrodes surrounding the measured EEG channel and uses the average signal as a reference (Fisch, 1999). For analysis of the EEG signal, any preferred montage can be constructed from the recorded signals in an effort to to clearly demonstrate waveform of EEG events as explained above.

For fMRI measurement, a conventional echo planar imaging (EPI) with the BOLD contrast is generally applied. However, some imaging parameters, such as repetition time (TR), should be carefully chosen to minimize the interference with EEG measurement (Mandelkow et al., 2006). In some cases where fMRI and EEG acquisition has to be recorded for an extended period of time, such as for sleep or epilepsy studies, the data size is too large that the data acquisition has to be performed in several separate sessions.

As briefly mentioned earlier, both the fMRI and the EEG signal can be contaminated when measured simultaneously. Thus, artefacts in the acquired data have to be eliminated before they can be analyzed. The types of artefacts encountered and the artefact reduction techniques that can be applied will be discussed in the following sections.

3. EEG artefacts and their reduction algorithms

When EEG and fMRI are simultaneously measured, both fMRI and EEG signals are influenced by each other. For example, MR image quality may be degraded because the main static field (B0) and the transverse rotational magnetic field (B1) can be altered due to EEG equipment inside the MR room (Mullinger et al., 2008). However, the quality of the MR image is not adversely degraded if the EEG equipment is properly designed and manufactured so that the field inhomogeneities caused by the EEG instrument are minimized. What should be more carefully investigated is the effect of fMRI measurement on the EEG signals, as the EEG quality can be significantly degraded with simultaneous fMRI acquisition, which can induce several types of artefacts, such as (i) image acquisition artefact (IAA); (ii) ballistocardiogram (BCG) artefact; and (iii) quantization error of the analogue-to-digital converter (ADC) (Garreffa et al., 2004). Therefore, when EEG is measured in combination with fMRI, a number of artefact reduction processes have to be employed before it can be used for clinical or research applications.

The two main EEG artefacts are IAA and BCG artefact. The IAA, caused by applied imaging gradient fields during fMRI measurements, is usually removed using periodicity and consistency of the applied gradient fields (Garreffa et al., 2004). The exact cause of the BCG artefacts is not figured out but it is generally known to be added to the EEG signal due to subtle movements of the subject's scalp or abrupt changes of the blood flow in the aortic arch during heartbeats (Ives et al., 1993). The IAA is easier to be removed than the BCG artefact because the former is relatively constant over time when the same imaging gradient is applied for every scan. However, it is rather difficult to remove the BCG artefact because the frequency, shape, and amplitude of the artefact vary from case to case. The third type of artefact is the quantization error. As the amplitude of the IAA can be more than two orders of magnitude higher than that of the EEG signal, the physiological signal in the EEG measurement may be lost if EEG is not measured with sufficient range (Allen et al., 2000).

In the following sections, a detailed explanation of the two main artefacts will be presented and the solutions for these two major artefacts will be discussed.

3.1. Image acquisition artefact (IAA)

The IAA is caused by the changes in the magnetic field during the scanning process, resulting from various factors such as the RF pulses, B^0 field inhomogeneities, body motion, and gradient switching. The switching gradient field, which is inevitable as manipulation of the applied gradient fields plays the main role in acquiring MR images, induces strong artefacts in EEG with an extremely large amplitude. Since the amplitude of IAA is 10~100 times larger than the amplitude of EEG signal, the actual EEG signal is almost completely obscured (Vanderperren et al., 2010). For that reason, earlier studies have performed aperiodic fMRI, where image acquisition is triggered after an EEG event of interest (Krakow et al., 2001). However, EEG-triggered fMRI or interleaved EEG-fMRI measurement is not an optimal solution because it reduces the flexibility of experimental design (Allen et al., 2000).

To remove the IAA from the EEG signal, researchers have focused on the properties of applied gradient fields. Since an MR imaging sequence, mostly the EPI sequence, is repeated during an fMRI experiment, identical changes take place in the gradient fields, inducing the IAA with a consistent shape for each EPI scan. Thus, most algorithms try to eliminate the IAA using the reproducibility and consistency of the IAA shape (Allen et al., 2000).

One of the first IAA reduction algorithms calculated the average IAA spectrum and subtracted the average IAA spectrum from the EEG spectrum (Sijbers et al., 1999; Hoffman et al., 2000). This artefact removal technique is integrated in FEMR software (Schwarzer GmbH, Munich, Germany), which eliminates unwanted signals that are outside the frequency range of the EEG (0.1-40Hz) using band-pass filtering. The artefacts within this frequency range have to be selectively removed. Hoffman's algorithm initially selects 10 different 10s-long sections of EEG acquired inside the magnet, which are unaffected by any artefacts, and uses them as baseline. Then, the frequency spectrum of the baseline is subtracted from the IAA-related spectrum embedded in the EEG signal (Hoffmann et al., 2000). Since IAA is periodic and its frequency range is limited, the removal can be performed in the frequency domain. However, there can be spectral overlap of the IAA and EEG signals in some cases, resulting in an excessive subtraction of the artefact spectrum from the EEG signal.

The other type of IAA reduction algorithm is based on Allen's algorithm (Allen et al., 2000), which is integrated in BrainVision Analyzer (Brain Products GmbH, Munich, Germany). Allen's IAA reduction algorithm consists of two stages: (i) the artefact waveform is averaged over a fixed number of gradient artefact epochs and subtracted from each epoch in the EEG signal; and (ii) the residual IAA is attenuated by a noise cancelling algorithm (Allen et al., 2000). Since template-based removal algorithms typically leave considerable residual noise, further reduction steps should be followed.

More recently, Allen's algorithm has been integrated in parts of many other IAA removal algorithms, including Niazy's algorithm (Niazy et al, 2005), which combines Allen's method with principal component analysis (PCA), and Mantini's algorithm (Mantini et al., 2007), which combines Allen's algorithm with independent component analysis (ICA). A new method to develop a more precise template using a time-continuous cubic spline model has been also presented (Koskinen et al. 2009). Figure 2 shows a typical example of EEG signal recorded inside a 3T MRI scanner (ISOL Technology, Korea). Fig.2 shows the EEG signal with IAA (top) and the signal after the IAA reduction using the BrainVision Analyzer (bottom).

In addition to the above-mentioned algorithms, triggering can be used in combination for detecting the starting point of every scan, which is then used as a marker for more precise averaging of the artefact waveform. Another approach is to perform an interleaved MRI acquisition, where MR acquisition is suspended at regular intervals, resulting in periods free of IAA on the EEG (Ritter et al, 2010).

In general, currently available hardware and software approaches to remove IAA from EEG signal provide satisfactory EEG signals. Moreover, it is less complicated than the removal of the cardiac pulse related artefacts which we discuss below because the timing and shape information of the IAA can be inferred from the applied gradients of MRI.

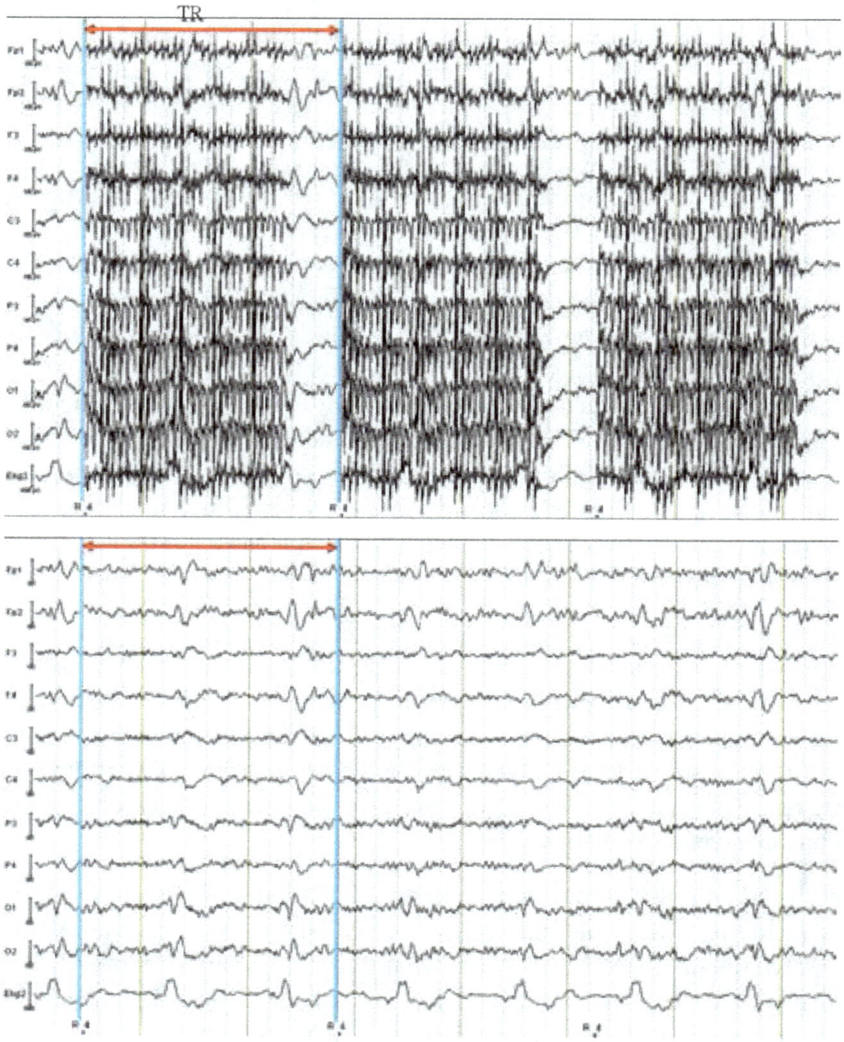

Figure 2. EEG signals recorded from 10 different channels (Fp1, Fp2, F3, F4, C3, C4, P3, P4, O1, O2) and ECG signal with the image acquisition artefact (top) and after the IAA reduction (bottom)

3.2. Cardiac-related artefact

Another EEG artefact that makes the interpretation of the EEG signal rather intricate is the ballistocardiogram artefact (BCG artefact), which is caused by alteration in physiological status. Although the exact cause of the BCG artefact is still being investigated, it is known to be induced by the movement of the patient's body as a result of acoustic vibrations due to the scanner as well as voluntary subject movements (Reilly, 1987). In this chapter, however, we refer to the small involuntary cardiac-related body movements (ballistocardiogram). The BCG artefact can be observed from the EEG signals measured outside an MR scanner but it is small and can be easily removed (Debener et al., 2008). However, the BCG artefact becomes much greater inside the scanner because of the interaction between the active cardiovascular system and the main static field (B0) (Allen et al., 1998). Consequently, it is observed in the EEG signals measured inside an MR scanner, even when EPI sequences are not applied.

A BCG artefact follows the shape of a cardiac cycle (Fig.3). In fact, the BCG artefact closely follows the cardiac cycle with a delay of approximately 210ms between the R peak of the ECG and the BCG artefact (Allen et al., 1998). Fig.3 also shows that the amplitude of the BCG artefact is comparable, if not slightly larger, to the EEG signal. However, it was predicted that the amplitude of the BCG artefact is proportional to the B0 field (Tenforde et al., 1983), and has been confirmed later (Debener et al., 2008). Debener et al. (2008) showed that the amplitude of the BCG artefact is a function of the static magnetic field strengthand the spatial variability of the BCG artefact substantially increased at higher magnetic field strengths. In reference to various BCG artefacts, Debener et al. has also demonstrated that individual subjects have different heart rates, peak latencies, and shapes (Debener et al., 2008). Moreover, the shapes of the BCG artefact of different EEG channels also vary. As a result, it is difficult to distinguish an 'event' from the EEG signal when the signal is distorted by the BCG artefact.

If the frequency of the BCG artefact is constrained in a certain range distinct from that of the EEG signal, one can think of filtering the artefact in the frequency domain. Although the frequency range of the BCG artefact is mainly in the theta (4-8 Hz) band, however, it can extend to the alpha (8-13 Hz) and delta (0.5-4 Hz) bands, thus overlapping with the EEG signals (Garreffa et al., 2004).

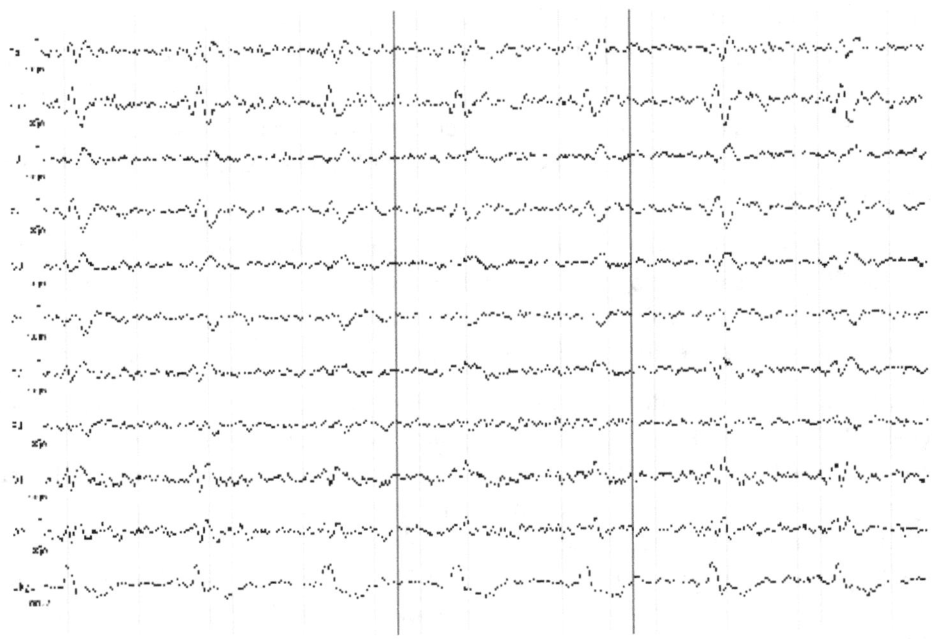

Figure 3. Shows ECG and EEG signals measured inside an MRI scanner without applying the imaging gradients. The BCG artefacts are embedded in each channel.

3.2.1. Average artefact subtraction (AAS)

There are also algorithms that remove the BCG artefacts from the EEG signal based on properties other than the frequency characteristic. One approach to remove the BCG artefact is based on the average artefact subtraction (AAS) algorithm (Allen et al., 1998), which creates an average BCG artefact template/waveform and subtracts it from the EEG signal. It is based on the observation that the shape and the occurrence rate of the BCG artefact is quite consistent across a number of successive heartbeats in each channel of the EEG. Thus, the AAS algorithm consists of two steps: generating an averaged BCG artefact template and subtracting it from the BCG artefact occurrences. First, reference points for each BCG artefact have to be defined. The average waveform is calculated for each referential EEG signal on a second-by-second basis and requires the previous 10 seconds of EEG and ECG signals. The R peak in the QRS complex of the ECG is detected for every heartbeat by thresholding the amplitude of the measured ECG signal using a predefined value and the onset of each BCG artefact is identified using a predefined delay (Allen et al., 1998). Once the onset of every cardiac cycle is detected, a BCG artefact template is generated by averaging the EEG signal over a predefined window size for each EEG channel as the BCG artefact exhibits different shapes in different EEG channels. Finally, the average BCG artefact template is subtracted from the measured EEG signal.

One of the most important steps for the AAS-based algorithms is to find the correct onset points of the BCG artefact because variations of the subject's heartbeat may alter the time delay between the R peak of the QRS complex in the ECG signal and the BCG artefact in the EEG signal. If the onset points are not correct, it is difficult to find the precise average artefact template and the exact reference point for subtraction and this leaves too much residual artefact after subtraction from the EEG signal. Although the AAS method assumes that the shape and occurrence of the BCG artefacts have little variance over time and the condition of the subject's heartbeat is stable, these assumptions may not be necessarily true. Thus, the AAS algorithm has a limitation that the corrected EEG signal can still have residual artefacts due to an inaccurate BCG artefact template.

To account for the shape variations of the BCG artefacts, more algorithms have been introduced to generate BCG artefact templates using other approaches, such as Gaussian weighted averaging (Goldman et al., 2000), median filtering (Sijbers et al., 2000; Ellingson et al., 2004), and wavelet-based adaptive filtering (Kim et al., 2004).

For the AAS-based methods, defining the template length is also an important issue. Since the actual R-R interval is not consistent, the BCG artefact can be subtracted twice if the R-R interval is shorter than the template length and insufficiently subtracted in the other case. To reduce the dependency of the AAS based algorithms on the template length, alternative algorithms have been introduced. One of these scales the template length to a certain percentage of the mean R-R period (Ellington et al. 2004). A plug-in for EEGLAB in FMRIB (http://www.fmrib.ox.ac.uk/eeglab/fmribplugin/), incorporates the BCG artefact data for all R-R period lengths in the current moving average window and the template is adaptively applied to each QRS period based on its R-R period (Brain Vision Analyzer software, http://www.brain-products.com/). Other algorithms account for the template duration problem using the Kalman filter (Bonmassar et al., 2002), the EOG signals (In et al., 2006), the recursive least squares motion recording (Masterton et al., 2007), and a moving general linear model (mGLM) (Vincent et al., 2007).

More recently, the optimal basis set (OBS) (Niazy et al., 2005) method was proposed to use a few principal components as representations of several distinct pulse artifact templates. Since these templates include most of the BCG artefact in any given EEG channel and can be used to regress the BCG artefact, the OBS method can account for a greater temporal variation in the BCG artefact shape (Debener et al., 2010). For the OBS method, however, the number of principal components that create the template have to be selected by the user, and thus, affect the performance of this method.

The major advantage of the AAS based algorithms, in comparison with the blind source separation (BSS) algorithm, is low complexity. However, obtaining satisfactory results can be quite difficult because finding the precise onset points of the cardiac cycle for an accurate template is rather complicated as demonstrated by the variants of the AAS method mentioned above.

3.2.2. Blind source separation (BSS)

The AAS based and the OBS based algorithms focus on the fact that the BCG artefact of each EEG-channel has different shapes. However, the BCG artefact can be also characterized by a number of typical topographies (Bénar et al., 2003). Thus, another algorithm to remove the BCG artefacts is based on the blind source separation (BSS) algorithm, which assumes that the characteristics of the BCG artefacts are independent from or orthogonal to the EEG signals (Bénar et al., 2003). The principal or independent components are obtained using the orthogonal or independent characteristics, respectively, between the BCG artefact and EEG activity of the brain. There are several ways to perform the separation of the BCG artefacts and the EEG signal. Early approaches of BSS algorithms are based on manual selection of the independent components, including the original algorithm using ICA (Bénar et al., 2003). In Bénar's algorithm, the components contributing to the BCG artefact are manually identified and taken out from the components. Then, reconstruction of the EEG signal with the remaining free of artefact components can produce EEG signal with reduced artefacts.

More ICA algorithms have been introduced, including Informax ICA, which uses the minimization of the mutual information (Bell & Sejnowski, 1995), FastICA, which uses the maximization of the non-Gaussianity (Hyvärinen & Oja, 2000), joint approximate diagonalization of eigenmatrices (JADE) (Cardoso & Souloumiac, 1993), and second order blind identification (Belouchrani et al., 1993). ICA methods are implemented in the EEGLAB software (http://sccn.ucsd.edu/eeglab/). Since the ICA algorithms reduce the BCG artefact by removing the subjectively defined components that are correlated to the BCG artefact after the ICA processing, the performance may depend on users.

To solve this problem, algorithms for automatic identification of components related to the BCG artefact have been also proposed. Some of the selection criteria for the automatic identification include correlation with the ECG signal (Srivastava et al., 2005; Mantini et al.,

2007), frequency content related to the heartbeat rate and its harmonics (Vanderperren et al., 2007), and autocorrelation of the EEG signal (Deburchgrave et al., 2008; Vandersperren et al., 2010). The BCG-related components can be distinguished by the peaks in their autocorrelation. In case of frequency related component selection, the fact that BCG artefacts can be characterized by peaks at the heart rate frequency and its harmonics is used. This property can be exploited as a tool to select the artifact-related components from the ICA decomposition, where the heart rate frequency is determined by computing the inverse of the average distance between consecutive QRS peaks. However, these algorithms require a delicate selection of parameters to achieve better performance (Vanderperren et al., 2010). Moreover, ICA method is inefficient to account for the spatial variation of the BCG artefact since independent components are obtained from EEG signals measured at different positions of the brain. As an alternative, OBS-ICA method can be used, which initially removes a major part of the BCG artifact using the OBS method and then removes the residual BCG artefact using the ICA method. (Debener et al., 2007)

The main advantage of the BSS algorithms is that, unlike the AAS based algorithms, the exact onset of the BCG artefact is not required to be identified. However, the BSS algorithms have higher computational complexity than the AAS algorithms. In addition, the BSS algorithms may not work properly for the EEG signals measured in higher field MRI scanners, i.e., 3T and 7T, as deviations in the spatial information of the BCG artefact become greater in higher field MRI systems (Debener et al., 2008).

3.2.3. Modified average artefact subtraction (MAAS)

As discussed in the previous sections, both ASS and BSS algorithms have advantages and disadvantages. However, for 3T or higher field MRI systems, the ASS algorithms can be more efficient (Vanderperren et al., 2010). To optimize the ASS algorithm for higher field MRI systems, a modified AAS (MAAS) algorithm has been proposed to improve the construction and the subtraction of the BCG template using a fully automatic process (Oh et al., 2012). The MAAS algorithm is composed of two steps; it initially finds an accurate reference point based on the ECG signal to use for the BCG artefact subtraction and the template generation. Then, an accurate BCG artefact subtraction algorithm is applied, which adaptively subtracts the BCG artefact template using different delay and window sizes.

To find the reference points for the BCG artefacts, R peaks of the ECG signal have to be accurately identified. According to Debener (Debener et al., 2007), a negative swing occurs between the S and T states of the P_QRS_T wave due to an axial blood flow momentum when the ECG signal is recorded in a high field MR system. This negative swing is used to automatically identify the R peak from ECG in the MAAS algorithm (Oh et al., 2012). Since an R peak and the following negative peak produce the maximum signal difference, the difference of positive and negative peaks is calculated to deduce the R peak. For each segment of the ECG signal with a predefined duration, a sliding window of 0.3s duration is defined to reflect the physiological characteristic (Debener et al., 2007). Within the sliding window, a positive peak and the following negative peak are identified and the difference between the peaks is calculated. After eliminating the positive and negative peak pairs whose difference is smaller than the average, the maximum peak among the remaining positive peaks is selected as the R peak candidate of the current window. Then, the false R peaks are eliminated from the candidate peaks using the resting heartbeat rate (Sharieff, 2006). Since the distances between adjacent R peaks should be within 0.5-1.3 seconds (for 46-120 bpm), the R peak candidate is eliminated if its distance from the previous R peak or the following R peak does not lie in this range. After elimination, the point which has the maximum ECG signal is assigned as a new R peak in sections where the distance of adjacent R peaks is larger than 1.3 seconds.

To detect the BCG artefact from the contaminated EEG signal, a BCG clip is defined for the EEG signal using the R peak as shown in Fig.4. After extracting the BCG clips from the current EEG segment, the BCG clips suitable for a correlation template (CT) generation are classified; if the absolute mean of a BCG clip is larger than the absolute mean of BCG from all previous EEG segments, it is not used for CT generation. Then, the remaining BCG clips are averaged to generate the CT, and then correlation coefficients between each BCG clip and the CT are calculated to figure out the true peak of the current BCG artefact. By considering the delay time between an R peak and the following BCG artefact, the BCG artefact is classified into a normal and a deformed BCG artefact.

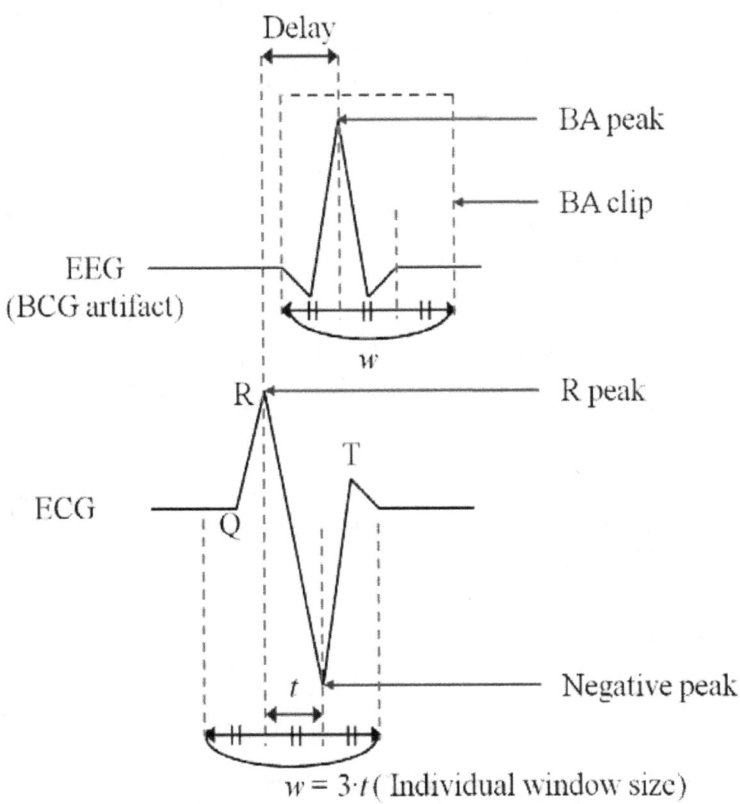

Figure 4. An illustration of the ballistocardiogram (BCG) artifact.

The BCG artefact template is simply obtained by averaging more than two normal BCG artefacts within the current segment, and its length is defined by the maximum window size of the normal BCG artefacts. For a normal BCG artefact, the contaminated EEG signal is corrected by subtracting the BCG artefact template using the individual delay and the individual window size. In case of a deformed BA artefact, the BCG artefact template is subtracted using the average window size and the average delay.

Figure 5 shows the contaminated EEG signal with the BCG artefact and the EEG signal after applying BCG reduction using the OBS, ICA, and MAAS algorithms. Since the MAAS algorithm detects R peaks accurately and uses variable window and delay properties, it can neatly remove the BCG artefacts. Since the OBS method uses the mean R-R interval as the window size of the BCG artefact template, it can result in distortion if the current R-R interval is shorter than the mean R-R interval. In this study, some of the epilepsy signals are overly removed since the mean R-R interval is used. The error is also partly due to the fact that the selected components of the OBS are related to epilepsy signals. For ICA, the estimated BCG artefact cannot handle the variation of the BCG artefacts for every EEG channel and the correction results can have residual artefacts.

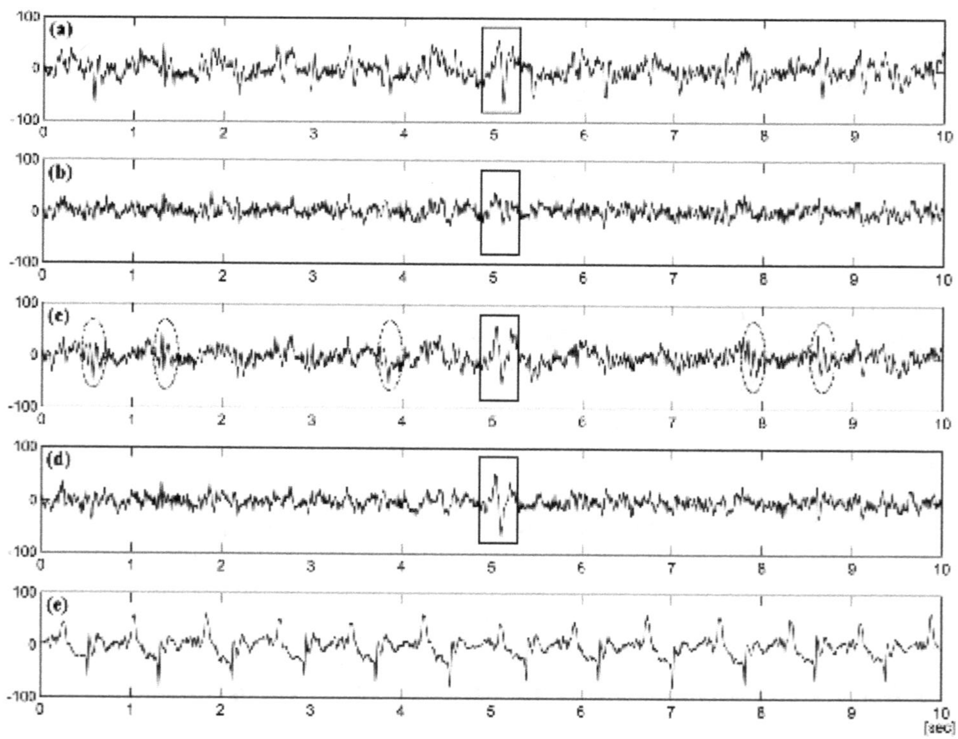

Figure 5. The BCG artefact and its corrected signals. (a) EEG signal on the F7 channel before correction, (b) corrected EEG signal by OBS, (c) corrected EEG signal by ICA, (d) corrected EEG signal by MAAS, and (e) scaled ECG signal. In this study, some of the epilepsy signals are overly removed when the OBS algorithm is used (marked with squares) and the ICA algorithm leaves too much residual BCG artefacts (marked with dotted ovals).

4. Application of fMRI+EEG measurements

The possibility of recording the EEG inside an MR scanner has opened a wide variety of new research areas. Generally, there are three application areas for simultaneous fMRI and EEG studies: neurovascular coupling, cognitive and systems neuroscience, and clinical studies. However, the most straightforward application would be to search for brain activation and deactivation areas related to specific events of the EEG signal. This type of research has been carried on via correlation between the BOLD time series and a postulated EEG-derived model of haemodynamic changes, generated by the general linear models (GLM). In other words, the temporal information acquired from the EEG signals can be used as timing information for the stimulus cue in fMRI. Then, the fMRI analysis can be performed using the MR images corresponding to the cue timing as images of stimulus conditions and the rest as images of reference conditions.

Typical application areas of simultaneous fMRI-EEG experiments include resting state studies such as sleep studies, brain rhythm studies, and activation studies for pain research, auditory research, visual research, and cognition research (Horovits et al., 2008; Christmann et al., 2007; Laufs et al., 2003). In this section, a practical example of a simultaneous fMRIEEG experiment for epilepsy patient is demonstrated. Moreover, three different BCG artefact reduction algorithms are compared using fMRI analysis results.

The development of simultaneous EEG and fMRI measurement was initially motivated out of interest in identifying the BOLD changes related to interictal epileptiform discharges (IED) (Rosenkranz et al., 2010). Although the timing and the shape of epilepsy waveform can be acquired using EEG, spatial information of EEG is not as accurate because the EEG signal is measured at certain locations on the surface of a brain only. Thus, fMRI analysis is used to provide more accurate spatial information of an epilepsy patient by providing not only the cortical but also the subcortical information.

In this experiment, three patients with intractable partial epilepsy were recruited and a written consent was signed by every patient prior to the experiments. A neurologist supervised the experiments to ensure the safety of the patients. EEG recording was performed inside a 3T MRI system (ISOL Technology, South Korea) using BrainAmp and BrainCap (BrainProducts GmbH, Germany). With BrainCap, 21 EEG channels (Fp1, Fp2, F3, F4, C3, C4, P3, P4, O1, O2, F7, F8, T7, T8, P7, P8, Fz, Cz, Pz, TP9, and TP10 in the 10-20 channel system), two ECG channels, and an EOG were recorded during 5 to 7 sessions, each lasting for 11 minutes. The international 10-20 system is an electrode placement scheme mostly applied for epilepsy studies, which is based on the relationship between the location of an electrode and the underlying area of the cerebral cortex. The 10 and 20 represent the distances between adjacent electrodes which are 10% and 20% of the total front-back and right-left distance of the skull (Fisch, 1999). The reference electrode of the cap was located at the mid-points (Cz and Fz), and EEG/ECG signals were recorded with a sampling rate of 5kHz to prevent aliasing.

At the same time, fMRI data was simultaneously acquired using the following imaging parameters: gradient-echo echo-planar-imaging (GE-EPI) sequence, TR/TE=3000/37 msec, matrix size=64×64, FOV=220×220 mm^2, slice thickness=4 or 5mm, number of slices=20 or 30, and flip angle=70°.

After the measurement, the EEG signals were filtered by a phase-shift-free Butterworth filter having a band-pass range of 0.5 to 55 Hz. IAA was then eliminated using the BrainVision Analyzer (BrainProducts) and the filtered signals were down-sampled to 500 Hz (Mandelkow et al., 2006). To remove the BCG artefacts, ICA, OBS and MAAS algorithms were separately applied to the EEG signals. For fMRI analysis, Statistical Parameter Mapping (SPM8, http://www.fil.ion.ucl.ac.uk/spm/) was used with the pre-processing steps of 'realign' and 'smoothing with a Gaussian filter having a full width at half maximum of 8mm'. For the t-test, p-value of 0.001 and a cluster analysis of 4mm was applied.

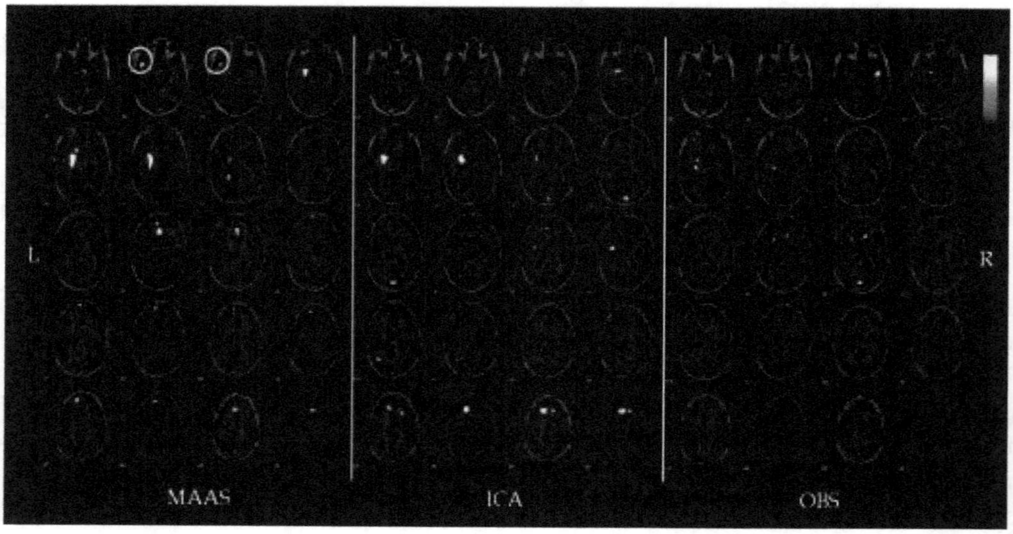

Figure 6. Activation regions from fMRI analysis after removing the BCG artefacts from the measured EEG signal using the MAAS, ICA, and OBS algorithms. The activation regions corresponding to the PEZ is marked with circles.

After post-processing, neurologists detected IEDs from the BCG-artefact removed EEG signals. To localize the IED regions in the brain, fMRI analysis was performed using SPM8 with the detected IED timing information. Then, the activated regions from the fMRI were compared to the presumed epileptogenic zone (PEZ), which was also determined by analyzing the EEG signals, PET images and anatomical MR images.

Since the activated regions from the fMRI are analyzed using the detected IEDs, the performance of the BCG artefact removal algorithms can be indirectly evaluated by comparing the fMRI activation regions. In this experiment, the IED regions in the subjects' brain were localized using the regions revealed by the fMRI analysis (Fig.6). IED regions of subject A is shown in Fig. 6. The localized activation regions of three subjects are shown in Table 1. While the detected fMRI activation regions from all three methods produced the same results for subjects B and C, coincident with PEZ, data of subject A produced different results when the

MAAS algorithm was applied. As shown in Fig.6, the left temporal pole of subject A could be only detected when the BCG artefact of the EEG signal was removed by the MAAS algorithm. When the fMRI activation results were compared to the PEZ of subject A, the activation region was coincident with the PEZ only when the MAAS algorithm was applied.

sub	PEZ	activated regions from fMRI		
		MAAS	ICA	OBS
A	l. ant -mid temporal area	l. limbic lobe, parahipocamppal gyrus	l. frontal lobe, superior frontal gyrus	r. temporal lobe, superior temporal lobe
		l. temporal pole	l. limbic lobe, parahipocamppal gyrus	r. limbic lobe, anterior cingulate
		r. limbic lobe, anterior cingulate	r. frontal lobe, superior frontal gyrus	l. limbic lobe, parahipocamppal gyrus
		l. frontal lobe, inferior frontal gyrus	r. occipital lobe, lingual gyrus	l. occipital lobe, cuneus
		left frontal lobe, superior frontal gyrus		
B	r. mid - temporal area	r. frontal lobe, middle frontal gyrus		
		r. frontal lobe, inferior frontal gyrus		
		r. temporal lobe, middle temporal gyrus		
C	bifrontal area	r. frontal lobe, middle frontal gyrus		
		r. frontal lobe, superior frontal gyrus		

Table 1. Localization of the IEDs based on the fMRI activation regions

As the results demonstrate, the MAAS algorithm outperforms the other algorithms in this study with epilepsy patients. In spite of its complex calculation, the ICA algorithm cannot clearly detect and remove the BCG artefacts because it cannot sufficiently account for the deviations of spatial information of the BCG artefacts (Debener et al., 2007). On the other hand, the timing information of every R peak is used to estimate the onset and duration of the corresponding BCG artefact more accurately in the MAAS algorithm. Since variation of a subject's heartbeat may alter the delay time of the BCG artifact in the EEG signal from the R peak in the ECG signal (Shin, et al., 2009; Assecondi et al., 2009), the BCG artefacts cannot be fully removed if a fixed delay is used for the BCG artefact detection, such as in the OBS method. Another advantage of the MAAS algorithm is that it uses individual window sizes when subtracting the BCG artefact template from the EEG signal. Since the OBS method uses the mean R-R interval as the window size for the BCG template, the correction result can be distorted if the current R-R interval is shorter than the mean R-R interval. In other words, some regions may be subtracted twice as it experiences an overlapping of successive subtraction windows.

The simultaneous fMRI-EEG experiment for epilepsy patient enables various types of analysis for research and diagnosis. In clinical fields, simultaneous fMRI-EEG measurement can be used for localization of the epileptic source in presurgical evaluation (Zijlmans et al., 2007) or in epilepsy surgery (Thornton et al., 2010). For research purposes, it can be used to study absence seizures (Moeller et al., 2009), temporal lobe interictal spikes heterotopias (Kobayashi et al, 2006a), startle epilepsy (Fernández et al., 2011), and gray matter heterotopias (Kobayashi et al, 2006b). However, the BOLD changes are related to the detected IEDs with only about 67% accuracy (Al et al. 2003; Krakow, et al., 2001; Salek-Haddadi et al., 2006), possibly due to significant difference in hemodynamic response function (HRF) of epilepsy and the standard HRF model (Bénar et al., 2001). To account for this problem, various HRFs have been developed for epilepsy (Bagshaw et al., 2004; Grouiller et al., 2010).

5. Conclusion

In this chapter, principles and applications for simultaneous fMRI and EEG measurement were discussed. The simultaneous fMRI and EEG measurements can both provide high spatial and temporal resolution, and thus, can generate valuable data for experimental and clinical neuroscientists. However, there are certain problems, such as the IAA and the BCG artefacts, which have to be carefully handled to make a full use of the methodology. If a proper elimination method is employed to reduce possible artefacts in the fMRI and EEG signals, the simultaneous measurement can become a useful tool in various clinical and system neuroscience studies. Thus, a combined analysis of fMRI and EEG will provide a more promising future for elucidating the mechanisms of brain than the separate application of these two tools.

Acknowledgements

This work was partly supported by National Research Foundation of Korea (NRF) grant funded by the Korea government (MEST) (No. 2012-0000125).

Author details

Yeji Han[1], Sung Suk Oh[1], Joong Koo Kang[2] and HyunWook Park[1]

1 Korea Advanced Institute of Science and Technology, Republic of Korea

2 Asan Medical Center, Republic of Korea

References

[1] Al-Asmi, A., Benar, C.G., Gross, D.W., Khani, Y.A., Andermann, F., Pike, B., Dubeau, F., & Gotman, J. (2003). fMRI Activation in Continuous and Spike-Triggered EEG-fMRI Studies of Epileptic Spikes. *Epilepsia,* Vol.44, pp.1328–1339, ISSN 0013-9580

[2] Allen, P.J., Polizzi, G., Krakow, K., Fish, D.R., & Lemieux, L. (1998). Identification of EEG Events in the MR Scanner: the Problem of Pulse Artefact and a Method for its Subtraction. *NeuroImage,* Vol.8, No.3, pp.229-239, ISSN 1053-8119

[3] Allen, P.J., Josephs, O., & Turner, R. (2000). A Method for Removing Imaging Artifact from Continous EEG Recorded During Functional MRI. *Neuroimage,* Vol.12, pp.230–9, ISSN 1053-8119

[4] Assecondi, S., Hallez, H., Staelens, S., Bianchi, A.M., Huiskamp, G.M., & Lemahieu, I. (2009). Removal of the Ballistocardiographic Artifact from EEG-fMRI Data: a Canonical Correlation Approach. *Physics in Medicine and Biology,* Vol.54, pp.1673-1689, ISSN 0031-9155

[5] Bagshaw, A.P., Aghakhani, Y., Bénar C.G., Kobayashi, E., Hawco, C., Dubeau, F., Pike, G.B., & Gotman, J. (2004). EEG-fMRI of Focal Epileptic Spikes: Analysis with Mmultiple Haemodynamic Functions and Comparison with Gadolinium-Enhanced MR Angiograms, *Human Brain Mapping,* Vol.22, pp.179–192, ISSN 1065-9471

[6] Bell, A.J. & Sejnowski, T.J. (1995). An Information-Maximization Approach to Blind Separation and Blind Deconvolution. *Neural Computation,* Vol.7, No.6, pp.1129-1159, ISSN 0899-7667

[7] Belouchrani, A., Abed-Meraim, K., Cardoso, J.F., & Moulines, E. (1993). Second-Order Blind Separation of Temporally Correlated Sources. *Proceedings of International Conference on Digital Signal Processing,* Cyprus, pp.346-351.

[8] Bénar, C.G., Gross, D.W., Wang, Y., Petre, V., Pike, B., Dubeau, F., & Gotman, J. (2001). The BOLD Resoponse to Interictal Epileptiform Discharge, *NeuroImage,* Vol. 17, pp.1182-1192, ISSN 1053-8119

[9] Bénar, C., Aghakhani, Y., Wang, Y., Izenberg, A., Al-Asmi, A., Dubeau, F., & Gotman, J. (2003). Quality of EEG in Simultaneous EEG-fMRI for Epilepsy. *Clinical Neurophysiology,* Vol.114, No.3, pp.569-580, ISSN 1388-2457

[10] Bonmassar, G., Purdon, P.L., Jaaskelainen, I.P., Chiappa, K., Solo, V., Brown, E.N., & Belliveau, J.W. (2002). Motion and Ballistocardiogram Artifact Removal for Interleaved Recording of EEG and EPs during MRI. *NeuroImage,* Vol.16, No.4, pp. 1127-1141, ISSN 1053-8119

[11] Cardoso, J.F. & Souloumiac, A. (1993). Blind Beamforming for Non-Gaussian Signals. *IEE Proceedings F Radar and Signal Processing,* Vol.140, No.6, pp.362-370, ISSN 0956-375X

[12] Debener, S., Strobel, A., Sorger, B., Peters, J., Kranczioch, C., Engel, A.K., & Goebel, R. (2007). Improved Quality of Auditory Event-Related Potentials Recorded Simultaneously with 3T fMRI: Removal of the Ballistocardiogram Artefact. *NeuroImage*, Vol. 34, pp.587–597, ISSN 1053-8119

[13] Debener, S., Mullinger, K.J., Niazy, R.K., & Bowtell, R.W. (2008). Properties of the Ballistocardiogram Artefact as Revealed by EEG Recordings at 1.5, 3 and 7 Tesla Static Magnetic Field Strength. *International Journal of Psychophysiology*, Vol.67, No.3, pp. 189–199, ISSN 0167-8760

[14] Debener, S., Kranczioch, C., & Gutberlet, I. (2010). EEG Quality: Origin and Reduction of the EEG Cardiac-Related Artefact, In: *EEG-fMRI Physiological Basis, Technique, and Applications*, Christoph Mulert and Louis Lemieux, pp.135-151, ISBN 978-3-540-87918-3, Germany

[15] Deburchgraeve, W., Cherian, P.J., De Vos, M., Swarte, R.M., Blok, J.H., Visser, G.H., Govaert, P., & Van Huffel, S. (2008). Automated Neonatal Seizure Detection Mimicking a Human Observer Reading EEG. *Clinical Neurophysiology*, Vol.119, No.11, pp. 2447–2454, ISSN 1388-2457

[16] Ellingson, M.L., Liebenthal, E., Spanaki, M.V., Prieto, T.E., Binder, J.R., & Ropella, K.M. (2004). Ballistocardiogram Artifact Reduction in the Simultaneous Acquisition of Auditory ERPS and fMRI. *NeuroImage*, Vol.22, No.4, pp.1534-1542 ISSN 1053-8119

[17] Fernández, S., Donaire, A., Maestro, I., Seres, E., Setoain, X., Bargalló, N., Rumià, J., Boget, T., Falcón, C., & Carreño, M. (2011). Functional Neuroimaging in Startle Epilepsy: Involvement of a Mesial Frontoparietal Network. *Epilepsia*, Early View, ISSN 0013-9580

[18] Fisch, B. J. (1999). *Fisch and Spehlmann's EEG Primer: Basic Principles of Digital and Analog EEG* (3rd Edition), Elsevier, ISBN 978-0-444-82148-5, Amsterdam.

[19] Garreffa, G., Bianciardi, M.D., Hagberg, G.E., Macaluso, E., Marciani, M.G., Maraviglia, B., Abbafati, M., Carni, M., Bruni, I., & Bianchi, L. (2004). Simultaneous EEG–fMRI Acquisition: How Far Is It from Being a Standardized Technique?. *Magnetic Resonance Imaging*, Vol.22, No.10, pp.1445-1455, ISSN 0730-725X

[20] Goldman, R.I., Stern, J.M., Engel Jr., J., & Cohen, M.S. (2000). Acquiring Simultaneous EEG and Functional MRI. *Clinical Neurophysiology*, Vol.111, No.11, pp.1974-1980, ISSN 1388-2457

[21] Grouiller, F., Vercueil, L., Krainik, A., Segebarth, C., Kahane, P., & David, O. (2010). Characterization of the Hemodynamic Modes Associated with Interictal Epileptic Activity Using a Deformable Model-Based Analysis of Combined EEG and Functional MRI Recordings. *Human Brain Mapping*, Vol.31, pp.1157–1173 ISSN 1065-9471

[22] Hoffmann, A., Jaejer, L., Werhahn, K.F., Jaschke, M., Noachtar, S., & Reiser, M. (2000). Electroencephalography During Functional Echo-Planar Imaging: Detection

of Epileptic Spikes Using Post-processing Methods. *Magnetic Resonance in Medicine,* Vol.44, pp.791-798, ISSN 0740-3194

[23] Huang-Hellinger, F., Breiter, H. C., McCormack, G., Cohen, M. S., Kwong, K. K., Sutton, J. P., Savoy, R. L., Weisskoff, R. M., Davis, T. L., Baker, J. R., Belliveau, J. W., & Rosen, B. R. (1995). Simultaneous Functional Magnetic Resonance Imaging and Electrophysiological Recording. *Human Brain Mapping,* Vol.3, pp.13–23, ISSN 1065-9471

[24] Hyvärinen, A. & Oja, E. (2000). Independent Component Analysis: Algorithms and Applications. *Neural Networks,* Vol.13, No.4-5, pp.411-430 ISSN 0893-6080

[25] In, M.H., Lee, S.Y., Park, T.S., Kim, T.S., Cho, M.H., & Ahn, Y.B. (2006). Ballistocardiogram Artifact Removal from EEG Signals Using Adaptive Filtering of EOG Signals. *Physiological Measurement,* Vol.27, pp.1227-1240

[26] Ives, J.R., Warach, S., Schmitt, F., Edelman, R.R., & Schomer, D.L. (1993). Monitoring the Patient's EEG During Echo Planar MRI. *Electroencephalography and Clinical Neurophysiology,* Vol.87, No.6, pp.417–20, ISSN 1388-2457

[27] Kim, K.H., Yoon, H.W., & Park, H.W. (2004). Improved Ballistocardiac Artifact Removal from the Electroencephalogram Recorded in fMRI. *Journal of Neuroscience Methods,* Vol.135, No.1-2, pp.193-203

[28] Kobayashi, E., Bagshaw, A.P., Benar, C.G., Aghakhani, Y., Andermann, F., Dubeau, F., & Gotman, J. (2006a). Temporal and Extratemporal BOLD Responses to Temporal Lobe Interictal Spikes. *Epilepsia,* Vol.47, pp.343–354, ISSN 0013-9580

[29] Kobayashi, E., Bagshaw, A.P., Grova, C., Gotman, J., & Dubeau, F. (2006b). Grey Matter Heterotopia: What EEG-fMRI Can Tell Us About Epileptogenicity of Neuronal Migration Disorders, *Brain,* Vol.129, pp.366–374.

[30] Koskinen, M. & Varitiainen, N. (2009). Removal of Imaging Artifacts in EEG during Simultaneous EEG/fMRI Recording: Reconstruction of a High-Precision Artefact Template. *Neuroimage,* Vol.46, pp.160-167, ISSN 1053-8119

[31] Krakow, K., Lemieux, L., Messina, D., Scott, C.A., Symms, M.R., Duncan, J.S., & Fish, D.R. (2001). Spatio-Temporal Imaging of Focal Interictal Epileptiform Activity Using EEG-Triggered Functional MRI. Epileptic Disorders, Vol.3, pp.67–74, ISSN 1950-6945

[32] Lemieux, L., Allen, P.J., Franconi, F., Symms, M.R., & Fish, D.R. (1997). Recording of EEG During fMRI Experiments: Patient Safety. *Magnetic Resonance in Medicine,* Vol. 38, No.6, pp.943–52, ISSN 0740-3194

[33] Mantini, D., Perrucci, M.G., Cugini, S., Ferretti, A., Romani, G.L., & Del Gratta, C. (2007). Complete Artifact Removal for EEG Recorded During Continuous fMRI Using Independent Component Analysis. *NeuroImage,* Vol.34, pp.598–607, ISSN 1053-8119

[34] Masterton, R.A., Abbott, D.F., Fleming, S.W., & Jackson G.D. (2007). Measurement and Reduction of Motion and Ballistocardiogram Artefacts from Simultaneous EEG and fMRI Recordings. *Neuroimage*, Vol.37, pp.202-211, ISSN 1053-8119

[35] Moeller, F., LeVan, P., Muhle, H., Stephani, U., Dubeau, F., Siniatchkin, M., & Gotman, J. (2010). Absence Seizures: Individual Patterns Revealed by EEG-fMRI, *Epilepsia*, Vol.51, No.10, pp.2000-10, ISSN 0013-9580

[36] Mullinger, K., Debener, S., Coxon, R., Bowtell, R. (2008). Effects of Simultaneous EEG Recording on MRI Data Quality at 1.5, 3 and 7 tesla. *International Jounal of Psychophysiology*, Vol.67, No.3, pp.178-188, ISSN 0167-8760

[37] Niazy, R.K., Beckmann, C.F., Iannetti, G.D., Brady, J.M., & Smith, S.M. (2005). Removal of FMRI Environment Artifacts From EEG Data Using Optimal Basis Sets. *NeuroImage*, Vol.28, pp.720–737, ISSN 1053-8119

[38] Reilly, E.L. (2005). EEG Recording and Operation of the Apparatus. In: *Electroencephalography: Basic Principles, Clinical Applications and Related Fields*. Ernst Niedermeyer and Frenando Lopes da Silva, pp.139-160, Lippincott Williams & Wilkins, ISBN 0-7817-5126-8, Philadelphia.

[39] Ritter, P., Becter, R., Freyer, F., & Villringer, A. (2010). EEG Quality: The Image Acquisition Artefact, In: *EEG-fMRI Physiological Basis, Technique, and Applications*, Christoph Mulert and Louis Lemieux, pp.153-171, ISBN 978-3-540-87918-3, Germany

[40] Rosenkranz, K. & Lemieux, L. (2010). Present and Future of Simultaneous EEG-fMRI. *Magnetic Resonance Materials in Physics, Biology and Medicine*, Vol.23. pp.309-316, ISSN 0968-5243

[41] Salek-Haddadi, A., Diehl, B., Hamandi, K., Merschhemke, M., Liston, A., Friston, K., Duncan, J.S., Fish, D.R., & Lemieux, L. (2006). Hemodynamic Correlates of Epileptiform Discharges: An EEG-fMRI Study of 63 Patients with Local Epilepsy. *Brain Research*, Vol.1088, No.1, pp.148-166, ISSN 0006-8993

[42] Sharieff, G.Q. & Rao, S.O. (2006). The Pediatric ECG, *Emergency Medicine Clinics of North America*, Vol.24, pp.195-208, ISSN 0733-8627

[43] Shin, J.H., Lee, K.M., & Park, K.S. (2009). Non-Constrained Monitoring of Systolic Blood Pressure on a Weighing Scale, *Phyiological Mesurement*, Vol.30, pp.679-693, ISSN 0967-3334

[44] Sijbers, J., Michiels, I., Verhoye, M., Van Audekerke, J., Van der Linden, A., & Van Dyck, D. (1999). Restoration of MR-Induced Artifacts in Simultaneously Recorded MR/EEG Data. *Magnetic Resonance Imaging*, Vol.17, No.9, pp.1383–1391, ISSN 0730-725X

[45] Sijbers, J., Van Audekerke, J., Verhoye, M., Van der Linden, A., & Van Dyck, D. (2000). Reduction of ECG and Gradient Related Artifacts in Simultaneously Recorded

Human EEG/fMRI Data. *Magnetic Resonance Imaging,* Vol.18, No.7, pp.881-886, ISSN 0730-725X

[46] Srivastava, G., Crottaz-Herbette, S., Lau, K.M., Glover, G.H., & Menon, V. (2005). ICA-Based Procedures for Removing Ballistocardiogram Artifacts from EEG Data Acquired in the MRI Scanner. *NeuroImage,* Vol.24, No.1, pp.50-60, ISSN 1053-8119

[47] Tenforde, T.S., Gaffey, C.T., Moyer, B.R., & Budinger, T.F. (1983). Cardiovascular Alterations in Macaca Monkeys Exposed to Stationary Magnetic Fields: Experimental Observations and Theoretical Analysis. *Bioelectromagnetics,* Vol.4, No.1, pp.1-9, ISSN 1521-186X

[48] Thornton, R., Laufs, H., Rodionov, R., Cannadathu, S., Carmichael, D.W., Vulliemoz, S., Salek-Haddadi, A., McEvoy, A.W., Smith, S.M., Lhatoo, S., Elwes, R.D., Guye, M., Walker, M.C., Lemieux, L., & Duncan, J.S. (2010). EEG Correlated Functional MRI and Postoperative Outcome in Focal Epilepsy. *Journal of Neurology, Neurosurgery, and Psychiatry,* Vol.81, pp.922–927, ISSN 0022-3050

[49] Vanderperren, K., De Vos, M., Ramauter, J., Novitskiy, N., Mennes, M., Assecondi, S., Vanrumste, B., Stiers, P., Van den Bergh, B., Wagemans, J., Lagae, L., Sunaert, S. & Van Huffel, S. (2010). Removal of BCG Artifacts from EEG Recordings Inside the MR Scanner: A Comparison of Methodological and Validation-Related Aspects. *NeuroImage,* Vol.50, No.3, pp.920-934, ISSN 1053-8119

[50] Vincent, J.L., Larson-Prior, L.F., Zempel, J.M., Snyder, A.Z. (2007). Moving GLM Ballistocardiogram Artifact Reduction for EEG Acquired Simultaneously with fMRI. *Clinical Neurophysiology,* Vol.118, No.5, pp.981-998, ISSN 1388-2457

[51] Zijlmans, M., Huiskamp, G., Hersevoort, M., Seppenwoolde, J.H., van Huffelen, A.C., & Leijten, F.S. (2007). EEG-fMRI in the Preoperative Work-Up for Epilepsy Surgery. Brain, Vol.130, pp.2343–2353, ISSN 1460-2156

3

Brain Functional Networks in the Developing Brain Using Resting BOLD

Wei Gao, Hongtu Zhu, Kelly S. Giovanello,
J. Keith Smith, Dinggang Shen, John H. Gilmore and
Weili Lin

1. Introduction

One of the most astounding transformations that takes place in the living world is the transformation of human brain from an earthworm like neural tube in the embryo to a well organized system consisting of billions of neurons, trillions of synapses, as well as supporting cells/structures. Equally astounding is the emergence of various complex functions that accompany this remarkable structural transformation. In the long query to shed light on brain's functional development process, two questions – (1) how and when specific functional modules emerge; and (2) how different functional modules integrate/coordinate to form an efficient brain system, lie in the core. Traditional behavioral studies (Amsterdam, 1972; Cepeda et al., 2001; Diesendruck et al., 2004) have provided valuable information about the developmental process, but such studies do not offer insights into the anatomical and functional development of the brain in relation to the observed behavioral maturation. Neuroimaging studies, in contrast, (including positron emission tomography (PET), magnetic resonance imaging (MRI), etc) enable either direct or indirect elucidation of the underlying neuronal activity, potentially, unveiling the neurophysiological mechanisms guiding the developmental process. Insights from such studies are also critical for better understanding of the neuropathology underlying various developmental disorders, whose early diagnosis/intervention/treatment may benefit greatly from the quantitative and objective nature of these investigations.

Traditional task-based functional magnetic resonance imaging (fMRI) techniques have been a powerful and non-invasive tool for adult brain imaging for decades (Bandettini et al., 1992

Belliveau et al., 1991; Ogawa et al., 1990) and its application in developmental investigation has also been long practiced. The feasibility of fMRI in newborns was first demonstrated by Born et al in 1996 (Born et al., 1996), who reported a differential visual activation pattern between infants and older children. Next, Hykin et al (Hykin et al., 1999) successfully conducted fMRI experiments in fetuses in 1999. Other groups have subsequently reported different functional activation patterns during both pre-and postnatal periods (Anderson et al., 2001; Born et al., 1998; Dehaene-Lambertz et al., 2002; Fulford et al., 2003). However, constrained by the inability to "perform tasks," only visual, auditory or tactile stimuli could be applied in such investigations, greatly limiting the scope of brain functions that were explored using this technique.

The recent advance of resting state functional connectivity MRI (fcMRI) technique (Biswal et al., 1995; Lowe et al., 1998), however, has greatly expanded the scope of fMRI beyond taskbased approaches and provided a unique opportunity to answer fundamental questions about the brain's functional network organization. Initially described in Biswal et al's seminal paper (Biswal et al., 1995), fcMRI measures temporal synchronization of spontaneous blood oxygen level dependent (BOLD) fluctuations at rest, eliminating the need for external stimuli/tasks. Thus, fcMRI greatly simplifies the experimental design and provides unique information regarding the brain's functional organization that is not available through traditional task-based fMRI analysis. In adult subjects, various resting state functional networks (RSNs) have been consistently reported including a motor-sensory network (Biswal et al., 1995), a visual network (Lowe et al., 1998), attention networks (Fox et al., 2006), a memory network (Vincent et al., 2006), and a network mediating self-related thinking (i.e., the brain's default-mode network) (Greicius et al., 2003; Raichle et al., 2001; Shulman GL, 1997). Results from these RSNs are highly consistent with the known anatomical connection and/or functional coactivation patterns (Biswal et al., 1995). More importantly, fcMRI is particularly suited for studies where the target population is not able to perform specific cognitive tasks as required by traditional fMRI, such as studies of early brain development and neurological diseases (Greicius et al., 2004; Liu et al., 2008; Seeley et al., 2009).

Although fcMRI has been successfully applied in numerous studies aimed at unveiling the brain's functional organization (e.g., development, aging, disease), several issues could affect the robustness/interpretation of the obtained results. Among them, the physiological underpinnings of fcMRI signal remain elusive. Since the BOLD signal provides only an indirect measure of the underlying neuronal activity, a pressing need for understanding of the neuronal correlates of the fMRI signal has been widely recognized. The consensus is that task-driven BOLD signal is highly correlated with local field potential (LFP), which is a complex signal arising from integrated electrical activity in the pre-and postsynaptic terminals recorded in the vicinity of embedded microelectrodes in the cortex (Logothetis, 2003; Logothetis et al., 2001; Raichle and Mintun, 2006). However, neuronal dynamics resulting from external tasks are likely fundamentally different from that observed in fcMRI signal. As a result, a direct translation from the previous findings of task-driven fMRI to fcMRI interpretation may be untenable. To directly delineate the underlying neural correlates of spontaneous BOLD signal fluctuations, several groups have made important discoveries. First, using an anesthetized monkey model, Shmuel and Leopold (Shmuel and Leopold, 2008) demonstrated a significant, time-lagged correlation between spontaneous BOLD fluctuations and the power of neuronal activity in the local filed potential gamma band, multi-unit activity, and spiking activity, directly supporting the notion that fcMRI correlation reflects the underlying neuronal interplay between remote cortical regions. Second, by extracting signal from the depth electrodes placed in the auditory cortex of epilepsy patients, Nir et al (Nir et al., 2008) found significant inter-hemispheric correlations in the slow modulations of neuronal firing rates and gamma (40~100Hz) LPF power with a clear spatial selectivity, further revealing the underlying neuronal correlates of fcMRI signal. Additionally, He et al (He et al., 2008) also examined the correlation structure of slow cortical potential (SCP) signal recorded from the implanted electrodes in a similar epilepsy patient study and showed a consistent correlation structure with that from fcMRI signals, providing evidence of the possible contribution of SCP in the observed fcMRI correlation structure. Overall, although some discrepancies exist among the studies examining the neuronal correlates of the observed fcMRI signal, the common finding of significant neuronal activity correlation strongly supports the notion that functional organization structures observed in fcMRI experiments reflect underlying neuronal interplay. Future studies are still needed to further discern the physiological origins of fcMRI signal.

While fcMRI has been utilized to examine a wide variety of neurological diseases (Fair et al., 2010; Greicius et al., 2004), aging (Achard and Bullmore, 2007), as well as brain development (Fair et al., 2008; Fransson et al., 2007; Gao et al., 2009), emphasis in this chapter is given to how fcMRI can be used to explore temporal and spatial evolution of early brain functional development. In particular, we will focus on the first two years of life – the most critical time period for postnatal brain development (Tau and Peterson, 2010). As early as the fifth week after conception, the first synapses begin forming in the fetus's spinal cord which permits the first fetal movements such as spontaneous arches and curls of the whole body (Joseph, 1999). More complicated and coordinated movements such as stretching, yawning, sucking, swallowing, and grasping soon follow in the first and second trimesters. Toward the end of the prenatal period, fetuses begin to respond to familiar odors and sounds (Joseph, 1999). It is clear that nature ensures such vital and basic bodily functions are in place by the time a baby emerges from the supporting womb.

After prenatal development, the first two years of life are commonly viewed as the most critical time period for postnatal brain development (Tau and Peterson, 2010). At birth, the brain is approximately one-quarter of its adult size and quickly grows to an adult-like volume (around 80%) by the end of the second year. The dramatic increase in the number of dendrites and synapses is partly responsible for such a fast volume increase. In fact, the first two years of life are an exuberant period for synapse growth and cerebral cortex produces most of its synaptic connections. By the end of the second year, a toddler's cerebral cortex contains more than one thousand trillions of synapses, which are far more than that in an adult's brain (around 50 percent more) and will experience a prolonged, experiencedependent pruning process to achieve its matured configuration (Johnson, 2000, 2001; Tau and Peterson, 2010). Axonal elongation, thickening, and myelination processes are also important growth factors during this period (Gao et al., 2008; Haynes et al., 2005). It has been documented that long axonal connections are nearly complete around 9 months of age (Conel, 1939-1963; Tau and Peterson, 2010). Moreover, continuous myelination of white matter during the first two years of life greatly improves the brain's electrical signal transfer efficiency (Haynes et al., 2005). Concurrent with the above mentioned dramatic structural development is the parallel improvement in brain function. Decasper and Fifer (DeCasper and Fifer, 1980) demonstrated that the sensorimotor experiences of fetus and voice of mother (Kolata, 1984) can be recognized. Additionally, Fivush and Hamond (Fivush, 1990) showed that 2yr olds can already retrieve much detail about a trip to the zoo. Studies on toddlers also revealed that 18-to 24-month-olds are able to use speaker's gaze direction (Baldwin, 1993) and affective expression (Tomasello et al., 1996) as cues leading to speaker's communicative purposes. Akhtar and Tomasello (Akhtar, 2000) further proposed that children are able to infer the meaning of words through an understanding of people's minds (Diesendruck et al., 2004). More importantly, one of the unique properties of human self-awareness has also been documented to undergo major development during the first two years of life (Amsterdam, 1972). The gradual emergence of such higher order cognitive functions leads to the hypothesis of parallel establishment of corresponding functional networks during this critical period. Moreover, as more complex functions emerge, the brain's information transfer efficiency is also expected to improve. Leveraging on graph theory analysis (Bullmore and Sporns, 2009), brain's information transfer efficiency can be effectively measured based on fcMRI time series data.

Although this chapter primarily focuses on the applications of fcMRI in normal brain development, fcMRI studies in developmental disorders are also briefly reviewed. This chapter is organized as follows: Section 2 provides a review of data acquisition, preprocessing and various analysis approaches for fcMRI study; Section 3 illustrates recent findings on the emergence of various functional networks; Section 4 shifts attention from individual networks to the whole brain network; Section 5 reviews recent applications of fcMRI on various developmental disorders; Section 6 provides a discussion of the limitations and future directions of the use of fcMRI in developmental studies; and finally, Section 7 provides a conclusion.

2. Data acquisition and analysis

The acquisition of resting state fcMRI data is identical to that of traditional task-based fMRI (except no task/stimuli are required during the acquisition) for which echo planer imaging (EPI) is the most frequently used imaging sequence due to its fast scan time. Using an EPI sequence, a 2D slice can be acquired in approximately 40 to 100ms and 2 to 3 seconds for whole brain coverage, which alleviates motion-related artifacts during imaging. However, this sequence is prone to other artifacts related to either hardware (e.g., eddy current effect) or imaging sample (e.g., T2* related susceptibility effect). Moreover, although EPI is already a fast imaging technique, the time resolution (~2 seconds) is still far from sufficient to characterize the dynamic of underlying neuronal activity and unable to faithfully sample several physiological factors such as respiratory/cardiac cycles resulting in potential noise contamination. Therefore, further improvement in imaging acquisition methods for faster scanning is greatly desired (Feinberg et al., 2010). Another important factor in fcMRI experiments is the required duration of acquisition. Van Dijk et al. (Van Dijk et al., 2010) compared the correlation strengths resulting from different lengths of data acquisitions (from ~4min to ~12min) and reported that they stabilized at 5-6 min of data acquisition. More recently, Whitlow et al. (Whitlow et al., 2011) reported similar findings and further proposed that graph theory metrics of network connectivity might be accurately calculated from as little as 1.5~2 min of fcMRI data. Besides these technical considerations, fcMRI study requires that subjects are at a "resting" state. In adult studies, different ways of keeping subjects at resting are utilized such as fixation, eyes closed resting (ECR), and eyes open resting (EOR). Van Dijk et al. (Van Dijk et al., 2010) compared the functional connectivity strength within default and attention networks during these different resting states and reported significant differences between ECR and fixation, as well as between ECR and EOR, but not between EOR and fixation, indicating a significant effect of eyes opening versus eyes closing. However, similar comparisons on other functional networks are lacking and the conclusion might not be directly generalized. In developmental studies, keeping the subjects "resting" and still within the scanner at wake condition proves to be extremely challenging. Therefore, most developmental studies, especially those focusing on the first two years of life, scan their subjects during sleeping state (either natural sleeping or sedation-induced sleeping). For older children, as keeping them sleeping within the scanner becomes harder, watching movie is an alternative for keeping them still in the scanner, but the brain state difference between sleeping and movie watching should be considered (Gao and Lin, 2012).

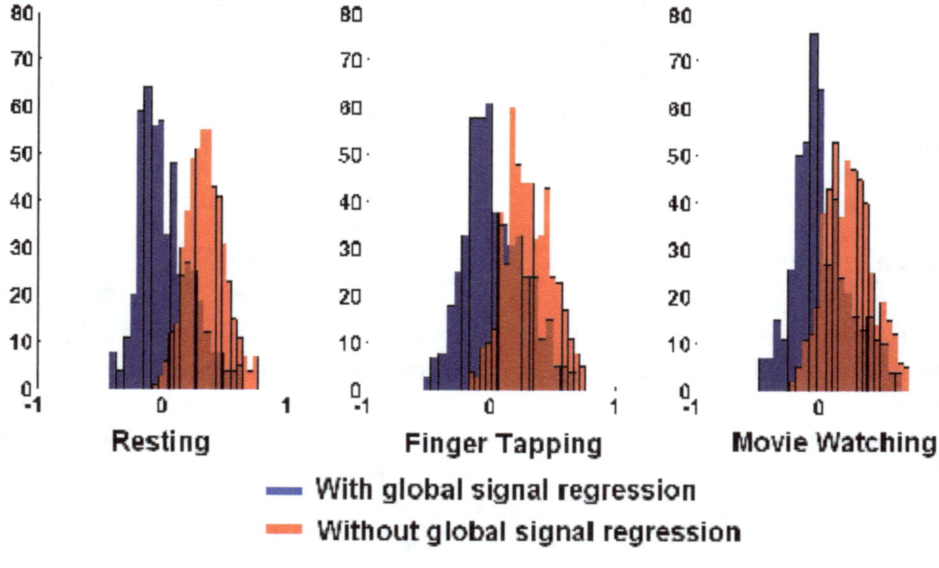

Figure 1. The histograms of the group mean correlation matrices (16 subjects, 32 ROIs covering five predefined functional networks, 496 correlations) with (blue) and without (red) global signal regression during three experimental conditions-resting, finger tapping, and movie watching. This figure was reproduced with the permission from Gao and Lin. (2012).

While acquiring fcMRI images is rather straightforward and EPI is the most widely employed imaging sequence, the means through which fcMRI data is processed to discern brain functional connectivity is less consistent across different research labs. Typically, fcMRI is preprocessed, including time shifting, motion correction, spatial smoothing, linear trend removal, low pass filtering (typically <0.1Hz) and nuisance signal regression. Although minor discrepancies exist regarding the pre-processing procedures among different researchers, most of the steps are fairly consistent and widely accepted with the exception of nuisance signal regression, especially global signal removal, which is designed to minimize the potential sources of physiological noise such as respiration and cardiac motion (Chang and Glover, 2010; Fox et al., 2009; Murphy et al., 2009). Such a regression forces the resulting correlation strength distribution (from a seed-based analysis) to be bellshaped centered at zero. Fig. 1 shows the distribution of correlation coefficients with and without global signal removal during three different experimental conditions-resting, finger tapping, and movie watching (Gao and Lin, 2012). It is immediately apparent that the removal of global signal leads to the presence of negative correlations. One immediate question is whether the observed negative correlation is "introduced" by global signal removal or is "brought" into light after removing the nuisance factors (global signal) obscuring the true relationships. Great controversy exists concerning the interpretation of negative correlations (Fox et al., 2009; Murphy et al., 2009). Fox et al (Fox et al., 2009) have shown that after removing the networks in question from the global signal mask (essentially eliminating the mathematical constraints on the two systems), certain anti-correlation can still be observed. Moreover, in an independent study, Chang and Glover (Chang and Glover, 2010) showed evidence of the presence of anti-correlation between the default network and the task-positive dorsal attention network, both with and without controlling for physiological noise variation induced by respiration and heart beating (although physiological noise correction did increase the spatial extent and magnitude of negative correlations). Such findings partially support the "authenticity" of the observed negative correlation, but future studies are needed to further delineate the nature of the global signal and the interpretation of the negative correlations after their removal.

After the pre-processing steps, three categories of methods generally exist for further processing fcMRI data to examine brain functional connectivity: (1) seed-based method; (2) independent component analysis based method; and (3) graph-theory analysis based method. The seed-based approach is the most widely adopted likely due to its simplicity in both implementation and interpretation. By designating a seed region for obtaining the reference signal, a voxel-wise whole brain correlation analysis can be conducted to acquire individual-based functional connectivity maps, which can then be pooled together to obtain a group map after statisitcal testing of each voxel's connectivity strength. Such a map represents the architecture of the functional network dictated by the seed region, enabling easy interpretation of the results. However, this approach could potentially be biased by the choice of the seed region and can only determine the brain functional connectivity specifically associated with the chosen seed. Most of the reported studies detemine the seed region either based on anatomical features or published coordinates of previous fMRI activation studies. Then a spherical ROI is defined centered at the seed with a certain radius, where both the location and size can vary from study to study. This variability poses a potential problem for direct comparisons between different studies. This problem is worsened in developmental studies since both the structural and functional brain organization might differ from those of adults, making the choice of seed regions based on the readily available adult literatures impractical. Mathematically, seed-based correlation analysis measures only the pair-wise correlation between a seed region and the voxel in question while ignoring the multivariate relationship among all brain voxels, which may be suboptimal especially when one intends to define the architectures of several networks simultaneously (Joel et al., 2011).

The independent component analysis (ICA) approach, on the other hand, largely alleviates the above mentioned problems. First, since it does not need pre-specified seed regions but extracts spatially/temporally independent components in a data-driven fashion, the biases associated with choosing seed regions are largely avoided. Second, depending on whether spatial or temporal ICA is applied, this approach maximizes the spatial/temporal independence among all identified components simultaneously by considering all voxel's time courses together, thus alleviating the "pair-wise" correlation problem embedded in the seed-based approach. Given these advantages, numerous studies (Damoiseaux et al., 2006; Fransson et al., 2010; Gao et al., 2009) have applied ICA and the results are fruitful. However, these advantages come at a cost. Since there is no inherent "ranking" available for ICA-extracted components, selecting components reflecting brain functions is a matter of subjectivity through either visual inspection or template matching. Although quantitative methods (De Martino et al., 2007; Perlbarg et al., 2007; Tohka et al., 2008) aiming to solve this issue are emerging, their effectiveness and robustness need to be validated by independent studies.

Another widely used strategy is to parcellate the entire brain into a set of ROIs and to perform graph-theory based analyses to delineate the whole brain's functional topology. More detailed reviews of graph theory based analysis can be found in Bullmore and Sporns (Bullmore and Sporns, 2009). The small-world related measures (Latora and Marchiori, 2001; Watts and Strogatz, 1998) are especially popular and have been used to quantify the brain's development (Supekar et al., 2009), aging (Achard and Bullmore, 2007), as well as various disease processes (Liu et al., 2008). However, similar to a seed-based approach, there is no standard approach as to how the whole brain should be parcellated. In practice, different anatomical feature based parcellation schemes including AAL (Tzourio-Mazoyer et al., 2002), ANIMAL (Collins et al., 1995) have been used. However, as described by Fornito et al (Fornito et al., 2010) and Wang et al. (Wang et al., 2009), different graph analytic measures may arise from different parcellation resolutions, making direct comparisons between studies untenable. Moreover, anatomical parcellation approaches do not explicitly consider functional similarity within the defined regions. As a result, spatial intra-region inhomogeneity of the BOLD signals may lead to spuriously averaged signals, and hence, inaccurate graph analytic measures. Data driven functional similarity based brain parcellation schemes are particularly desired in studies where the architecture of brain functional regions may deviate from that in normal adults. Such methods (Nelson et al., 2010; Neumann et al., 2006; Shen et al., 2010) directly utilize Pearson's correlation or canonical correlation between BOLD time series as similarity measure aiming at defining functionally sensible parcellations. As such strategies could effectively address the functional inhomogeneity concern inherent in anatomical-defined parcellation schemes, potential issues also exist. Among them, the most challenging one might be the number of regions to define. As most current methods relying on predefining a fixed number based on prior information, more data-driven approaches are highly desired and deserve further effort.

In addition, another limit for graph-theory based methods is that there is currently no optimal way to compare networks with different number of nodes and/or edges (van Dijk et al., 2010). A summary of different fcMRI analysis methods can be found in Table. 1.

Methods	Brief Description	Advantage	Disadvantage
Seed-based method	By designating a seed region for obtaining the reference signal, a voxel-wise whole brain correlation analysis is conducted to define a particular functional network.	Easy implementation ; Straightforward Interpretation.	Seed choice bias; Focusing on pair-wise correlation while ignoring multivariate relationship among multiple networks.
Independent component analysis (ICA)	Functional networks are extracted through blind source separation technique-ICA.	Data-driven way to define functional networks; Simultaneous extraction of multiple functional networks based on their multivariate relation.	Subjective selection of independent components for subsequent analysis.
Graphtheory based analysis	The brain is first pacellated into a set of ROIs after which graphtheory based analysis is performed to evaluate brain's functional topology using various network measures.	Whole brain analysis enabling assessment of brain's overall information transferring property through various graph-theory based measures.	Anatomically defined parcellation; Currently no standard ways to compare networks with different numbers of nodes and/or edges.

Table 1. Typical methods applied in fcMRI study.

3. The emergence of individual functional networks during the first two years of life

A mature brain works as a unified system involving various functionally specialized networks each dealing with an array of specialized functions. Generally, depending on the nature of the functions, brain networks are classified into primary functional networks such as sensory, motor, and visual networks or higher order cognitive networks such as attention, memory, executive control, emotion, etc. The developmental trajectory of each individual functional network is of great interest. Successful interaction with the outside world rests on the proper functioning of the primary networks and it has been suggested that they are essential for the tuning and establishment of the higher order cognitive networks (Johnson, 2000, 2001). Therefore, it is anticipated that primary functional networks will develop faster and earlier than those higher order cognitive functional networks.

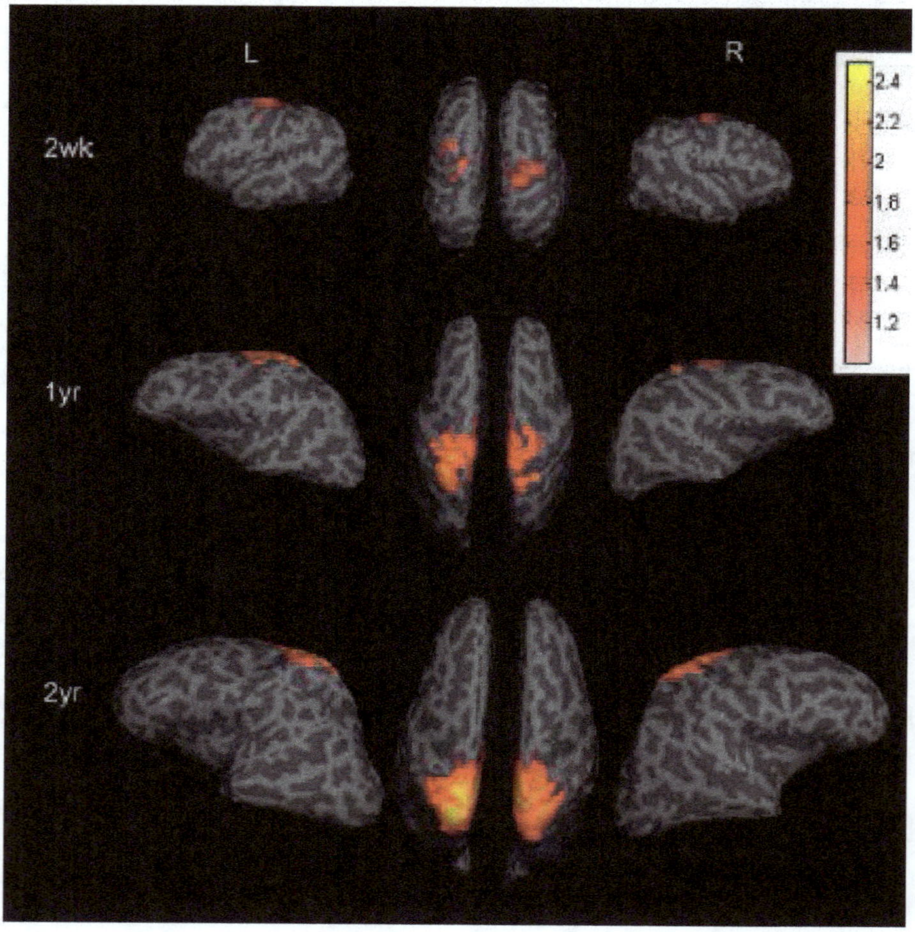

Figure 2. The functional connectivity maps of motor-sensory network at 2wks, 1yr and 2yrs of age, respectively. The color bar represents z-score values. This figure was reproduced with the permission from Lin et al. (2008).

Using a seed-based approach, we (Lin et al., 2008) have reported the developmental patterns of both the motor-sensory and visual networks during the first two years of life (Fig. 2 and Fig. 3). The seeds were manually drawn around bilateral motor-sensory cortex and visual cortex for the two networks, respectively. The most noticeable feature is that starting at neonates, the two networks already demonstrate a bilateral-symmetric functional connectivity pattern similar to that of 2yr olds, which is also reasonably consistent with their adult configuration (Biswal et al., 1995). Consistent with this finding, Fransson et al (Fransson et al., 2007) also reported the existence of adult-like motor-sensory, visual, as well as auditory networks in preterm infants scanned at term equivalent age. A longitudinal study by Smyser et al (Smyser et al., 2010) further delineated the dramatic development of such primary sensory networks during the prenatal period from 26 weeks postmenstrual age to the term equivalent age supporting the network structures observed in neonatal subjects. The early synchronization of these primary sensory functional networks most likely indicates an evolutional optimization to ensure early survival as well as effective interaction with the outside world for proper experience-based tuning of other higher order networks. However, despite of the common feature of early synchronization, Fig. 2 and 3 show that the motor-sensory network demonstrates more development during the first year of life, while visual network shows more increase during the second year of in terms of normalized volume of cortical connectivity, which indicates certain level of differential growth trajectories for different primary networks.

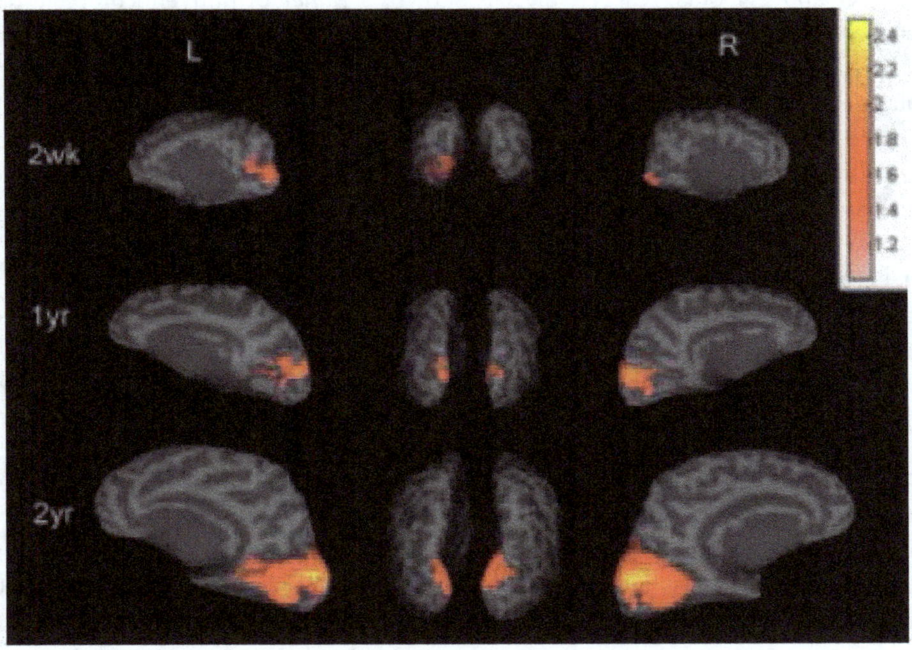

Figure 3. The functional connectivity maps of visual network at 2wks, 1yr and 2yrs of age, respectively. The color bar represents z-score values. This figure was reproduced with the permission from Lin et al. (2008).

While the primary brain functional networks appear to be reasonably developed immediately after birth, the growth trajectories of other higher order cognitive functional networks likely differ. Recently, a novel brain functional network was proposed by Raichle et al (Raichle et al., 2001) where the involved brain regions exhibit down-regulated activity during various goal-directed external tasks but up-regulated activity during uncontrolled resting state (Shulman GL, 1997). Various studies have been conducted in an attempt to probe the exact function of this network (Buckner et al., 2008; Buckner and Carroll, 2007; Greicius and Menon, 2004; Gusnard et al., 2001; Gusnard and Raichle, 2001). Among them, the consensus is that this network mainly supports self-related internal cognition (Andrews-Hanna et al., 2010; Buckner et al., 2008; Buckner and Carroll, 2007; Gusnard et al., 2001). From a developmental perspective, the establishment of self-consciousness has to be the preface of such self-referential thinking process and hence is likely related to the integrity of this network. Interestingly, Amsterdam (Amsterdam, 1972) vividly documented the emerging process of self-consciousness during the first two years of life. He showed that neonates could not recognize themselves from their mirror images but infants from 6 through 12 months of age demonstrate prolonged and repeated reaction to their mirror images as a sociable playmate. Wariness, withdrawal, self-admiring, and embarrassed behaviors start at 14 months and have been observed in 75% of the children after 20 months of age. From 20 to 24 months of age, the majority of subjects demonstrate recognition of their mirror images. If the default network is indeed responsible for the self-consciousness based internal thinking process, we would expect a gradual orchestration of this network during the first two years of life. Fig. 4 shows the default network of 3wks, 1yr and 2yr olds, respectively. As shown, a rather primitive/incomplete default network consisting of 6 brain regions is observed in neonates, among which only medial prefrontal cortex (MPFC) and posterior cingulate cortex (PCC) regions are typically observed in its adult configuration. The finding of an "incomplete" default network is consistent with results from several other studies (Fransson et al., 2007; Smyser et al., 2010). However, at 1yr old, a total of 13 regions are observed and 10 of them are consistent with that observed in adults, including ventral/dorsal MPFC, PCC/retrosplenial (Rsp), bilateral lateral temporal cortex (LTC), bilateral inferior parietal lobule (IPL), and the hippocampal formation (HF) (Buckner et al., 2008). Such dramatic synchronization reflects fast orchestration of this network during the first year of life. In 2yr olds, the default network continues to grow by covering more regions (13 regions) consistent with adult's configuration. However, 6 non-typical regions including the orbital frontal, anterior cingulate cortex (ACC), right and medial parietal, and bilateral superior temporal regions are also observed.

The spring embedding plots (Ebbels et al., 2006) further demonstrate the topology of the default network throughout the first two years of life (Fig. 5). These graphs are arranged such that the most strongly connected regions were drawn close to each other and placed in the center of the graph and vice versa. One notable feature is that both PCC/Rsp and MPFC are consistently located in the center of each graph with the exception of the neonate group (only PCC/Rsp), implying that these two regions are most strongly connected with other regions. Moreover, the PCC/Rsp and MPFC reliably exhibit the highest mean connection strengths across all ages (Fig. 6). Such finding is consistent with adult studies (Buckner et al., 2008) reporting the "hub" role of these two regions in this distributed network. The betweenness centrality (BC) (Brandes, 2001) – a measure of node importance in graph theory further confirm that PCC/RSp and MPFC indeed serve as the hubs in the pediatric default network (Fig. 7). These results suggest that the PCC/Rsp may be the major hub of the default network whereas the MPFC subsequently emerges, potentially, as the secondary hub starting at 1yr of age.

Overall, a gradual emergence of the default network is observed during the first two years of life and the PCC/Rsp and MPFC emerge as two potential hubs. This finding is consistent with previous reports of the emergence of self-consciousness (Amsterdam, 1972), as well as other

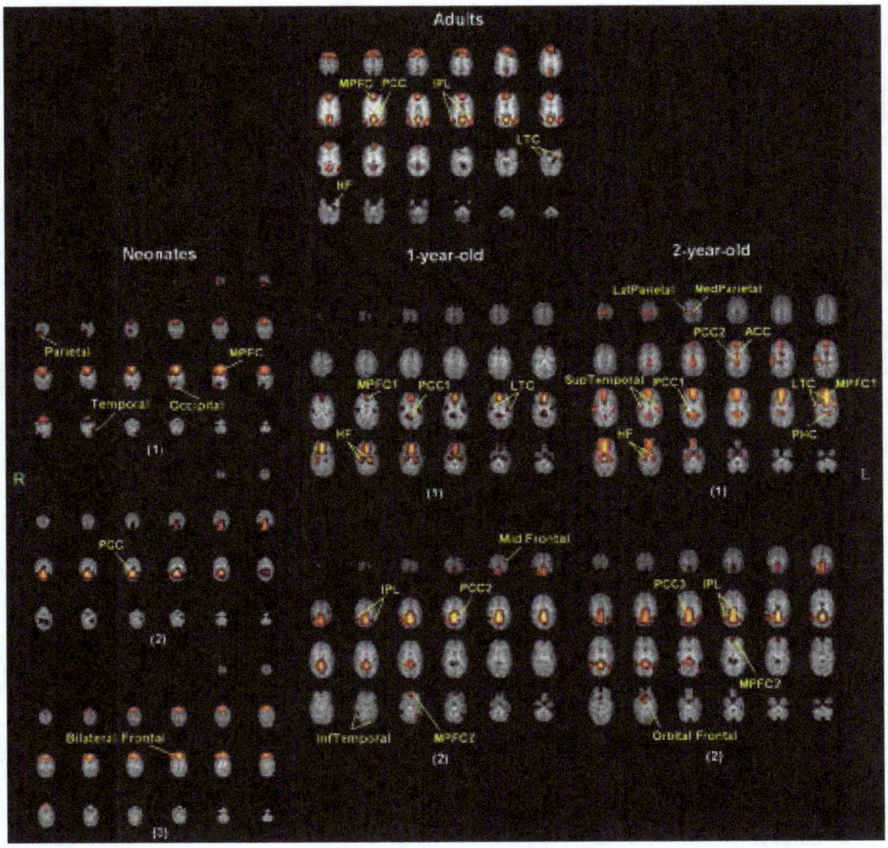

Figure 4. The independent components associated with brain's default network for neonates, 1yr olds, 2yr olds and adults. Individual regions are labeled for each map. ACC: anterior cingulate cortex; HF: hippocampal formation; InfTemporal: inferior temporal cortex; IPL: inferior parietal lobule; LTC: lateral temporal cortex; LatParietal: lateral parietal cortex; MedParietal: medial parietal cortex; MidFrontal: middle frontal cortex; MPFC: medial prefrontal cortex; PCC: posterior cingulate cortex; PHC: para-hippocampal cortex; SupTemporal: superior temporal cortex. This figure was reproduced with the permission from Gao et al. (2009).

default network related functions such as episodic memory (Fivush, 1990; Kolata, 1984). Moreover, the appearance of non-typical regions in all three pediatric groups' default network indicates further pruning/specialization process needed for final maturation. Therefore, in contrast to the primary networks (e.g., motor-sensory, visual) for which the major development is done prenatally, the establishment of the higher order default network takes prolonged postnatal development to achieve its functioning configuration.

Up to now, the discussions are largely focused on individual network level. As our brain is an integrated system consisting of many functionally specialized networks, it is of critical importance to further understand the interaction among different networks. Five networks including the previously described motor-sensory, visual, default network and two other higher order networks-dorsal attention and fronto-parietal control network (Vincent et al., 2008) were simultaneously studied based on an extended dataset including 51 neonates (27

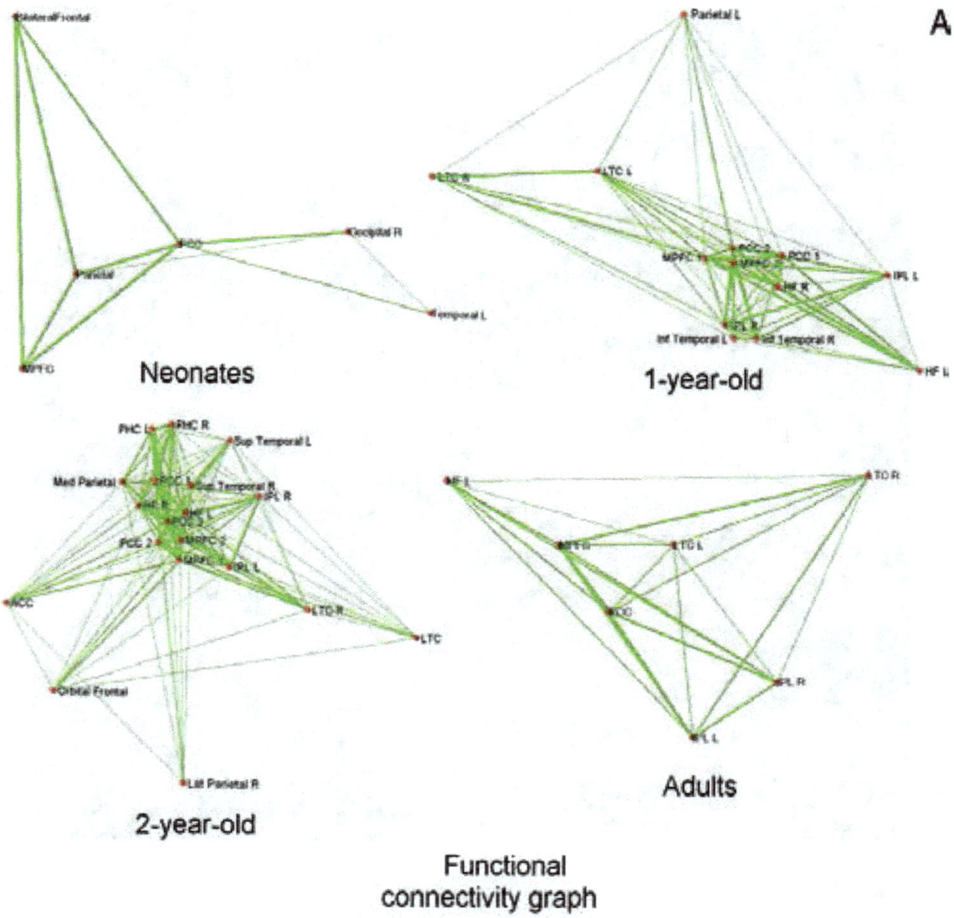

Figure 5. The spring embedding plots of the group-mean functional correlation patterns within the default network for neonates, 1yr olds, 2yr olds and adults. This figure was reproduced with the permission from Gao et al. (2009).

male, 23± 12days (SD)), 50 1yr olds (27 male, 13± 1 months) and 46 2yr olds (28 male, 24± 1 months). Specifically, 5, 6, 6, 6, and 9 ROIs (8mm-radius sphere, altogether 32 ROIs) were defined based on the MNI coordinates published in adult studies (Vincent et al., 2008) to construct the five networks, respectively, from which the group mean correlation matrices were constructed (32×32) and visualized using spring-embedding plot (Fig. 8). In this figure, the segregation/synchronization of the five networks across the first two years of life can be simultaneously characterized. In neonates, except for the motor-sensory network (red) and the visual network (blue), which are already well organized into cohesive clusters, the remaining three higher-order cognitive networks are rather scattered (i.e., three separated clusters for default network (yellow); two for the dorsal attention network (magenta) and two for fronto-parietal control network (brown).

This finding is highly consistent with results shown in Fig. 2-4, which again indicates early maturation of primary functional networks. In fact, the motor-sensory and visual networks

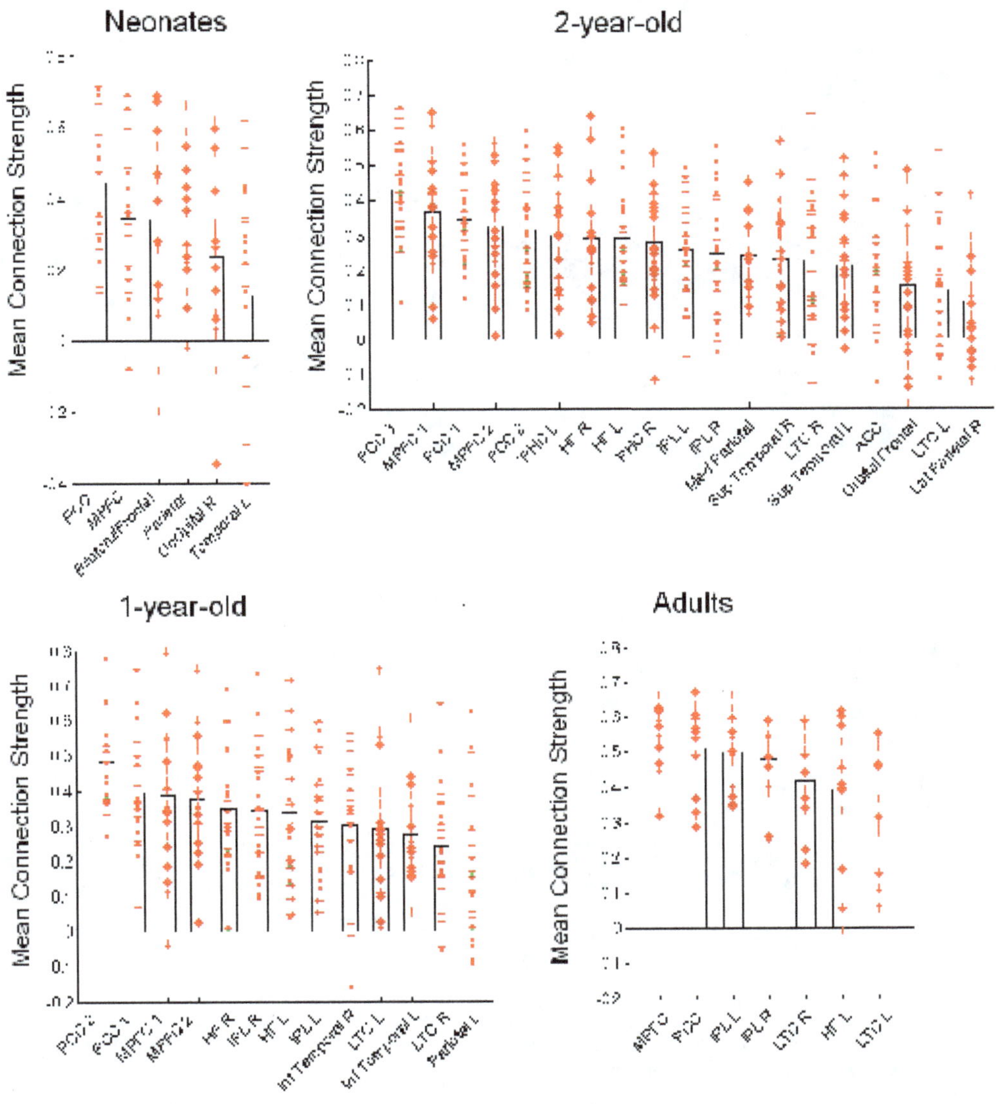

Figure 6. The mean connectivity strength of each node within the default mode network for neonates, 1yr olds, 2yr olds and adults. Each bar represents the group mean of each node's mean connectivity strength within the default network. Each asterisk represents an individual subjects' value. This figure was reproduced with the permission from Gao et al. (2009).

remain as cohesive clusters throughout the different age groups examined (i.e., neonates, 1yr olds, 2yr olds, and adults, Fig. 8). In great contrast, the synchronization of higher-order cognitive networks takes a more prolonged time. Specifically, the default network starts to be synchronized into one cluster in 1yr olds and remains so thereafter. However, although the other two networks (i.e., the dorsal attention network and the fronto-parietal control network) demonstrate certain long-distance synchronization during the first two years of life (Fig. 8), it

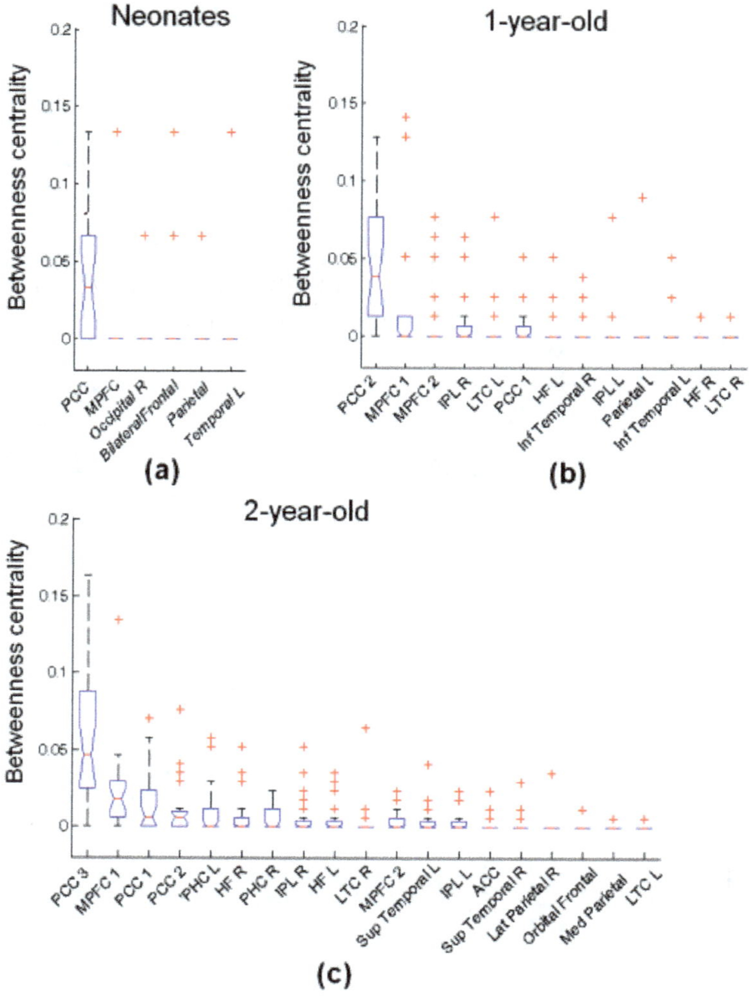

Figure 7. The betweenness centrality value for each node in the default network for neonates, 1yr olds, and 2yr olds. This figure was reproduced with the permission from Gao et al. (2009).

is not until adults are they organized into selfcontained clusters. Clearly, more quantitative characterization, as well as additional sampling between 2yr olds and adults, is highly desirable for more specific delineation of the complete growth trajectories of these five networks. Nevertheless, one trend is again clear in Fig. 8; primary networks such as motor-sensory and visual are wired prenatally while the synchronization of higher-order cognitive networks is achieved during postnatal life (Fransson et al., 2007; Lin et al., 2008; Smyser et al., 2010). Interestingly, from a spatial perspective, higher order cognitive networks are usually spatially distributed but primary sensory networks are mostly locally wired. This local organization might partially contribute to their early synchronization. Specifically, it is likely that long distance connections are not established immediately after birth (discussed below) and that the anatomical proximity facilitates formation of short-distance connections so close

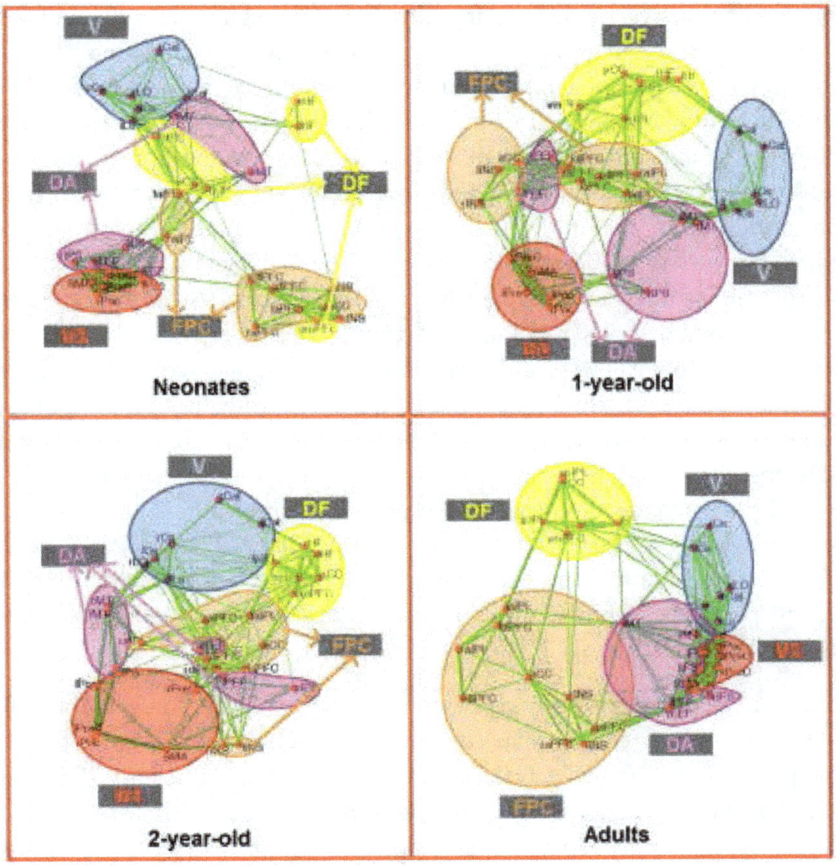

Figure 8. Spring embedding plots of the group-mean correlation pattern among five predefined functional networks: motor-sensory, visual, default, dorsal attention, and fronto-parietal control network. The spatial evolution of each network is highlighted by different colors. DA: dorsal attention network; DF: default network; FPC: fronto-parietal control network; MS: motor-sensory network; V: visual network.

interaction immediately after birth can be achieved. This property is likely attributed by evolutional optimization so that early survival can be ensured. Moreover, this evolution process promotes the development of experience based fine tuning and maturation of higher order networks (Johnson, 2000, 2001). Overall, existing results support the notion that brain's matured organization is optimized according to the developmental process which not only ensures early functioning of primary functions but also allows sufficient environmental tuning of higher order functions for better adaptation.

4. The evolution of whole brain's efficient topology

The examination of individual functional networks provides vital information about the early development of brain's sub-systems. Yet, how the whole brain topology evolves during this critical time remains elusive. By designating different brain regions as nodes and connections between them as edges, recent graph theory advancement, especially the smallworld topology (Watts and Strogatz, 1998) appears well suited to quantitatively characterize the complex network structure of the human brain. Small world topology is characterized by a high level of local cliquishness as well as sufficient long-range direct connections bridging the local clusters, leading to excellent local and global wiring efficiency for information transfer. The regions that bridge disparate and local clusters are important information transfer portals, usually termed network hubs (Barabasi and Albert, 1999). While many studies have confirmed the existence of small world characters in matured brain networks (Achard et al., 2006; Hilgetag et al., 2000; Salvador and E., 2005; Watts and Strogatz, 1998), Fransson et al (Fransson et al., 2010) showed that the infant (1 week old) brain also exhibits a small world topology. However, how the whole brain network topology continues to evolve during the first years of life remains elusive. In particular, given the dramatic axonal elongation/thickening and myelination during this period (Conel, 1939-1963; Fair et al., 2008; Tau and Peterson, 2010), the resulting enhancement in long-distance connections must have profound implications in achieving a highly efficient brain network. To test these hypotheses, 51 neonates (27 male, 23±12days (SD)), 50 1yr olds (27 male, 13± 1 months) and 46 2yr olds (28 male, 24± 1 months) with successful fcMRI scan were retrospectively identified and graph theoretical analyses were conducted (same as the data used in Fig. 7) (Gao et al., 2011).

A whole brain parcellation approach (as described above) was employed by parcellating the brain into 90 ROIs and correlation matrices from individual subjects were constructed after standard preprocessing (Section 2). Local efficiency (LE), global efficiency (GE) (Latora and Marchiori, 2001), and betweenness centrality measures (Brandes, 2001) were calculated. The significant correlation matrices ($p<0.05$, FDR corrected) are presented in Fig. 9 for neonates, 1yr and 2yr olds. Dramatically increased connection density (Fig. 9b) can be observed from neonates to 1yr olds. Moreover, the anatomical distance histogram plot (Fig. 9c) of these significant connections clearly demonstrates a rightward shift, suggesting increased longrange connections. More importantly, those connections exhibiting increased strength with age are always associated with significantly longer connection distances than those decreasing strength with age (Fig. 9d).

To further examine the topological changes as resulting from the emerging long-distance connections, the top 15% of most significant connections from the group mean correlation matrices were visualized on a brain surface in Fig. 10. Imposing a fixed cost ensures that the topological changes arise not from different number of connections but instead from the rearrangement of connections. Different nodes are classified into different functional modules (represented by different colors) based on modularity analysis of their functional relationship (Newman, 2006). Interestingly, the neonates group's modules are largely local and agree well with the boundaries of different lobes. However, 1yr and 2yr olds' modular structures become dramatically more distributed. For example, in 1yr olds, the cyan-colored module spans across temporal and parietal lobes; the red-colored module covers both the parietal and subcortical regions; while the magenta-colored module includes regions from the parietal, frontal, and temporal lobes. Similarly, the red-colored module covers parietal and subcortical regions; the

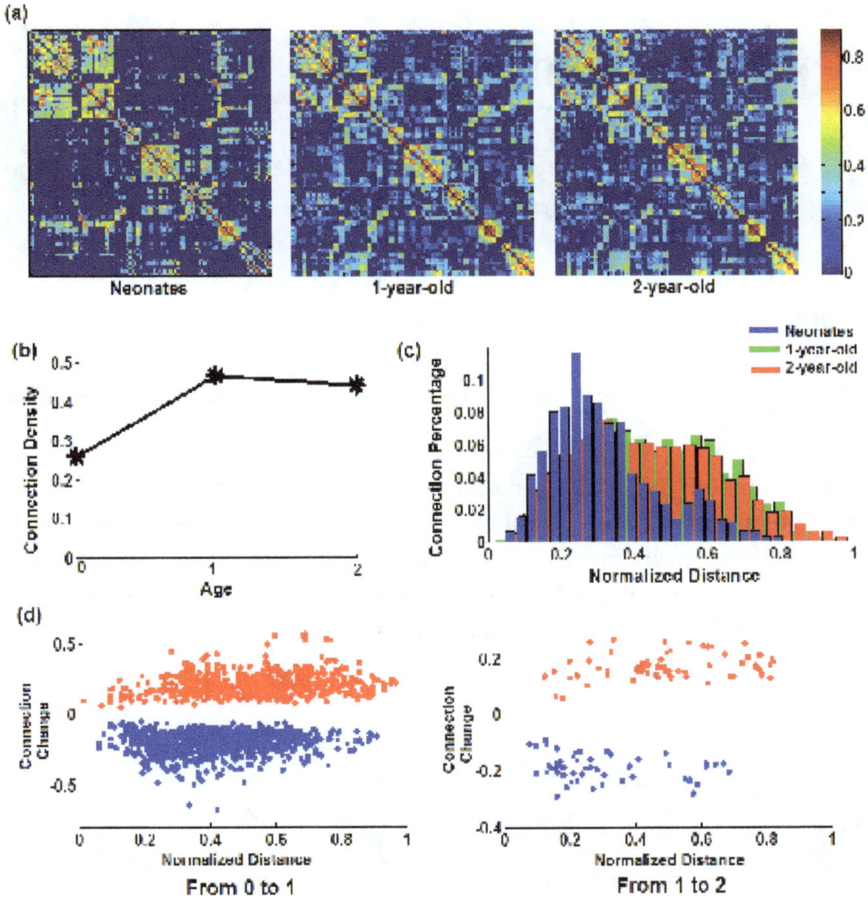

Figure 9. Assessment of age-dependent change of brain network topology. (a) significant connectivity matrices ($p<0.05$, FDR corrected) for neonates, 1yr and 2yr olds; (b) connection density change in the three age groups; (c) the histogram of the normalized anatomical distance associated with the significant connections in each age group's network; (d) comparison of the anatomical distances associated with connections showing age-dependent increase/decrease in strength. Increasing connections with age (red) consistently possess longer anatomical distances than decreasing connections (blue, $p<1e-10$ from 0 to 1and $p=1e-6$ from 1 to 2).

cyan-colored module spans across the frontal and temporal lobes; while the blue-colored module is distributed between the frontal and parietal lobes in 2yr olds, demonstrating a largely distributed functional modular structure. The apparent increase of long-range connections (shown in Fig. 10) highlights the modular structure changes from local to distributed network during the first two years of life.

One of the main characteristics of graph theory analysis is the determination of brain functional hubs for information transfer. The brain's functional hubs (top 10 regions showing highest betweenness centrality values at cost 15%) demonstrate an interesting evolution pattern during the first two years of life (see Fig. 11). There are two apparent clusters of hubs, anterior and posterior clusters, in neonates, suggesting that major functional developments may have

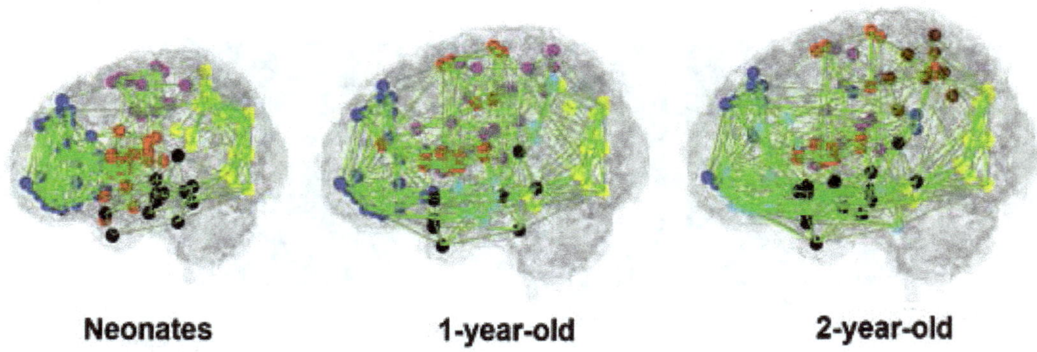

Figure 10. Changes of modular structure during the first two years of life. Different colors represent different modules in each age group.

already occurred in both the frontal and occipital lobes. In addition, most of the connections between the hubs are interhemispherical with no clear connections between the two clusters. In 1 yr olds, the hubs are well connected and more anatomically centered with few hubs located in the anterior and posterior areas of the brain. Finally, the distribution of hubs becomes more spatially uniform in 2yr olds and the connections associated with the hubs provide a fairly uniform covering of the whole brain (Fig. 11).

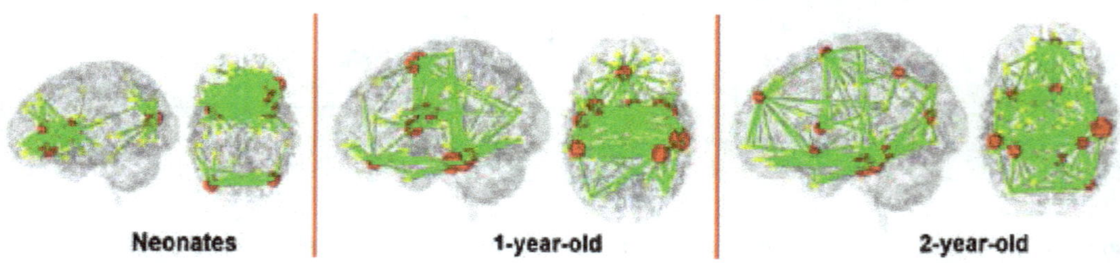

Figure 11. The distribution of functional hubs in the three age groups based on connection matrices at cost 15%. Hub regions together with connections (at cost 15%) are visualized on the corresponding brain surface.

Together, with the aforementioned brain functional network development during the first two years of life, it is highly plausible that brain efficacy for information transfer also undergoes a similar evolution process. To quantitatively examine the efficiency improvement resulting from such dramatic topological changes, local (LE) and global efficiency (GE) for the whole network were calculated for each individual subject at the same cost of 15%. The results are presented in Fig. 12. Significant increases of LE and GE are observed from 3wks to 1yr of age (red asterisks, p=4e-7 and 6e-8 for LE and GE, respectively) but neither measure is statistically different between 1 and 2 yrs of age. Note when comparing neonates with 2yr olds, 2yr olds also demonstrate significantly higher LE (p=1e-8) and GE (p=7e-9).

In summary, the results reported in the literature have consistently indicated that the neonatal brain already exhibits a small-world network with reasonable information transfer efficiency

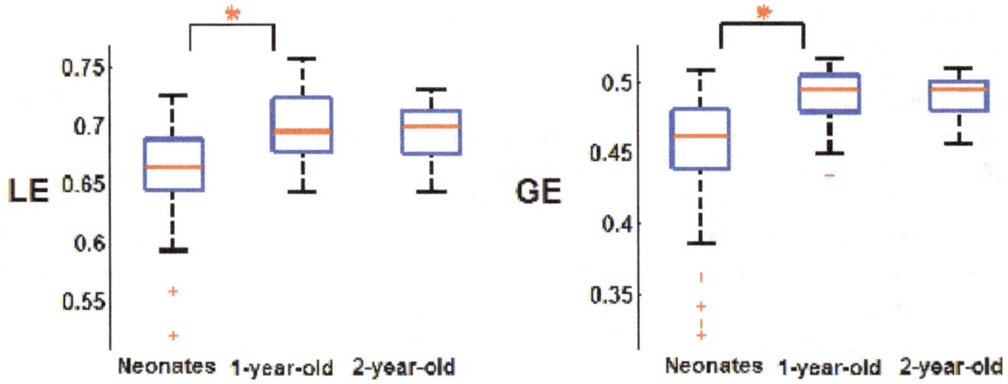

Figure 12. Quantitative measures of whole brain network's local efficiency (LE) and global efficiency (GE) at cost 15% based on individual subject's correlation matrices. Red asterisks represent significant difference at $p<0.05$ (FDR corrected).

(Fransson et al., 2010; Gao et al., 2011). The well documented prenatal axonal development (Haynes et al., 2005) might set the foundation for an efficient connectivity network hence explains this finding. However, significant improvements of both LE and GE are observed from neonates to 1yr olds, whereas no statistical difference between 1 and 2yr olds is observed (Fig. 12). This non-linear developing pattern of brain wiring efficiency, particularly GE, is intriguing. Neonates demonstrate an anatomically ordered architecture (Fig. 10), in which neighboring clusters are largely sequentially connected, leading to a longer path length, while 1 and 2yr olds show considerably better wired brain topologies with abundant bridging connections even between distant clusters, suggesting that anatomical long-range connections may play a critical role in the observed improvement. Indeed, quantitative compassions of connectivity strength show remarkable growth of longdistance connections (Fig. 9) strongly supporting the anatomical basis of network efficiency and suggesting that the establishment of a higher GE rests critically on the development of long-distance connections. An increase in long-distance connections has been reported when comparing school-aged children with adults (Fair et al., 2008; Fair et al., 2009; Kelly et al., 2009). Nevertheless, given the age differences between our study cohort and that reported in the literature, the biological underpinnings associated with the observed increased longrange connections most likely differ. Specifically, since the axonal properties (e.g., length, diameter, density) are most likely well established in school-aged children, the observed increase in long-range connectivity strength might primarily arise from the continuing myelination process, improving information transfer efficiency between distant brain regions (Tau and Peterson, 2010). In contrast, although some of the major long-range axonal connections (especially callosal fibers) are present in neonates (Fransson et al., 2007; Tau and Peterson, 2010), continuing axonal elongation/thickening is expected at this age to facilitate forming connections with other distant brain functional areas (e.g., in the anterior-posterior direction), especially during the first year of life (Tau and Peterson, 2010). Moreover, the myelination process is also documented to experience the most dramatic growth during the first two years of life (Gao et al., 2008; Haynes et al.,

2005; Tau and Peterson, 2010). Therefore, a combination of axonal growth and myelination likely accounts for the changes observed in our study.

The observation of no significant changes between 1yr and 2yr olds in whole brain smallworld properties echoes the findings by Supekar et al (Supekar et al., 2009) and Fair et al (Fair et al., 2009), who also failed to detect significant whole brain efficiency changes when comparing school-aged children with adults. However, significant regional wiring changes (LE/GE) have been documented in previous studies (Fair et al., 2009; Supekar et al., 2009; Gao et al., 2011). In considering these findings, it is plausible that the whole brain reaches an adultlike "small-world" topology from 1-year-old on while after that although significant local changes continue to reshape the brain for the development of specific functions, the whole brain efficiency property remains un-disturbed.

5. Explorations into developmental disorders

Studies utilizing fcMRI to discern potential neuropathological underpinnings of various developmental disorders are emerging (Church et al., 2009; Di Martino et al., 2010; Dickstein et al., 2010; Fair et al., 2010; Liston et al., 2011; Qiu et al., 2010; Uddin et al., 2008). For example, Church et al (Church et al., 2009) examined youth subjects (aged between 9 to 15) with Tourette syndrome (TS), a developmental disorder characterized by irresistible stereotyped movements and vocalizations called "tics". They specifically evaluated functional connectivity associated with two putative control networks – a "fronto-parietal network" likely involved in online control and a "cingulo-opercular network" important for set-maintenance. Specifically, they found that most of the connections with abnormal connection strengths (less-matured) were associated with the fronto-parietal network indicating more pronounced disruption of adaptive online control function in TS subjects. Di Martino et al (Di Martino et al., 2010) investigated autism spectrum disorders (ASD), a developmental disorder characterized by impaired social interaction and communication. They compared the striatal functional connectivity between children with ASD (aged between 7-and 13-year-old) and normal controls and found widespread hyper-connectivity among all striatal regions as well as between striatal regions and other associative regions such as insular and right superior temporal gyrus. Based on these findings, they postulated that developmental derangement rather than immaturity of functional circuits might underlie ASD. Dickstein et al (Dickstein et al., 2010) studied pediatric bipolar disorder (BD) in youth subjects between the age of seven and seventeen and found greater negative functional connectivity between left dorsal lateral prefrontal cortex and right superior temporal gyrus in BD subjects when compared with normal controls, indicating abnormal development of this important circuit for working memory and learning.

Attention-deficit/hyperactivity disorder (ADHD) characterized by attentional problems and hyperactivity has also attracted great interest in resting-state fMRI studies (Liston et al., 2011). Among these, Fair et al (Fair et al., 2010) examined the functional connectivity within the default network and found generally reduced connectivity in children with ADHD comparing with normal controls, reflecting atypical circuit maturation of this network. Interestingly, using the independent component analysis approach, Qiu et al (Qiu et al., 2010) reported both decreased and increased functional connectivity within this network (i.e., increased functional connectivity in anterior cingulate cortex, posterior cingulate cortex, lateral prefrontal cortex, precuneus and thalamus but increased connectivity in posterior medial frontal cortex). In a separate study, Uddin et al (Uddin et al., 2008) also found decreased network homogeneity in the precuneus node of the default network. Besides default network, other studies targeting at ADHD have also investigated into abnormal functional connectivity in other parts of the brain. For a recent review of fcMRI studies on ADHD, please refer to Liston et al (Liston et al., 2011).

As described above, most of existing studies focused on the population of children no younger than 7-year-old. However, the first two years of life is perhaps a critical time period where certain developmental disorders start to develop such as autism syndrome disorder ASD (Levy et al., 2009). Other disorders such as ADHD may have a late onset as school-aged children but the underlying neurophysiologic changes may occur well before the onset of behavioral symptoms (Ilott et al., 2010; Kieling et al., 2008). Hence the understanding of the underlying neuropathology during the first years of life is vital to early diagnosis and potential treatment of such disorders. As a result, resting-state fMRI studies focusing on a much younger age period are highly warranted for successful delineation of the underlying neurophysiological mechanisms of different developmental disorders. In addition, most of the existing studies focus on specific circuits/connections, potentially limiting the findings of novel abnormal circuits/connections that may underlie such disorders. Therefore, more studies with an exploratory nature are greatly needed in future research.

6. Technical issues in the application of fcMRI for early brain development

There are potential issues that are of particular importance for the utilization of fcMRI in the developmental brain. The first and foremost is the definition of ROIs for pediatric subjects, especially for those younger than 1 year of age when both brain's structural morphology and functional organization is largely different from its matured configuration. The current practice of applying either a parcellation template or functional activation coordinates from adult studies to the pediatric populations facilitates direct comparison between the two populations. However, such a practice may lead to potential bias against pediatric subjects given the known organizational difference. To a certain extent, this may be a circular problem since it is this development related reorganization that we are studying. Fortunately, the utilization of a data-driven method such as ICA could potentially alleviate this problem given that no prior ROIs are needed. However, as mentioned previously, the choice of components reflecting functional connectivity is subjective. Thus, quantitative comparisons of connection strength are less straightforward for ICA-based approaches. Clearly, methodological improvements are greatly needed to solve such issues.

But before that, developmental studies should choose different strategies according to the specific question(s) involved and the results should be interpreted with these issues in mind.

Viewing the brain's functional organization at the network level has been shown to be important in brain disease studies (Greicius et al., 2004; Seeley et al., 2009). For example, Seely et al (Seeley et al., 2009) proposed the "network degeneration hypothesis" where they reported that neurodegeneration may be related to network-level dysfunction and suggested the need for developing new network-based diagnostic assays. Logically, the interaction between different functional networks might also have significant influence on the developmental process. Different methods aimed at directly quantifying network-level interactions are emerging. Jafri et al (Jafri et al., 2008) described a method to calculate the functional connectivity between networks defined by spatial ICA and examined the differences between Schizophrenia and normal subjects. Gao et al (Gao et al., 2010) have proposed a different method based on canonical correlation to directly quantify the mutual dependence between two functional networks and applied it to delineate the dynamics of network level interactions under different brain states. In the future, we expect an increasing interest in both the development and application of network based analysis due to the intrinsic organization of the brain as individual functional modules.

Finally, in most cases the infants are sleeping inside the scanner with or without sedation in developmental investigations. The effect of sedation on resulting connectivity measurement should be better addressed. Even without sedation, different stages of sleep could also have an effect on the resulting functional connectivity measures. Therefore, studies incorporating sleep stage monitoring (e.g., through simultaneous EEG recording) would be beneficial to minimize experimental variability.

7. Conclusion

In this chapter, we have reviewed several results delineating the normal brain functional development process during the first two years of life using resting state functional connectivity. The application of fcMRI in various developmental disorders was also discussed. The uncertainty of the physiological underpinnings of fcMRI signal, as well as other technical issues related to its practical application are also briefly discussed pointing to the pressing need for improvement in future studies. The results support the notion that the brain's primary functional networks are in place and partially functioning immediately after birth, but the maturation of higher order cognitive networks takes prolonged experience based tuning during postnatal life. Moreover, dramatic evolution of the brain's functional topology is observed during this critical period, which greatly changes the brain's modular structure and distribution of hubs, as well as improves whole brain information transfer efficiency at both local and global levels. Finally, the evidence shows that less maturation and/or derangement of certain functional circuits might underlie different developmental disorders.

Author details

Wei Gao[1], Hongtu Zhu[2], Kelly S. Giovanello[3], J. Keith Smith[4], Dinggang Shen[1], John H. Gilmore[5] and Weili Lin[1]

1 Department of Radiology and Biomedical Research Imaging Center, UNC-Chapel Hill, USA

2 Department of Biostatistics and Biomedical Research Imaging Center, UNC-Chapel Hill, USA

3 Department of Psychology and Biomedical Research Imaging Center, UNC-Chapel Hill, USA

4 Department of Radiology, UNC-Chapel Hill, USA

5 Department of Psychiatry, UNC-Chapel Hill, USA

References

[1] Achard, S., Bullmore, E., 2007. Efficiency and cost of economical brain functional networks. PLoS Comput Biol 3, e17.

[2] Achard, S., Salvador, R., Whitcher, B., Suckling, J., Bullmore, E., 2006. A resilient, low-frequency, small-world human brain functional network with highly connected association cortical hubs. J Neurosci 26, 63-72.

[3] Akhtar, N., & Tomasello, M., 2000. The social nature of words and word learning. Oxford University Press., Oxford.

[4] Amsterdam, 1972. Mirror self-image reactions before age two. Developmental Psychology. Psychology 5, 297-305.

[5] Anderson, A.W., Marois, R., Colson, E.R., Peterson, B.S., Duncan, C.C., Ehrenkranz, R.A., Schneider, K.C., Gore, J.C., Ment, L.R., 2001. Neonatal auditory activation detected by functional magnetic resonance imaging. Magn Reson Imaging 19, 1-5.

[6] Andrews-Hanna, J.R., Reidler, J.S., Sepulcre, J., Poulin, R., Buckner, R.L., 2010. Functional-Anatomic Fractionation of the Brain's Default Network. Neuron 65, 550-562.

[7] Baldwin, D.A., 1993. Early referential understanding: young children' s ability to recognize referential acts for what they are. Developmental Psychology 29, 832-843.

[8] Bandettini, P.A., Wong, E.C., Hinks, R.S., Tikofsky, R.S., Hyde, J.S., 1992. Time course EPI of human brain function during task activation. Magn Reson Med 25, 390-397.

[9] Barabasi, A.L., Albert, R., 1999. Emergence of scaling in random networks. Science 286, 509-512.

[10] Belliveau, J.W., Kennedy, D.N., Jr., McKinstry, R.C., Buchbinder, B.R., Weisskoff, R.M., Cohen, M.S., Vevea, J.M., Brady, T.J., Rosen, B.R., 1991. Functional mapping of the human visual cortex by magnetic resonance imaging. Science 254, 716-719.

[11] Biswal, B., Yetkin, F.Z., Haughton, V.M., Hyde, J.S., 1995. Functional connectivity in the motor cortex of resting human brain using echo-planar MRI. Magn Reson Med 34, 537-541.

[12] Biswal, B.B., Mennes, M., Zuo, X.N., Gohel, S., Kelly, C., Smith, S.M., Beckmann, C.F., Adelstein, J.S., Buckner, R.L., Colcombe, S., Dogonowski, A.M., Ernst, M., Fair, D., Hampson, M., Hoptman, M.J., Hyde, J.S., Kiviniemi, V.J., Kotter, R., Li, S.J., Lin, C.P., Lowe, M.J., Mackay, C., Madden, D.J., Madsen, K.H., Margulies, D.S., Mayberg, H.S., McMahon, K., Monk, C.S., Mostofsky, S.H., Nagel, B.J., Pekar, J.J., Peltier, S.J., Petersen, S.E., Riedl, V., Rombouts, S.A., Rypma, B., Schlaggar, B.L., Schmidt, S., Seidler, R.D., Siegle, G.J., Sorg, C., Teng, G.J., Veijola, J., Villringer, A., Walter, M., Wang, L., Weng, X.C., Whitfield-Gabrieli, S., Williamson, P., Windischberger, C., Zang, Y.F., Zhang, H.Y., Castellanos, F.X., Milham, M.P., 2010. Toward discovery science of human brain function. Proc Natl Acad Sci U S A 107, 4734-4739.

[13] Born, P., Leth, H., Miranda, M.J., Rostrup, E., Stensgaard, A., Peitersen, B., Larsson, H.B., Lou, H.C., 1998. Visual activation in infants and young children studied by functional magnetic resonance imaging. Pediatr Res 44, 578-583.

[14] Born, P., Rostrup, E., Leth, H., Peitersen, B., Lou, H.C., 1996. Change of visually induced cortical activation patterns during development. Lancet 347, 543.

[15] Brandes, U., 2001. A faster algorithm for betweenness centrality. J Math Sociol 25, 163-177.

[16] Buckner, R.L., Andrews-Hanna, J.R., Schacter, D.L., 2008. The brain's default network: anatomy, function, and relevance to disease. Ann N Y Acad Sci 1124, 1-38.

[17] Buckner, R.L., Carroll, D.C., 2007. Self-projection and the brain. Trends Cogn Sci 11, 49-57.

[18] Bullmore, E., Sporns, O., 2009. Complex brain networks: graph theoretical analysis of structural and functional systems. Nat Rev Neurosci 10, 186-198.

[19] Cepeda, N.J., Kramer, A.F., Gonzalez de Sather, J.C., 2001. Changes in executive control across the life span: examination of task-switching performance. Dev Psychol 37, 715-730.

[20] Chang, C., Glover, G.H., Time-frequency dynamics of resting-state brain connectivity measured with fMRI. Neuroimage 50, 81-98.

[21] Church, J.A., Fair, D.A., Dosenbach, N.U., Cohen, A.L., Miezin, F.M., Petersen, S.E., Schlaggar, B.L., 2009. Control networks in paediatric Tourette syndrome show immature and anomalous patterns of functional connectivity. Brain 132, 225-238.

[22] Collins, D.l., Holmes, C.J., Peters, T.M., Evans, A.C., 1995. Automatic 3-D model-based neuroanatomical segmentation. Hum Brain Mapp 3, 190-208.

[23] Conel, J.L., 1939. The Postnatal Development of Human Cerebral Cortex. Harvard University Press, Cambridge.

[24] Damoiseaux, J.S., Rombouts, S.A., Barkhof, F., Scheltens, P., Stam, C.J., Smith, S.M., Beckmann, C.F., 2006. Consistent resting-state networks across healthy subjects. Proc Natl Acad Sci U S A 103, 13848-13853.

[25] De Martino, F., Gentile, F., Esposito, F., Balsi, M., Di Salle, F., Goebel, R., Formisano, E., 2007. Classification of fMRI independent components using IC-fingerprints and support vector machine classifiers. Neuroimage 34, 177-194.

[26] DeCasper, A.J., Fifer, W.P., 1980. Of human bonding: newborns prefer their mothers' voices. Science 208, 1174-1176.

[27] Dehaene-Lambertz, G., Dehaene, S., Hertz-Pannier, L., 2002. Functional neuroimaging of speech perception in infants. Science 298, 2013-2015.

[28] Di Martino, A., Kelly, C., Grzadzinski, R., Zuo, X.N., Mennes, M., Mairena, M.A., Lord, C., Castellanos, F.X., Milham, M.P., 2010. Aberrant striatal functional connectivity in children with autism. Biol Psychiatry 69, 847-856.

[29] Dickstein, D.P., Gorrostieta, C., Ombao, H., Goldberg, L.D., Brazel, A.C., Gable, C.J., Kelly, C., Gee, D.G., Zuo, X.N., Castellanos, F.X., Milham, M.P., 2010. Fronto-temporal spontaneous resting state functional connectivity in pediatric bipolar disorder. Biol Psychiatry 68, 839-846.

[30] Diesendruck, G., Markson, L., Akhtar, N., Reudor, A., 2004. Two-year-olds' sensitivity to speakers' intent: an alternative account of Samuelson and Smith. Dev Sci 7, 33-41.

[31] Ebbels, T.M., Buxton, B.F., Jones, D.T., 2006. springScape: visualisation of microarray and contextual bioinformatic data using spring embedding and an 'information landscape'. Bioinformatics 22, e99-107.

[32] Fair, D.A., Cohen, A.L., Dosenbach, N.U., Church, J.A., Miezin, F.M., Barch, D.M., Raichle, M.E., Petersen, S.E., Schlaggar, B.L., 2008. The maturing architecture of the brain's default network. Proc Natl Acad Sci U S A 105, 4028-4032.

[33] Fair, D.A., Cohen, A.L., Power, J.D., Dosenbach, N.U., Church, J.A., Miezin, F.M., Schlaggar, B.L., Petersen, S.E., 2009. Functional brain networks develop from a "local to distributed" organization. PLoS Comput Biol 5, e1000381.

[34] Fair, D.A., Posner, J., Nagel, B.J., Bathula, D., Dias, T.G., Mills, K.L., Blythe, M.S., Giwa, A., Schmitt, C.F., Nigg, J.T., 2010. Atypical default network connectivity in youth with attention-deficit/hyperactivity disorder. Biol Psychiatry 68, 1084-1091.

[35] Feinberg, D.A., Moeller, S., Smith, S.M., Auerbach, E., Ramanna, S., Glasser, M.F., Miller, K.L., Ugurbil, K., Yacoub, E., 2010. Multiplexed echo planar imaging for sub-second whole brain FMRI and fast diffusion imaging. PLoS One 5, e15710.

[36] Fivush, R., Hamond, N.R, 1990. Autobiographical memory across the preschool years: Toward reconcepualizing childhood amnesia. In: J.A.Hudson, R.F.a. (Ed.), Knowing and remembering in young children. Cambridge Univ. Press, New York:.

[37] Fornito, A., Zalesky, A., Bullmore, E.T., 2010. Network scaling effects in graph analytic studies of human resting-state FMRI data. Front Syst Neurosci 4, 22.

[38] Fox, M.D., Corbetta, M., Snyder, A.Z., Vincent, J.L., Raichle, M.E., 2006. Spontaneous neuronal activity distinguishes human dorsal and ventral attention systems. Proc Natl Acad Sci U S A 103, 10046-10051.

[39] Fox, M.D., Zhang, D., Snyder, A.Z., Raichle, M.E., 2009. The global signal and observed anticorrelated resting state brain networks. J Neurophysiol 101, 3270-3283.

[40] Fransson, P., Aden, U., Blennow, M., Lagercrantz, H., 2010. The Functional Architecture of the Infant Brain as Revealed by Resting-State fMRI. Cereb Cortex.

[41] Fransson, P., Skiold, B., Horsch, S., Nordell, A., Blennow, M., Lagercrantz, H., Aden, U., 2007. Resting-state networks in the infant brain. Proc Natl Acad Sci U S A 104, 15531-15536.

[42] Fulford, J., Vadeyar, S.H., Dodampahala, S.H., Moore, R.J., Young, P., Baker, P.N., James, D.K., Gowland, P.A., 2003. Fetal brain activity in response to a visual stimulus. Hum Brain Mapp 20, 239-245.

[43] Gao, W., Lin, W., 2011. Frontal parietal control network regulates the anti-correlated default and dorsal attention networks. Hum Brain Mapp (In Press).

[44] Gao, W., Lin, W., Chen, Y., Gerig, G., Smith, J.K., Jewells, V., Gilmore, J.H., 2008. Temporal and Spatial Development of Axonal Maturation and Myelination of White Matter in the Developing Brain. AJNR Am J Neuroradiol.

[45] Gao, W., Zhu, H., Giovanello, K., Lin, W., 2010. Multivariate network-level approach to detect interactions between large-scale functional systems. Med Image Comput Comput Assist Interv 13, 298-305.

[46] Gao, W., Zhu, H., Giovanello, K.S., Smith, J.K., Shen, D., Gilmore, J.H., Lin, W., 2009. Evidence on the emergence of the brain's default network from 2-week-old to 2-year-old healthy pediatric subjects. Proc Natl Acad Sci U S A 106, 6790-6795.

[47] Greicius, M.D., Krasnow, B., Reiss, A.L., Menon, V., 2003. Functional connectivity in the resting brain: a network analysis of the default mode hypothesis. Proc Natl Acad Sci U S A 100, 253-258.

[48] Greicius, M.D., Menon, V., 2004. Default-mode activity during a passive sensory task: uncoupled from deactivation but impacting activation. J Cogn Neurosci 16, 1484-1492.

[49] Greicius, M.D., Srivastava, G., Reiss, A.L., Menon, V., 2004. Default-mode network activity distinguishes Alzheimer's disease from healthy aging: evidence from functional MRI. Proc Natl Acad Sci U S A 101, 4637-4642.

[50] Gusnard, D.A., Akbudak, E., Shulman, G.L., Raichle, M.E., 2001. Medial prefrontal cortex and self-referential mental activity: relation to a default mode of brain function. Proc Natl Acad Sci U S A 98, 4259-4264.

[51] Gusnard, D.A., Raichle, M.E., 2001. Searching for a baseline: functional imaging and the resting human brain. Nat Rev Neurosci 2, 685-694.

[52] Haynes, R.L., Borenstein, N.S., Desilva, T.M., Folkerth, R.D., Liu, L.G., Volpe, J.J., Kinney, H.C., 2005. Axonal development in the cerebral white matter of the human fetus and infant. J Comp Neurol 484, 156-167.

[53] He, B.J., Snyder, A.Z., Zempel, J.M., Smyth, M.D., Raichle, M.E., 2008. Electrophysiological correlates of the brain's intrinsic large-scale functional architecture. Proc Natl Acad Sci U S A 105, 16039-16044.

[54] Hilgetag, C.C., Burns, G.A., O'Neill, M.A., Scannell, J.W., Young, M.P., 2000. Anatomical connectivity defines the organization of clusters of cortical areas in the macaque monkey and the cat. Philos Trans R Soc Lond B Biol Sci 355, 91-110.

[55] Hykin, J., Moore, R., Duncan, K., Clare, S., Baker, P., Johnson, I., Bowtell, R., Mansfield, P., Gowland, P., 1999. Fetal brain activity demonstrated by functional magnetic resonance imaging. Lancet 354, 645-646.

[56] Ilott, N.E., Saudino, K.J., Asherson, P., 2010. Genetic influences on attention deficit hyperactivity disorder symptoms from age 2 to 3: a quantitative and molecular genetic investigation. BMC Psychiatry 10, 102.

[57] Jafri, M.J., Pearlson, G.D., Stevens, M., Calhoun, V.D., 2008. A method for functional network connectivity among spatially independent resting-state components in schizophrenia. Neuroimage 39, 1666-1681.

[58] Joel, S.E., Caffo, B.S., van Zijl, P.C., Pekar, J.J., 2011. On the relationship between seed-based and ICA-based measures of functional connectivity. Magn Reson Med.

[59] Johnson, M.H., 2000. Functional brain development in infants: elements of an interactive specialization framework. Child Dev 71, 75-81.

[60] Johnson, M.H., 2001. Functional brain development in humans. Nat Rev Neurosci 2, 475-483.

[61] Joseph, R., 1999. Fetal Brain & Cognitive Development. Developmental Review 20, 81-98.

[62] Kelly, A.M., Di Martino, A., Uddin, L.Q., Shehzad, Z., Gee, D.G., Reiss, P.T., Margulies, D.S., Castellanos, F.X., Milham, M.P., 2009. Development of anterior cingulate functional connectivity from late childhood to early adulthood. Cereb Cortex 19, 640-657.

[63] Kieling, C., Goncalves, R.R., Tannock, R., Castellanos, F.X., 2008. Neurobiology of attention deficit hyperactivity disorder. Child Adolesc Psychiatr Clin N Am 17, 285-307, viii.

[64] Kolata, G., 1984. Studying learning in the womb. Science 225, 302-303.

[65] Latora, V., Marchiori, M., 2001. Efficient behavior of small-world networks. Phys Rev Lett 87, 198701.

[66] Levy, S.E., Mandell, D.S., Schultz, R.T., 2009. Autism. Lancet 374, 1627-1638.

[67] Lin, W., Zhu, Q., Gao, W., Chen, Y., Toh, C.H., Styner, M., Gerig, G., Smith, J.K., Biswal, B., Gilmore, J.H., 2008. Functional connectivity MR imaging reveals cortical functional connectivity in the developing brain. AJNR Am J Neuroradiol 29, 1883-1889.

[68] Liston, C., Cohen, M.M., Teslovich, T., Levenson, D., Casey, B.J., 2011. Atypical prefrontal connectivity in attention-deficit/hyperactivity disorder: pathway to disease or pathological end point? Biol Psychiatry 69, 1168-1177.

[69] Liu, Y., Liang, M., Zhou, Y., He, Y., Hao, Y., Song, M., Yu, C., Liu, H., Liu, Z., Jiang, T., 2008. Disrupted small-world networks in schizophrenia. Brain 131, 945-961.

[70] Logothetis, N.K., 2003. The underpinnings of the BOLD functional magnetic resonance imaging signal. J Neurosci 23, 3963-3971.

[71] Logothetis, N.K., Pauls, J., Augath, M., Trinath, T., Oeltermann, A., 2001. Neurophysiological investigation of the basis of the fMRI signal. Nature 412, 150-157.

[72] Lowe, M.J., Mock, B.J., Sorenson, J.A., 1998. Functional connectivity in single and multislice echoplanar imaging using resting-state fluctuations. Neuroimage 7, 119-132.

[73] Murphy, K., Birn, R.M., Handwerker, D.A., Jones, T.B., Bandettini, P.A., 2009. The impact of global signal regression on resting state correlations: are anti-correlated networks introduced? Neuroimage 44, 893-905.

[74] Neumann, J., von Cramon, D.Y., Forstmann, B.U., Zysset, S., Lohmann, G., 2006. The parcellation of cortical areas using replicator dynamics in fMRI. Neuroimage 32, 208-219.

[75] Newman, M.E., 2006. Modularity and community structure in networks. Proc Natl Acad Sci U S A 103, 8577-8582.

[76] Nir, Y., Mukamel, R., Dinstein, I., Privman, E., Harel, M., Fisch, L., Gelbard-Sagiv, H., Kipervasser, S., Andelman, F., Neufeld, M.Y., Kramer, U., Arieli, A., Fried, I., Malach, R., 2008. Interhemispheric correlations of slow spontaneous neuronal fluctuations revealed in human sensory cortex. Nat Neurosci 11, 1100-1108.

[77] Ogawa, S., Lee, T.M., Nayak, A.S., Glynn, P., 1990. Oxygenation-sensitive contrast in magnetic resonance image of rodent brain at high magnetic fields. Magn Reson Med 14, 68-78.

[78] Perlbarg, V., Bellec, P., Anton, J.L., Pelegrini-Issac, M., Doyon, J., Benali, H., 2007. CORSICA: correction of structured noise in fMRI by automatic identification of ICA components. Magn Reson Imaging 25, 35-46.

[79] Qiu, M.G., Ye, Z., Li, Q.Y., Liu, G.J., Xie, B., Wang, J., 2010. Changes of Brain Structure and Function in ADHD Children. Brain Topogr.

[80] Raichle, M.E., MacLeod, A.M., Snyder, A.Z., Powers, W.J., Gusnard, D.A., Shulman, G.L., 2001. A default mode of brain function. Proc Natl Acad Sci U S A 98, 676-682.

[81] Raichle, M.E., Mintun, M.A., 2006. Brain work and brain imaging. Annu Rev Neurosci 29, 449-476.

[82] Salvador, R., Suckling, J., Coleman, M., Pickard, J. D., Menon, D., Bullmore,, E., 2005. Neurophysiological architecture of functional magnetic resonance images of human brain. Cerebral Cortex 34, 387-413.

[83] Seeley, W.W., Crawford, R.K., Zhou, J., Miller, B.L., Greicius, M.D., 2009. Neurodegenerative diseases target large-scale human brain networks. Neuron 62, 42-52.

[84] Shmuel, A., Leopold, D.A., 2008. Neuronal correlates of spontaneous fluctuations in fMRI signals in monkey visual cortex: Implications for functional connectivity at rest. Hum Brain Mapp 29, 751-761.

[85] Shulman GL, F.J., Corbetta M, Buckner RL, Miezin FM, 1997. Common blood flow changes across visual tasks: II.: decreases in cerebral cortex. J. Cogn. Neurosci 9, 648-663.

[86] Smyser, C.D., Inder, T.E., Shimony, J.S., Hill, J.E., Degnan, A.J., Snyder, A.Z., Neil, J.J., 2010. Longitudinal Analysis of Neural Network Development in Preterm Infants. Cereb Cortex.

[87] Supekar, K., Musen, M., Menon, V., 2009. Development of large-scale functional brain networks in children. PLoS Biol 7, e1000157.

[88] Tau, G.Z., Peterson, B.S., 2010. Normal development of brain circuits. Neuropsychopharmacology 35, 147-168.

[89] Tohka, J., Foerde, K., Aron, A.R., Tom, S.M., Toga, A.W., Poldrack, R.A., 2008. Automatic independent component labeling for artifact removal in fMRI. Neuroimage 39, 1227-1245.

[90] Tomasello, M., Strosberg, R., Akhtar, N., 1996. Eighteen-month-old children learn words in non-ostensive contexts. J Child Lang 23, 157-176.

[91] Tzourio-Mazoyer, N., Landeau, B., Papathanassiou, D., Crivello, F., Etard, O., Delcroix, N., Mazoyer, B., Joliot, M., 2002. Automated anatomical labeling of activations in SPM using a macroscopic anatomical parcellation of the MNI MRI single-subject brain. Neuroimage 15, 273-289.

[92] Uddin, L.Q., Kelly, A.M., Biswal, B.B., Margulies, D.S., Shehzad, Z., Shaw, D., Ghaffari, M., Rotrosen, J., Adler, L.A., Castellanos, F.X., Milham, M.P., 2008. Network homogeneity reveals decreased integrity of default-mode network in ADHD. J Neurosci Methods 169, 249-254.

[93] Van Dijk, K.R., Hedden, T., Venkataraman, A., Evans, K.C., Lazar, S.W., Buckner, R.L., 2010. Intrinsic functional connectivity as a tool for human connectomics: theory, properties, and optimization. J Neurophysiol 103, 297-321.

[94] Vincent, J.L., Kahn, I., Snyder, A.Z., Raichle, M.E., Buckner, R.L., 2008. Evidence for a frontoparietal control system revealed by intrinsic functional connectivity. J Neurophysiol 100, 3328-3342.

[95] Vincent, J.L., Snyder, A.Z., Fox, M.D., Shannon, B.J., Andrews, J.R., Raichle, M.E., Buckner, R.L., 2006. Coherent spontaneous activity identifies a hippocampal-parietal memory network. J Neurophysiol 96, 3517-3531.

[96] Wang, J., Wang, L., Zang, Y., Yang, H., Tang, H., Gong, Q., Chen, Z., Zhu, C., He, Y., 2009. Parcellation-dependent small-world brain functional networks: a resting-state fMRI study. Hum Brain Mapp 30, 1511-1523.

[97] Watts, D.J., Strogatz, S.H., 1998. Collective dynamics of 'small-world' networks. Nature 393, 440-442.

[98] Whitlow, C.T., Casanova, R., Maldjian, J.A., 2011. Effect of resting-state functional MR imaging duration on stability of graph theory metrics of brain network connectivity. Radiology 259, 516-524.

4

Big Challenges from the "Little Brain" – Imaging the Cerebellum

John Schlerf, Tobias Wiestler,
Timothy Verstynen and Jörn Diedrichsen

1. Introduction

The cerebellum is a compact structure that has about one-ninth of the volume of the neocortex, but comprises more than half of the neurons in the central nervous system. While the cerebellum has historically been understood to assist with movement and balance (e.g., Holmes, 1917, 1939), today we know that the cerebellum is also involved in non-motor functions (for review, see Stoodley & Schmahmann, 2009). Indeed, the cerebellum appears to play a role in nearly as many separate functions as the neocortex. This functional diversity within a restricted area poses unique challenges for the study of the cerebellum using functional magnetic resonance imaging (fMRI).

While no additional equipment or specialized pulse sequences are required to obtain fMRI data from the cerebellum, most so-called "whole brain" fMRI experiments focus on the study of the neocortex, often excluding inferior aspects of the cerebellum from data acquisition altogether. Furthermore, most common analysis methods are designed with the neocortex in mind and may be suboptimal for the analysis of cerebellar data, thus necessitating novel approaches to obtain insights about cerebellar function.

In this chapter we will highlight the current "best practices" to cerebellar fMRI experiments and address methodological challenges such as anatomical realignment, cerebellar atlases, cardiac artifacts on functional data, and the physiological source of the cerebellar blood-oxygen-level-dependent (BOLD) signal. We also review important research findings about the cerebellum, highlighting the role of fMRI studies in shaping our understanding of cerebellar function.

2. Methodological concerns for cerebellar imaging

2.1. Anatomical methods

Hypothesis testing using fMRI often requires data from multiple individuals; therefore we need a common anatomical frame of reference. Most widely-used normalization methods result in poor alignment of regions within the cerebellar cortex, which weakens statistical power (Diedrichsen, 2006). The deep cerebellar nuclei (the output of the cerebellum) are small and lie adjacent to the fourth ventricle and vascular supply, and therefore pose a special challenge to spatial normalization.

2.2. Localization within the cerebellar cortex

Like the neocortex, the cerebellar cortex is intricately folded. There are clearly defined lobules and sub-lobules within this cortex, separated by a number of fissures that can be reliably identified across individuals (Figure 1). Each lobule has its own pattern of connectivity with the neocortex (Kelly & Strick, 2003), and likely its own functional role (Stoodley & Schmahmann, 2009). Since each lobule is relatively small (5-10mm), inaccuracies in normalization will lead to functional data being averaged across neighboring structures. Indeed, if one uses standard spatial normalization procedures (which result in satisfactory overlap of structures within the cerebrum), the location of the primary fissure in the cerebellum (which forms the boundary between the anterior and posterior lobes) can be mis-localized by 1-2 cm (Diedrichsen, 2006). The top row of Figure 2 illustrates this overlap following the standard nonlinear SPM normalization to the MNI group template. When averaging anatomical scans across participants after normalization, most spatial details of the underlying anatomy are lost.

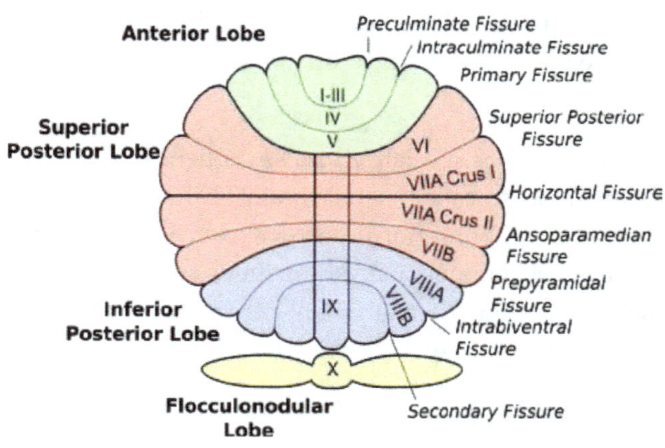

Figure 1. Anatomy of the cerebellar cortex. Traditionally, the cerebellum is split into the Anterior (green), Posterior (red and blue), and Flocculonodular (yellow) Lobes. Since the posterior lobe in the human cerebellum is large, researchers often subdivide it into Superior (red) and Inferior (blue) aspects. The cortex is subdivided longitudinally into lobules (Roman Numerals) by deep fissures. The current consensus on anatomical nomenclature is based on work by Larsell (1952, 1953), as laid out (along with excellent translations of prior nomenclature systems) by Schmahmann and colleagues (1999).

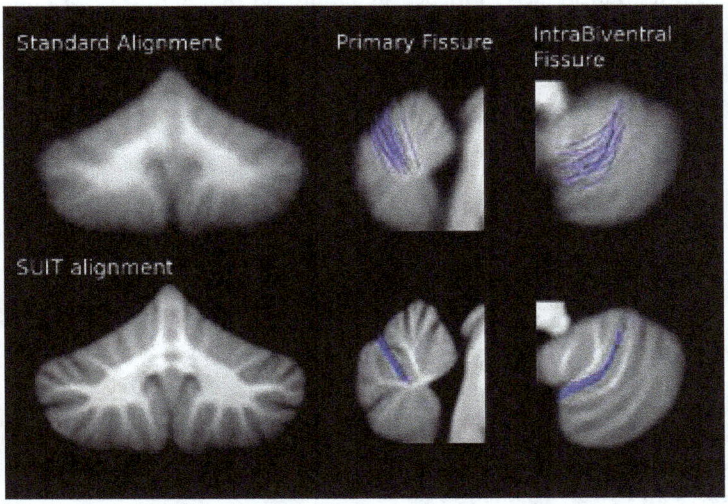

Figure 2. Comparison of normalization procedures. The top row demonstrates the normalization and coregistration of 21 individuals using the SPM standard normalization procedure to the MNI 152 template, which is not specialized for the cerebellum. Note the loss of detail, and the poor alignment of the Primary and Intrabiventral fissures. The second row shows the same 20 brains normalized using the SUIT template.

An equally serious problem is anatomical bias. Even within the same neuroimaging coordinate system (e.g., MNI152), different normalization methods may lead to substantially different locations of the same cerebellar structure in atlas space (Diedrichsen et al., 2009). For example, it has become common to identify the anatomical location of cerebellar coordinates using the MRI atlas of the human cerebellum (Schmahmann et al., 1999). While this atlas provides a framework for subdividing the structure into individual lobules, the atlas is based on a single individual with a unique anatomy. Examination of 20 participants after normalization in SPM suggests that coordinate-based assignment using this atlas is correct for only 38% of the voxels in the cerebellar cortex (Diedrichsen et al., 2009).

Better normalization should be achievable, as cerebellar fissures are stereotyped and consistent across individuals (Makris et al., 2003, 2005). This makes it possible to use higher resolution anatomical normalization methods combined with a template that preserves anatomical detail within the cerebellum, implemented in the SUIT toolbox (Diedrichsen, 2006). This template is spatially unbiased relative to the space defined by the MNI 152 template, so each cerebellar structure is located where it would end up – on average-after affine alignment to the MNI 152 template. Thus, the resultant coordinates can be directly compared to results obtained in other studies. The use of the toolbox dramatically improves overlap of individual fissures (Figure 2, bottom row).

Since the development of the SUIT method, other methods have been published that use similar high-resolution warps and detailed nonlinear templates. While these methods improve the alignment of cerebellar structures, SUIT still improves the overlap of individual lobules by about 8% (Diedrichsen et al., 2009). The advantage of the SUIT approach likely arises from the initial segmentation into cerebellum and neocortex, as only subtentorial structures drive the normalization. Segmentation also reduces the likelihood that activity from nearby neocortex will be misattributed to the cerebellum.

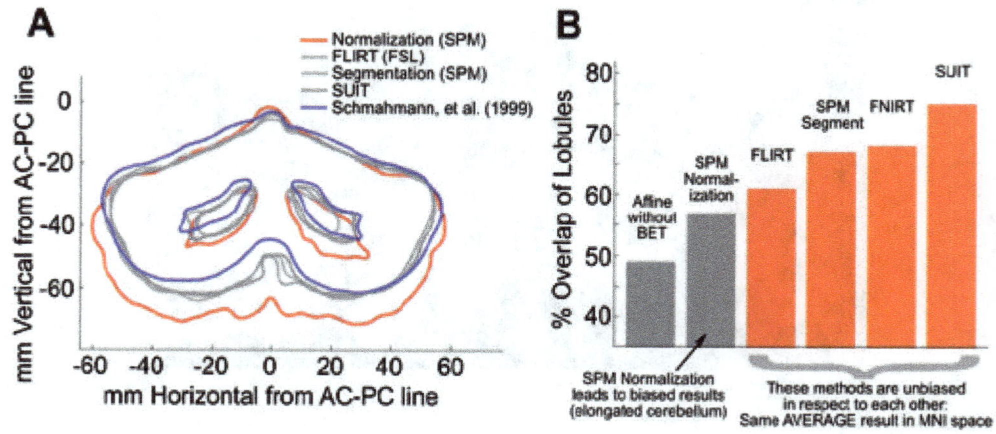

Figure 3. Overlap and bias of different normalization methods. A) When the outline of the cerebella are overlaid, the standard SPM normalization method (red outline) is clearly biased, particularly with respect to the Schmahmann atlas (blue outline). The other methods (including SUIT) are unbiased with respect to each other. B) Comparing the percent overlap of individual lobules, we can see some differences even among methods which result in the same overall spatial location.

To overcome bias in labeling the anatomical locations of activated regions, a probabilistic atlas for the cerebellum has been developed (Diedrichsen et al., 2009) to allow for accurate anatomical description of cerebellar activations observed in group analyses. This atlas can also facilitate analyses that eschew the group-overlap approach in favor of analysis based on anatomical regions of interest (ROIs). While it is possible to identify cerebellar lobules manually to constrain the anatomical extent of analysis (Makris et al., 2003, 2005), doing this by hand is tedious, and requires specialized knowledge to be reliable. The use of independently validated probabilistic atlases is much more efficient.

2.2.1. Imaging the nuclei

While SUIT-normalization and the associated probabilistic atlas provide sufficient accuracy for fMRI studies of the cerebellar cortex, more specialized techniques are required for the alignment of the deep cerebellar nuclei (DCN). These structures can be difficult to identify using conventional anatomical scans, as they can appear contiguous with the cerebellar white matter. Due to the high concentration of iron in these nuclei, they can be visualized more easily in T1-weighted images in older individuals (Dimitrova et al., 2002b) or by using T2-weighted images (Dimitrova et al., 2006).

Because the deep cerebellar nuclei are small, the inter-individual overlap using typical normalization methods is quite poor. Good superposition of the nuclei in group analyses is essential, especially because the T2* signal from the DCN is lower than the surrounding white matter and the nearby gray matter (Dimitrova et al., 2006). Since variability in fMRI is proportional to the average raw signal, this means that the functionally induced signal variations in the dentate nucleus are very low compared with functional activation in nearby gray matter. If these signals are averaged together with the signal from areas where both the raw signal and noise is twice as large (a consequence of spatial smoothing), it is extremely unlikely that they will be detected. This problem is exacerbated by high field strength, where the differences in T2* are even more pronounced.

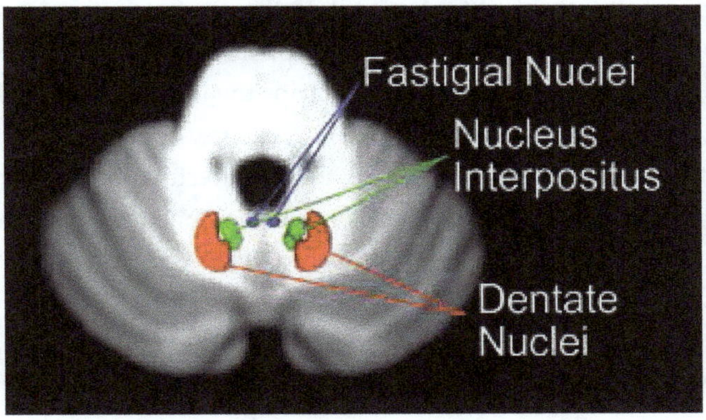

Figure 4. Overview and approximate location of the deep cerebellar nuclei. Adapted from (Diedrichsen et al., 2011).

A refined method for the normalization of the cerebellum and the dentate nucleus has recently been developed in conjunction with a probabilistic atlas for the DCN (Diedrichsen et al., 2011). As with the cerebellar cortical atlas (Diedrichsen et al., 2009), inter-individual anatomical variability depends on the normalization method chosen. Traditional MNI-alignment methods perform the worst, while segmentation-based methods perform slightly better (Diedrichsen et al., 2011). The best overlap for the deep cerebellar nuclei was obtained by using a variation of the SUIT-normalization method, combining white matter segmentation with an anatomical ROI that covers the deep cerebellar nuclei. Currently, this ROI must be traced by hand, and is most reliable when traced onto the phase image of susceptibility-weighted scans collected at 7T (Diedrichsen et al., 2011).

Using these techniques, Timmann and colleagues have shown that the dentate nucleus can be subdivided into cognitive and sensorimotor components (Küper et al., 2011a). They were able to demonstrate a somatotopic gradient between hand and foot movement in the motor portion of the dentate nucleus at 7T (Küper et al., 2011b). These studies provide important and exciting advances into our understanding of the human dentate nucleus. They also, however, highlight the limits of current fMRI techniques and the need for further development. Both magnetic inhomogeneity artifacts as well as physiological noise near arterial vessels make the detection of these weak signals challenging. As high-field scanners become more accessible and functional imaging at this field strength matures, we hope to see these techniques used for testing specific hypotheses about the deep cerebellar nuclei.

2.3. Interpretation of the cerebellar bold signal

FMRI involves repeatedly imaging the brain and analyzing small changes caused by variations in blood oxygenation. It is important to know which neurophysiological processes drive the cerebellar BOLD signal. Neural activity increases the cerebral metabolic rate of oxygen consumption ($CMRO_2$), which causes an increase in the local concentration of deoxy-hemoglobin, whose magnetic properties decrease BOLD. Neuronal activity also leads to a compensatory increase in cerebral blood flow (CBF), which raises the local concentration of oxygenated hemoglobin and thus increases the BOLD signal. In the neocortex, these two quantities have been measured and the relationship between them appears to be relatively fixed: the increased oxygenated hemoglobin from increased CBF outstrips the increased deoxy-hemoglobin from increased $CMRO_2$ by ratio of 2:1 (Hoge et al., 1999). As a result, neural activity in the cerebral cortex increases the BOLD signal. However, the architecture of the cerebellar cortex is dramatically different from that of the neocortex, and the same ratios may not apply. Careful thought and experimental work are needed to illuminate the relationship between neural activity and BOLD in the cerebellum.

2.3.1. Neural sources

There are two primary input systems to the cerebellar cortex (Figure 5). The first is the mossy fiber inputs that project to granule cells, which give rise to parallel fibers. Each parallel fiber synapses onto the dendritic trees of thousands of Punkinje cells-the only output cell of the cerebellar cortex. A single Purkinje cell can receive weak synapses from tens of thousands of parallel fibers. The second input system is the climbing fibers that arise from the inferior olive. Each Purkinje cell receives a very strong synaptic input from a single climbing fiber. Stimulation of each of these two pathways leads to time-locked increases in blood flow at the cerebellar cortex (Mathiesen et al., 2000), which by inference suggests that activity in both pathways may be contributing to the BOLD signal.

To understand the source of the cerebellar BOLD signal under physiologically plausible conditions, it is informative to understand how much energy (and hence oxygen) neural processes within the cerebellum demand. Calculations based on cell numbers, spontaneous firing rates and membrane potentials (Howarth et al., 2009) lead to the estimation that approximately 18% of the energy in the rat cerebellar cortex is consumed by Purkinje cells. In contrast, granule cells use 67% of the energy, most of which is consumed by the process of relaying mossy fiber input to cells in the cerebellar cortex. During sensory stimulation, mossy fibers have been shown to fire bursts of action potentials exceeding 700 Hz, compared to baseline firing rates at rest on the order of 3 Hz (Rancz et al., 2007). If the proportional increases of blood flow and energy use observed in the cerebral cortex hold for the cerebellum, we would be tempted to conclude that activity-dependent BOLD signal changes are mostly caused by increased signaling in the mossy fiber input pathway.

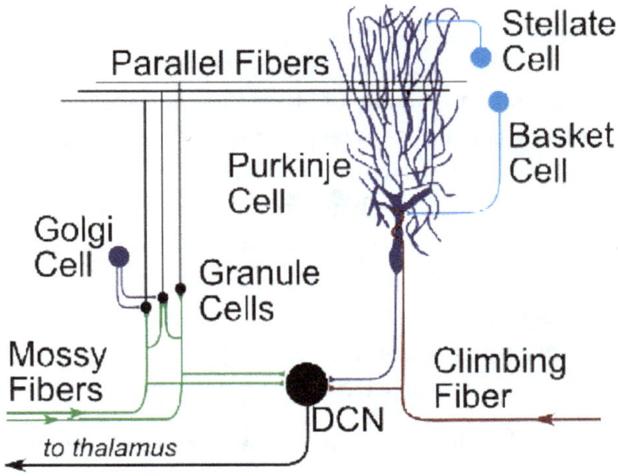

Figure 5. Overview of the cerebellar circuit. The input pathways are the mossy and climbing fibers, which are excitatory. Mossy fibers (green) synapse onto granule cells, which give rise to excitatory parallel fibers which synapse onto Purkinje cells, the output of the cerebellar cortex. Climbing fibers (red) synapse directly onto the Purkinje cells. Stellate, Basket, Golgi, and Purkinje cells are all inhibitory. Both input pathways, as well as Purkinje cells, synapse on the Deep Cerebellar Nuclei (DCN), the output of the cerebellum. (Adapted from Ito, 2001)

When the parallel fibers of anesthetized rats are electrically stimulated, blood flow to the region increases (Iadecola et al., 1996). This increased blood flow outstrips the increased $CMRO_2$, thereby leading to increased tissue oxygen (Thomsen et al., 2009). By inference, this suggests that increased activity in the mossy fiber/parallel fiber system will be tightly coupled with an increase in the BOLD signal. In line with energy use predictions outlined in the previous paragraph, increased neural activity within Purkinje cells alone does not seem to be strong enough to increase blood flow (Thomsen et al., 2004).

The possible response of the BOLD signal to activity within the climbing fiber system is less clear. After lesions of the inferior olive, stimulation of the whiskers of a rat produced only 42% of the blood flow increase observed in control animals (Zhang et al., 2003). This suggests that climbing fibers may be responsible for approximately half of the activity-dependent modulation of the BOLD signal. However, when complex (and simple) spike firing rates in Purkinje cells are increased by pharmacologically removing inhibitory input from interneurons, increases are observed in $CMRO_2$, but not in CBF (Thomsen et al., 2009). According to these results, increasing the complex spike rate by increasing the climbing fiber input could actually decrease the BOLD signal.

Clearly, the question of which neural processes are reflected in the cerebellar BOLD signal remains unanswered. While it appears likely that increased mossy/parallel fiber input would lead to robust increases in the BOLD signal at the cerebellar cortex, it remains unclear how climbing fiber input would modulate BOLD, if at all. Parallel electrophysiological recording and BOLD measurements would constitute an important step forward.

2.3.2. Physiological artifacts

Since the BOLD signal depends on the rate of blood flow and oxygenation, it should come as no surprise that it is sensitive to changes in respiration and cardiac function. This is especially true in the cerebellum and brainstem, which are surrounded by a dense vascular bed. Problematically, these physiological processes have been shown to change in response to behavior. Systematic heart rate changes are known to occur in many tasks involving the control of action (Damen & Brunia, 1987; Jennings et al., 1991, 1992, 1993; Jennings & van der Molen, 2002) as well as feedback processing in cognitive (Crone et al., 2004, 2005, 2006) and motor tasks (Schlerf et al., 2012). Thus, we may misinterpret BOLD signal changes caused by physiological processes as changes caused by neural activity.

Fortunately, physiological signals (respiration, heart rate) are easily recorded. The main challenge, then, becomes one of data analysis: how should one best remove physiological artifacts from the fMRI signals using these recordings? There are two principal ways that physiological processes can influence the BOLD signal. First, the time of slice acquisition relative to the physiological event is important (Figure 6A and B). The rate of blood flow varies for different phases of the cardiac cycle, and the brainstem shows movement with every heartbeat. The rise and fall of the chest during breathing induces subtle changes in the magnetic field. An efficient way to deal with changes related to the phase of these processes without any *a priori* knowledge of how the BOLD signal will change with these events is to use the RETROICOR method (Glover et al., 2000). This method deals with this by including both the sine and the cosine-and higher harmonics-of the phase of the physiological process as nuisance covariates within a standard GLM analysis. Thus, variability within a voxel's time series due to phasic changes of the signals measured will be modeled, instead of merely adding residual noise to the estimate of the BOLD response. This method was developed for the cerebral cortex, but provides efficient noise reduction for sub-tentorial structures as well. Within the brainstem, it has been demonstrated that the BOLD signal contains physiological noise which can be best modeled by three harmonics of respiration, two harmonics of heart rate, as well as a multiplicative term (Harvey et al., 2008). For areas around the cerebellum and brain stem, our own observations suggest that more than 30% of the variance in the raw fMRI signal can be explained by the first two harmonics of heart and breathing rate (Figure 6C). More recent methods have also been proposed for modeling other physiological artifacts in the BOLD signal, like spontaneous variations in breathing rate (Birn et al., 2006, 2008) and cardiac output (Chang & Glover, 2009). This approach can be quite important for correctly identifying neurally relevant portions of the cerebellar BOLD signal (Schlerf et al. 2012). While the proper balance between noise reduction and over-fitting has to be determined in each individual case, recording heart rate and breathing should become commonplace for cerebellar imaging studies to ensure that the effects of interest do not correlate systematically with physiological processes.

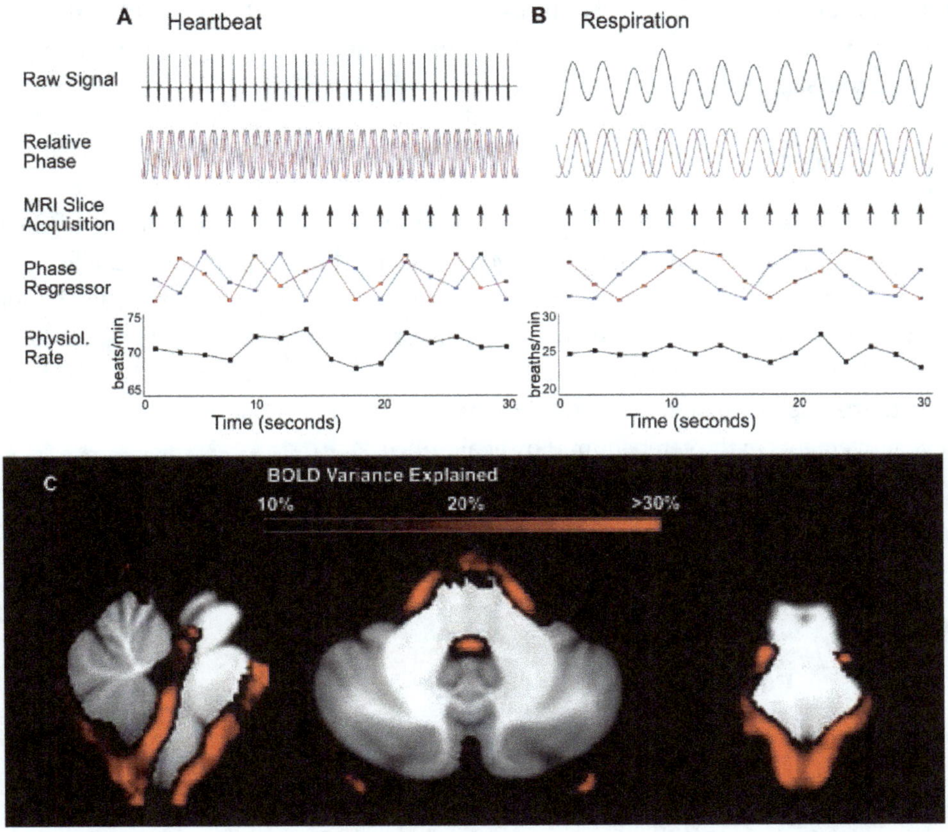

Figure 6. Influence of heart rate onto the BOLD signal. A) As a demonstration, a representative individual's heartbeat is shown. The top row shows the raw EKG trace of the hearbeat, and the next shows the first Fourier expansion (both sine and cosine waves) of the relative phase of the heartbets. Since fMRI data is acquired at regular intervals, BOLD artifacts may arise related to the phase of the heartbeat the data was acquired. The bottom row demonstrates heart rate effects. B) A representative individuals breathing is shown. The top row is the raw trace from a pneumatic compression belt, and the next rows show the instantaneous phase, as well as the phase and rate regressors. Note that breathing rate is substantially slower than heart rate. C) Data from a study conducted of the cerebellum (Schlerf et al., 2012) showing a high level of variability (greater than 30% of BOLD variance) accounted for by cardiac and respiratory phase regressors in CSF and arteries surrounding the cerebellum.

3. Functional studies of the cerebellum

3.1. Sensorimotor function

Because damage or removal of the cerebellum results first and foremost in movement impairments, the cerebellum has historically been categorized as a sensorimotor structure (Holmes, 1917, 1939). While it is now understood that the functional domain of the cerebellum extends beyond movement, sensorimotor processing remains one of the most active and important areas of cerebellar research.

Movement is one of the most efficient tasks for modulating BOLD-signal within the cerebellum. Below we review a few important fMRI results that have shaped our thinking of the function of this structure.

3.1.1. Maps of the body

Physiological work has suggested the presence of multiple body maps within the cerebellum. Two somatotopic maps were initially observed in the non-human primate cerebellum: one in the anterior lobe and the other in the inferior posterior lobe (Snider & Eldred, 1952). Both of these maps are somatotopically organized on a gross level (Figure 7). This organization has also been shown in humans using functional imaging. Indeed, the first published imaging study of the cerebellum (using PET) revealed spatially specific activations in response to finger and eye movements in the cerebellum (Fox et al., 1985).

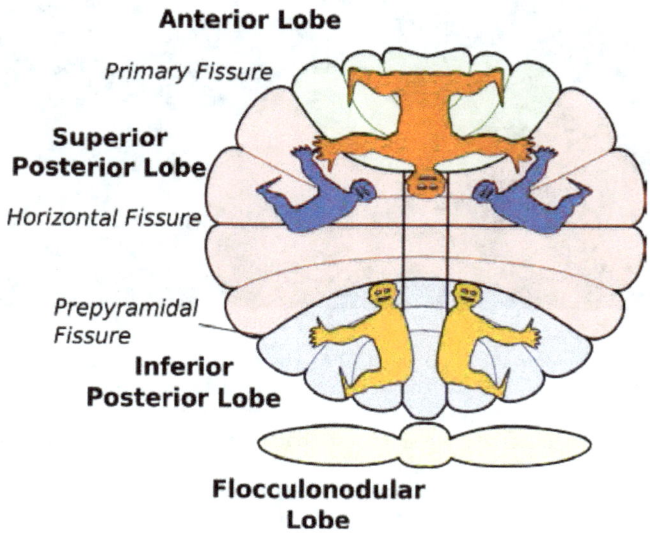

Figure 7. Multiple body representations within the cerebellum. The lobes are shaded to match the regions in Figure 1. Shown are the anterior (top, orange) and inferior posterior (bottom, yellow) body representations, as well as the newly identified superior posterior representation (blue). (Adapted from Snider & Eldred, 1952; Grodd et al., 2001; Schlerf et al., 2010)

Using fMRI, researchers have confirmed and extended these results. Rijntjes and colleagues (1999) confirmed that both sensory-motor representations show a somatopic gradient using finger and toe movements. Grodd et al. (2001) built upon this finding, demonstrating anterior and posterior representations for the hand, lips, tongue, and feet. These distinct maps were observed in the anterior and posterior lobes, in good agreement with animal physiology. The representation within the anterior lobe (lobules I-V; see Schmahmann et al., 1999) is generally unilateral, with each cerebellar hemisphere representing the movement of the ipsilateral limb. Within the somatomotor representation in the posterior lobe (chiefly lobule VIII), the observed activations are usually also stronger on the ipsilateral side, but bilateral activation is commonly observed (Grodd et al., 2001; Schlerf et al., 2010).

A number of studies have tried to dissociate the function of the anterior and posterior body maps. Thickbroom et al. (2003) explored the functional response to both active and passive movements of single fingers. Activation was observed to both types of movement in both the anterior lobe and the inferior aspect of the posterior lobe, suggesting that these regions have both sensory and motor functions. Habas et al. (2004a, 2004b) explored the response of the anterior map and the inferior posterior map during bimanual movements. Contrasting with the Thickbroom study, they found that passive bimanual movements did not activate the representation in lobule VIII, while active bimanual movements did (Habas et al., 2004a). A second study found that the inferior representation is more strongly activated by out-of-phase bimanual movements than in-phase movements, suggesting that this region may be specifically engaged by movements requiring the coordination of multiple effectors (Habas et al., 2004b).

A recent study, designed to explore the cerebellar response to coordination between individual fingers, tested simple rhythmic movements of all digits (fingers or toes) as well as complex sequential movements of individual digits (Schlerf et al., 2010). The body map within the anterior lobe was not strongly affected by movement complexity. Interestingly, there was evidence for a new map in lobules VI and VIIA Crus I, which was much more strongly activated for sequential movements of both the fingers (medially) and toes (laterally, see Figure 7). This suggests that these regions (thought to have cognitive functions) may be more involved in motor behavior than previously thought (Schlerf et al., 2010).

The aforementioned fMRI studies reveal somatotopic organization on a gross anatomical level, with neighboring voxels activating in response to different body parts. Physiological experiments, however, suggest that neighboring patches of cerebellar cortex respond to stimulation of quite different areas of the skin within the same bodypart. The term "fractured somatotopy" has been coined to capture this disjointed organization (Shambes et al., 1978; Bower & Woolston, 1983; Kassel et al., 1984). This organization poses a challenge to cerebellar imaging, as each voxel averages the activity over several of these patches of cerebellar cortex. Thus, conventional fMRI analyses will reach a resolution limit. A recent study was able to explore finer resolution maps of individual fingers using advanced analysis techniques (Wiestler et al., 2011). The analysis approach rests on the assumption that even if the average level of BOLD signal change across a region is not sensitive to individual finger movement, the spatial pattern of activity across multiple voxels may be specific for fingers and can be detected by multivariate analyses. The authors used local voxel patterns to train a linear classifier, and then predicted which finger was moved or stimulated in an independent test dataset. Better-than-chance prediction indicates that the region contains a finger representation. Two finger maps were identified: one in lobule V, and a second in lobule VIII. The activation patterns in these two representations were equally informative of finger identity for movement and tactile stimulation. This suggests that motor as well as sensory events are encoded with equal fidelity in the cerebellum. In contrast to the finger representations in the neocortex, which are ~3-4mm in size, the authors showed that the cerebellar representations are ~1-2mm in size, smaller than an individual voxel. Such "hyper-acuity" of multivariate analysis has also been demonstrated for the case of orientation columns in visual cortex (Swisher et al., 2010). Thus, multivariate analysis promises to be an excellent tool to study fractured somatotopy within the cerebellum.

3.1.2. Motor learning

In addition to studying topographic organization, fMRI has been used to explore the cerebellar involvement in motor learning. A large body of evidence shows that the cerebellum is involved in the process of error-based learning (Martin et al., 1996; Straube et al., 2001; Maschke et al., 2004; Pisella et al., 2005; Smith & Shadmehr, 2005; Morton & Bastian, 2006; Tseng et al., 2007; Alahyane et al., 2008). One example of such a task is saccade adaptation, in which the length of an eye-movement is adjusted on a trial-by-trial basis, based on whether the eye movement under-or over-shot the target during the previous saccade. This rapid learning process is impaired in cerebellar patients (Golla et al., 2008).

A seminal model proposed by Marr (1969) and Albus (1971) suggests that the architecture of the cerebellar cortex is ideally suited for such error-based learning. The model suggests that context information about the planned or ongoing movement is signaled over the mossy-fiber-parallel-fiber system. The climbing fiber input to the cerebellar cortex then provides an error signal that leads to plasticity at the parallel-fiber-Purkinje cell synapses. Through this mechanism, the cerebellar output associated with the same movement (parallel fiber input) is rapidly adjusted.

Researchers have used error-based learning tasks to test the involvement of the cerebellum in motor adaptation, albeit with mixed results. Generally, two types of learning responses can be predicted for the blood oxygenation level dependent (BOLD) signal. The first, based directly on the Marr/Albus model (Marr, 1969; Albus, 1971), is that the BOLD response should reflect an error-signal, and therefore should be high early in learning when errors are large and then taper off as performance improves. The second type of activity change is related to the storage of the learned representation. This idea predicts that as participants learn to produce more accurate movements (often referred to by motor control researchers as "acquiring an internal model") the BOLD response in regions that support those accurate movements should increase, because they perform more, or more accurate computations. Early-learning related activity was observed during a study of skill learning, with increased activity in the ipsilateral anterior lobe early during a pinch-force training task (Floyer-Lea & Matthews, 2005). An adaptation study conducted by Imamizu and colleagues (2000) reported activation patterns during a visuomotor adaptation task which were consistent with both error-processing and storage. With learning, activity decayed in broad regions throughout the anterior and lateral cerebellum, while the most lateral regions (bilaterally) increased in activation as the new rule was stored. A more recent study using a similar adaptation task observed chiefly storage related activity in the ipsilateral anterior lobe (Luauté et al., 2009). Storage related activity in PET has also been observed for saccade adaptation, with bilateral cerebellar lobules VI and VII showing increased activity when performing the adapted movement (Desmurget et al., 2000).

Learning is a slow process when compared with the time-course of the BOLD signal measured in fMRI, and it is not easy to repeat, which reduces the reliability of the measured brain response. Finally, many behavioral changes can be conflated with learning. For example, Seidler and colleagues (2002) argue that storage-related changes in cerebellar activation reflect performance parameters rather than learning per se. Similarly, the error-related component of the learning response may result from increased corrective movements when errors are prevalent. A study looking for signatures of error processing using a design containing random perturbations found no cerebellar regions which were significantly active in a contrast of trials containing errors and corrective movements against trials containing corrective movements without errors, while cerebral voxels in the postcentral gyrus were active in this contrast (Diedrichsen et al., 2005). A very recent study used a task in which corrective movements were impossible, and observed proprioceptive error-related activity in lobules V and VI (Schlerf et al., 2012).

The cerebellum may also play a role in other forms of learning. The serial reaction time task (SRTT) is a classic paradigm used to study motor sequence learning (Nissen & Bullemer, 1987). Typically, a set of stimuli appear on a computer screen, telling participants which keys to press. If these cues appear in a sequential order, responses will get faster as participants learn the sequence. Patients with cerebellar damage have consistently shown impairments in learning during the SRTT (Doyon et al., 1997; Molinari et al., 1997; Gómez-Beldarrain et al., 1998; Shin & Ivry, 2003). Yet, imaging studies using fMRI and PET have consistently shown either no change in cerebellar responses during learning (Seidler et al., 2002; van der Graaf et al., 2006) or slight decreases in the anterior lobe ipsilateral to the moving hand (Hazeltine et al., 1997; Doyon et al., 2002). Thus, while patient studies suggest some role of the cerebellum in sequence learning, evicence from brain imaging is much more limited.

3.1.3. *Timing and coordination*

Patients with cerebellar lesions show consistent impairment in tasks that require timing and coordination (in addition to deficits in error-based learning). The relationship between these two functions, and the cerebellar involvement in both, has been a very active area of research that has sparked substantial controversies in the last years.

There is a longstanding debate about the cerebellar contribution to movement timing, and fMRI has provided evidence for both sides. Work on eyeblink conditioning, where a tone is predictably delivered prior to an aversive stimulus delivered to the eyelid, has historically provided strong evidence for the role of the cerebellum in timing (Gellman & Miles, 1985; Steinmetz et al., 1986; Ivry & Keele, 1989). This task has been successfully adapted to the MR environment, revealing activation in lobules VI and VIIA Crus I during eye-blink conditioning (Ramnani et al., 2000; Dimitrova et al., 2002a; Miller et al., 2003; Gerwig et al., 2007; Cheng et al., 2008). Timed movement tasks, such as the production of rhythmic finger movements, reveal strong cerebellar activation (Lutz et al., 2000; Dhamala et al., 2003; Garraux et al., 2005; Jantzen et al., 2005; Spencer et al., 2007). Studies have also examined the response to timing without movement, and found cerebellar activation in response to sensory estimates of temporal delay in left lobules VI and VIIA Crus I (Harrington et al., 2004) and broad activation throughout the anterior lobe in response to deviations from predictable rhythmic sequences (Liu et al., 2008).

While the link between timing and the cerebellum may be somewhat controversial (Rao et al., 2001; Hinton et al., 2004), the link between the cerebellum and coordination is not. A cardinal symptom of cerebellar disease is ataxia, or the lack of movement coordination. This deficit is especially pronounced when the movement task involves the coordination of movement across multiple joints (Thach et al., 1992; Bastian et al., 1996; Thach, 1998). In healthy participants, increased cerebellar activation in fMRI studies is commonly observed when the coordination requirements of the task increase. For example, during eye-hand coordination the cerebellum increases its activation parametrically with increased temporal offset between the required eye and hand movements (Miall et al., 2001).

Many researchers assume that the precise sequential activation of separate muscles in the context of a coordinated movement relies on the same neural mechanisms that underlie explicit timing tasks (Ivry et al., 2002; Ivry & Spencer, 2004). In this view, deficits in timing are the cause of coordination deficits. Coordinating across effectors (e.g., the shoulder and hand muscles when pitching a baseball) would thus require accurately timing the serial order of events. Incorrect timing of the release of a baseball during the shoulder swing of a pitch would result in highly uncoordinated and inaccurate pitching. However, recent behavioral studies have shown that the motor system controls the moment of ball release based on a predictive estimate of the arm position, rather than "timing" the ball release based on the state of an internal clock triggered by a particular event (Hore & Watts, 2005). An imaging study comparing the role of the cerebellum in timing and coordination using a single task showed that these are dissociable processes with lateral lobule V being more strongly engaged during coordination than timing (Diedrichsen et al., 2007).

3.2. Nonmotor function

While the cerebral neocortex is divided into cytoarchitectonic regions that delineate functional specialization, the cerebellar cortex is nearly uniform. Functional specificity is likely determined by the connections between the cerebellum and other parts of the brain (Schmahmann, 2004). Virus tracer studies in primates have demonstrated connections between the cerebellum and cortical association areas, such as the prefrontal and parietal cortices (Strick et al., 2009). FMRI connectivity studies confirm the existence of these networks in humans (Krienen & Buckner, 2009; Buckner et al., 2011), with connections largely involving the lateral cerebellar hemispheres, especially lobules VI and VIIA (Crus I and II). Since the prefrontal and parietal association areas within the neocortex are believed to play important roles in executive function and language, connected regions within the cerebellum should contribute to these functions as well.

3.2.1. Executive control

FMRI has provided important evidence for the role of the cerebellum in executive functions such as attention and working memory. Attention is the cognitive process of focusing on a particular feature in the environment. Working memory is the short-term storage (on the order of seconds) of information for later processing. Humans with damaged cerebella have been observed to have deficits in both attention (e.g., Akshoomoff & Courchesne, 1992) and working memory (e.g., Ravizza et al., 2006).

An early fMRI study of the cerebellar role in attention asked participants to attend to visual stimuli and count certain targets, or make repetitive finger movements without attention (Allen et al., 1997). Motor responses were mostly contained within lobule V, while attentional responses were more posterior, chiefly lobules VI and VIIA, which are connected with the prefrontal cortex. A third task combined these processes (asking participants to press a button every time the target stimulus appeared), and revealed activation in both of these regions (Allen et al., 1997). This finding corroborated an early patient study of the cerebellar role in attention (Akshoomoff & Courchesne, 1992). At any given point, participants were asked to respond to either colored flashes or tones, detecting a target item in that series. During a "switch" condition, participants were asked to wait for a target in the other sensory modality following the successful identification of a target. Patients with damage to the cerebellum responded particularly slowly during this condition, suggesting that attention switching may be an important function of the cerebellum (Akshoomoff & Courchesne, 1992). An fMRI study was conducted using a similar task, asking participants to attend to either the shape or color of a visual stimulus. Increased and reproducible cerebellar activation near right lobule VI was observed during the attention switching condition compared to the sustained attention condition (Le et al., 1998). Bischoff-Grethe and colleagues (2002) pointed out that these switching tasks did not control for motor demands, as separate stimulus-response mappings must be maintained and switched in addition to attention. This study replicated the previous task of Le et al (1998), and included a control condition where participants performed the same attention switch but only responded to one of the two features. Since the control condition involved identical attentional processes, any differences would support a motor explanation of this effect. Analysis of this data found increased activity in right lobule VI when two response mappings were required, suggesting that response reassignment was more important than attention switching (Bischoff-Grethe et al., 2002).

Individuals with cerebellar damage have impaired verbal working memory, but intact spatial working memory (Ravizza et al., 2006). Transcranial magnetic stimulation over right lobule VI selectively impairs response time on verbal working memory tasks (Desmond et al., 2005). FMRI has also supported a cerebellar role in working memory. Studies have compared activation during the Sternberg working memory task (Sternberg, 1966) to a control task of silent rehearsal, where participants continuously read a list of items for later matching. Cerebellar activity in bilateral lobules VI and VIIa crus I is observed during both tasks, while Lobule VIII is specifically activated in response to working memory (Desmond et al., 1997; Chen & Desmond, 2005a). Activity in all of these regions, bilateral lobules VI and VIIa Crus I and right lobule VIII, increases parametrically with working memory load (Kirschen et al., 2005).

The Sternberg task (Sternberg, 1966) can be used in event-related fMRI studies, where distinct components of working memory can be explored. Lobules VI and VIIA Crus I are chiefly involved during the encoding phase, while lobules VIIB and VIIIA were involved in encoding as well as maintenance across delay (Chen & Desmond, 2005b).

3.2.2. Language

While overt language disturbances such as aphasia are not commonly observed following cerebellar damage, speech disturbances have been documented (e.g., Holmes, 1917), which may mask subtle linguistic effects. FMRI has become an important tool for exploring the cerebellar contribution to language.

The first study to observe cerebellar activation in a cognitive task detected activity in the right cerebellum during verb generation (Petersen et al., 1989). Verb generation has since been successfully used to demonstrate functional activation of bilateral lobules VI and right VIIA Crus I by a number of researchers (e.g., Seger et al., 2000; Frings et al., 2006). A similar task is word-stem completion, where words are generated to complete a command prompt of a few letters. An early study observed that the right cerebellum (chiefily lobule VIIA Crus I, extending into midline lobules VI through VIIB) is more active when there are a limited number of correct completions of the word compared to when there are many (Desmond et al., 1998). This suggests that the search for correct words requires more cerebellar computation than selection among a number of easily identified options.

Despite the ease of observing activation during linguistic tasks, the role of the cerebellum in language is not without controversy. Participants with cerebellar degeneration do not have impairments in verb-generation tasks (Richter et al., 2004). Furthermore, while most fMRI studies control for speech articulation using noun repetition tasks, some investigators argue that this is not a strong enough control. Ackermann and colleagues (1998) observed cerebellar activity in right lobule VI by asking participants to perform a self-guided repetition task by rehearsing the months of the year repeatedly. This suggests that the cerebellum's role may still be fundamentally articulatory, as well-learned sequences of words are not demanding to recite. While the cerebellar contribution to language is not the only example of the difficulty in reconciling brain imaging studies with clinical investigation, it does underscore the need for elegant experimental manipulations when exploring cerebellar activity.

4. Conclusion

This chapter has provided a brief overview of some of the specialized techniques for imaging this particular part of the brain. We discussed some specialized anatomical methods for normalization and inter-individual alignment, as well as region-of-interest identification. We also discussed the importance of removing physiological nuisance covariates, and the promise of future innovation by multivariate analysis methods. Brain scientists who are interested in the cerebellum should become familiar with these methods.

We also discussed literature covering the functional specificity of this structure. Cerebellar regions likely play a role in many different functions, ranging from sensorimotor functions to higher cognitive functions. We provided an overview of the major areas of research, attempting to highlight some of the current controversies with regard to the role of the cerebellum. As MRI scanners and pulse sequences improve and researchers make better use of specialized cerebellar analysis techniques, some of these controversies may be resolved. Fortunately, new controversies will undoubtedly emerge to take their place.

The cerebellum is a fascinating structure that poses unique challenges to MRI. As new solutions to some of these challenges come of age, we expect that imaging the "little brain" will continue to provide fresh and important insights to cerebellar function for years to come.

Author details

John Schlerf[1], Tobias Wiestler[3], Timothy Verstynen[2] and Jörn Diedrichsen[3]

1 Johns Hopkins University, USA

2 Carnegie Mellon University, USA

3 University College London, UK

References

[1] Ackermann H, Wildgruber D, Daum I, Grodd W. Does the cerebellum contribute to cognitive aspects of speech production? A functional magnetic resonance imaging (fMRI) study in humans. *Neurosci Let* 247: 187–190, 1998.

[2] Akshoomoff N, Courchesne E. A new role for the cerebellum in cognitive operations. *Behav Neurosci* 106: 731–738, 1992.

[3] Alahyane N, Fonteille V, Urquizar C, Salemme R, Nighoghossian N, Pelisson D, Tilikete C. Separate Neural Substrates in the Human Cerebellum for Sensory-motor Adaptation of Reactive and of Scanning Voluntary Saccades. *Cerebellum* 7: 595–601, 2008.

[4] Albus J. A theory of cerebellar function. *Math Biosci* 10: 25–61, 1971.

[5] Allen G, Buxton RB, Wong EC, Courchesne E. Attentional Activation of the Cerebellum Independent of Motor Involvement. *Science* 275: 1940 –1943, 1997.

[6] Bastian AJ, Martin TA, Keating JG, Thach WT. Cerebellar ataxia: abnormal control of interaction torques across multiple joints. *J Neurophysiol* 76: 492 –509, 1996.

[7] Bischoff-Grethe A, Ivry R, Grafton S. Cerebellar involvement in response reassignment rather than attention. *J Neurosci* 22: 546–553, 2002.

[8] Bower JM, Woolston DC. Congruence of spatial organization of tactile projections to granule cell and Purkinje cell layers of cerebellar hemispheres of the albino rat: vertical organization of cerebellar cortex. *J Neurophysiol* 49: 745 –766, 1983.

[9] Buckner RL, Krienen FM, Castellanos A, Diaz JC, Yeo BTT. The Organization of the Human Cerebellum Estimated by Intrinsic Functional Connectivity. *J Neurophysiol* 106: 2322–2345, 2011.

[10] Chen SHA, Desmond JE. Cerebrocerebellar networks during articulatory rehearsal and verbal working memory tasks. *NeuroImage* 24: 332–338, 2005a.

[11] Chen SHA, Desmond JE. Temporal dynamics of cerebro-cerebellar network recruitment during a cognitive task. *Neuropsychologia* 43: 1227–1237, 2005b.

[12] Cheng DT, Disterhoft JF, Power JM, Ellis DA, Desmond JE. Neural substrates underlying human delay and trace eyeblink conditioning. *PNAS* 105: 8108–8113, 2008.

[13] Crone E, Bunge S, de Klerk P, van der Molen M. Cardiac concomitants of performance monitoring: context dependence and individual differences. *Cog Brain Res* 23: 93–106, 2005.

[14] Crone E, Jennings R, Van der Molen M. Developmental change in feedback processing as reflected by phasic heart rate changes. *Dev Psych* 40: 1228–1238, 2004.

[15] Crone E, Somsen R, Zanolie K, Van der Molen M. A heart rate analysis of developmental change in feedback processing and rule shifting from childhood to early adulthood. *J Exp Child Psych* 95: 99–116, 2006.

[16] Damen E, Brunia C. Changes in Heart Rate and Slow Brain Potentials Related to Motor Preparation and Stimulus Anticipation in a Time Estimation Task. *Psychophysiol* 24: 700–713, 1987.

[17] Desmond J, Chen S, Shieh P. Cerebellar transcranial magnetic stimulation impairs verbal working memory. *Ann Neurol* 58: 553–560, 2005.

[18] Desmond J, Gabrieli J, Glover G. Dissociation of Frontal and Cerebellar Activity in a Cognitive Task: Evidence for a Distinction between Selection and Search. *NeuroImage* 7: 368–376, 1998.

[19] Desmond J, Gabrieli J, Wagner A, Ginier B, Glover G. Lobular patterns of cerebellar activation in verbal working-memory and finger-tapping tasks as revealed by functional MRI. *J Neurosci* 17: 9675–9685, 1997.

[20] Desmurget M, Pélisson D, Grethe JS, Alexander GE, Urquizar C, Prablanc C, Grafton ST. Functional adaptation of reactive saccades in humans: a PET study. *Exp Brain Res* 132: 243–259, 2000.

[21] Dhamala M, Pagnoni G, Wiesenfeld K, Zink C, Martin M, Berns G. Neural correlates of the complexity of rhythmic finger tapping. *NeuroImage* 20: 918–926, 2003.

[22] Diedrichsen J, Balsters JH, Flavell J, Cussans E, Ramnani N. A probabilistic MR atlas of the human cerebellum. *NeuroImage* 46: 39–46, 2009.

[23] Diedrichsen J, Criscimagna-Hemminger S, Shadmehr R. Dissociating Timing and Coordination as Functions of the Cerebellum. *J Neurosci* 27: 6291–6301, 2007.

[24] Diedrichsen J, Hashambhoy Y, Rane T, Shadmehr R. Neural correlates of reach errors. *J Neurosci* 25: 9919–9931, 2005.

[25] Diedrichsen J, Maderwald S, Küper M, Thürling M, Rabe K, Gizewski ER, Ladd ME, Timmann D. Imaging the deep cerebellar nuclei: A probabilistic atlas and normalization procedure. *NeuroImage* 54: 1786–1794, 2011.

[26] Diedrichsen J. A spatially unbiased atlas template of the human cerebellum. *NeuroImage* 33: 127–138, 2006.

[27] Dimitrova A, Weber J, Maschke M, Elles H, Kolb FP, Forsting M, Diener H, Timmann D. Eyeblink-related areas in human cerebellum as shown by fMRI. *Hum Brain Map* 17: 100–115, 2002a.

[28] Dimitrova A, Weber J, Redies C, Kindsvater K, Maschke M, Kolb F, Forsting M, Diener H, Timmann D. MRI atlas of the human cerebellar nuclei. *NeuroImage* 17: 240–255, 2002b.

[29] Dimitrova A, Zeljko D, Schwarze F, Maschke M, Gerwig M, Frings M, Beck A, Aurich V, Forsting M, Timmann D. Probabilistic 3D MRI atlas of the human cerebellar dentate/interposed nuclei. *NeuroImage* 30: 12–25, 2006.

[30] Doyon J, Gaudreau D, Laforce R Jr, Castonguay M, Bédard PJ, Bédard F, Bouchard JP. Role of the striatum, cerebellum, and frontal lobes in the learning of a visuomotor sequence. *Brain Cogn* 34: 218–245, 1997.

[31] Doyon J, Song AW, Karni A, Lalonde F, Adams MM, Ungerleider LG. Experience-dependent changes in cerebellar contributions to motor sequence learning. *PNAS* 99: 1017–1022, 2002.

[32] Floyer-Lea A, Matthews P. Distinguishable brain activation networks for short- and long-term motor skill learning. *J Neurophysiol* 94: 512–518, 2005.

[33] Fox P, Raichle M, Thach W. Functional mapping of the human cerebellum with positron emission tomography. *PNAS* 82: 7462–7466, 1985.

[34] Frings M, Dimitrova A, Schorn CF, Elles H-G, Hein-Kropp C, Gizewski ER, Diener HC, Timmann D. Cerebellar involvement in verb generation: An fMRI study. *Neurosci Let* 409: 19–23, 2006.

[35] Garraux G, McKinney C, Wu T, Kansaku K, Nolte G, Hallett M. Shared brain areas but not functional connections controlling movement timing and order. *J Neurosci* 25: 5290–5297, 2005.

[36] Gellman R, Miles F. A new role for the cerebellum in conditioning? *Trends Neurosci* 8: 181–182, 1985.

[37] Gerwig M, Kolb FP, Timmann D. The involvement of the human cerebellum in eye-blink conditioning. *Cerebellum* 6: 38–57, 2007.

[38] Glover G, Li T-Q, Ress D. Image-based method for retrospective correction of physiological motion effects in fMRI: RETROICOR. *Magn Reson Med* 44: 162–167, 2000.

[39] Golla H, Tziridis K, Haarmeier T, Catz N, Barash S, Thier P. Reduced saccadic resilience and impaired saccadic adaptation due to cerebellar disease. *Eur J Neurosci* 27: 132–144, 2008.

[40] Gómez-Beldarrain M, García-Moncó JC, Rubio B, Pascual-Leone A. Effect of focal cerebellar lesions on procedural learning in the serial reaction time task. *Exp Brain Res* 120: 25–30, 1998.

[41] van der Graaf FHCE, Maguire RP, Leenders KL, de Jong BM. Cerebral activation related to implicit sequence learning in a Double Serial Reaction Time task. *Brain Res* 1081: 179–190, 2006.

[42] Grodd W, Hülsmann E, Lotze M, Wildgruber D, Erb M. Sensorimotor mapping of the human cerebellum: fMRI evidence of somatotopic organization. *Hum Brain Map* 13: 55–73, 2001.

[43] Habas C, Axelrad H, Cabanis E. The cerebellar second homunculus remains silent during passive bimanual movements. *Neuroreport* 15: 1571–1574, 2004a.

[44] Habas C, Axelrad H, Nguyen T, Cabanis E. Specific neocerebellar activation during out-of-phase bimanual movements. *Neuroreport* 15: 595–599, 2004b.

[45] Harrington D, Boyd L, Mayer A, Sheltraw D, Lee R, Huang M, Rao S. Neural representation of interval encoding and decision making. *Cog Brain Res* 21: 193–205, 2004.

[46] Harvey A, Pattinson K, Brooks J, Mayhew S, Jenkinson M, Wise R. Brainstem functional magnetic resonance imaging: Disentangling signal from physiological noise. *J Magn Reson Imaging* 28: 1337–1344, 2008.

[47] Hazeltine E, Grafton ST, Ivry R. Attention and stimulus characteristics determine the locus of motor-sequence encoding. A PET study. *Brain* 120 (Pt 1): 123–140, 1997.

[48] Hinton S, Harrington D, Binder J, Durgerian S, Rao S. Neural systems supporting timing and chronometric counting: an FMRI study. *Cog Brain Res* 21: 183–192, 2004.

[49] Hoge R, Atkinson J, Gill B, Crelier G, Marrett S, Pike G. Linear coupling between cerebral blood flow and oxygen consumption in activated human cortex. *PNAS* 96: 9403–9408, 1999.

[50] Holmes G. The symptoms of acute cerebellar injuries due to gunshot injuries. *Brain* 40: 461–535, 1917.

[51] Holmes G. The cerebellum of man. *Brain* 62: 1–30, 1939.

[52] Hore J, Watts S. Timing Finger Opening in Overarm Throwing Based on a Spatial Representation of Hand Path. *J Neurophysiol* 93: 3189 –3199, 2005.

[53] Howarth C, Peppiatt-Wildman C, Attwell D. The energy use associated with neural computation in the cerebellum. *J Cereb Blood Flow Metab* 30: 403–414, 2009.

[54] Iadecola C, Li J, Xu S, Yang G. Neural mechanisms of blood flow regulation during synaptic activity in cerebellar cortex. *J Neurophysiol* 75: 940–950, 1996.

[55] Imamizu H, Miyauchi S, Tamada T, Sasaki Y, Takino R, Putz B, Yoshioka T, Kawato M. Human cerebellar activity reflecting an acquired internal model of a new tool. *Nature* 403: 192–195, 2000.

[56] Ito M. Cerebellar Long-Term Depression: Characterization, Signal Transduction, and Functional Roles. *Physiol Rev* 81: 1143–1195, 2001.

[57] Ivry R, Keele S. Timing Functions of The Cerebellum. *J Cogn Neurosci* 1: 136–152, 1989.

[58] Ivry R, Spencer R, Zelaznik H, Diedrichsen J. The cerebellum and event timing. *Ann N Y Acad Sci* 978: 302–317, 2002.

[59] Ivry R, Spencer R. The neural representation of time. *Curr Opin Neurbiol* 14: 225–232, 2004.

[60] Jantzen K, Steinberg F, Kelso J. Functional MRI reveals the existence of modality and coordination-dependent timing networks. *NeuroImage* 25: 1031–1042, 2005.

[61] Jennings J, van der Molen M, Brock K, Somsen R. Response inhibition initiates cardiac deceleration: evidence from a sensory-motor compatibility paradigm. *Psychophysiol* 28: 72–85, 1991.

[62] Jennings J, van der Molen M, Brock K, Somsen R. On the synchrony of stopping motor responses and delaying heartbeats. *J Exp Psychol [Hum Percept]* 18: 422–436, 1992.

[63] Jennings J, van der Molen M, Brock K, Somsen R. How are tonic and phasic cardiovascular changes related to central motor command? *Biol Psych* 35: 237–254, 1993.

[64] Jennings R, van der Molen M. Cardiac timing and the central regulation of action. *Psychol Res* 66: 337–349, 2002.

[65] Kassel J, Shambes GM, Welker W. Fractured cutaneous projections to the granule cell layer of the posterior cerebellar hemisphere of the domestic cat. *J Comp Neurol* 225: 458–468, 1984.

[66] Kelly R, Strick P. Cerebellar loops with motor cortex and prefrontal cortex of a nonhuman primate. *J Neurosci* 23: 8432–8444, 2003.

[67] Kirschen MP, Chen SHA, Schraedley-Desmond P, Desmond JE. Load- and practice-dependent increases in cerebro-cerebellar activation in verbal working memory: an fMRI study. *NeuroImage* 24: 462–472, 2005.

[68] Krienen F, Buckner R. Segregated fronto-cerebellar circuits revealed by intrinsic functional connectivity. *Cereb Cortex* 19: 2497, 2485, 2009.

[69] Küper M, Dimitrova A, Thürling M, Maderwald S, Roths J, Elles HG, Gizewski ER, Ladd ME, Diedrichsen J, Timmann D. Evidence for a motor and a non-motor domain in the human dentate nucleus -- An fMRI study. *NeuroImage* 54: 2612–2622, 2011a.

[70] Küper M, Thürling M, Stefanescu R, Maderwald S, Roths J, Elles HG, Ladd ME, Diedrichsen J, Timmann D. Evidence for a motor somatotopy in the cerebellar dentate nucleus—an fMRI study in humans. *Hum Brain Map*. .

[71] Larsell O. The morphogenesis and adult pattern of the lobules and fissures of the cerebellum of the white rat. *J Comp Neurol* 97: 281–356, 1952.

[72] Larsell O. The cerebellum of the cat and the monkey. *J Comp Neurol* 99: 135–199, 1953.

[73] Le TH, Pardo JV, Hu X. 4 T-fMRI Study of Nonspatial Shifting of Selective Attention: Cerebellar and Parietal Contributions. *J Neurophysiol* 79: 1535 –1548, 1998.

[74] Liu T, Xu D, Ashe J, Bushara K. Specificity of Inferior Olive Response to Stimulus Timing. *J Neurophysiol* 100: 1557–1561, 2008.

[75] Luauté J, Schwartz S, Rossetti Y, Spiridon M, Rode G, Boisson D, Vuilleumier P. Dynamic changes in brain activity during prism adaptation. *J Neurosci* 29: 169–178, 2009.

[76] Lutz K, Specht K, Shah NJ, Jäncke L. Tapping movements according to regular and irregular visual timing signals investigated with fMRI. *Neuroreport* 11: 1301–1306, 2000.

[77] Makris N, Hodge SM, Haselgrove C, Kennedy DN, Dale A, Fischl B, Rosen BR, Harris G, Caviness VS, Schmahmann JD. Human Cerebellum: Surface-Assisted Cortical Parcellation and Volumetry with Magnetic Resonance Imaging. *J Cogn Neurosci* 15: 584–599, 2003.

[78] Makris N, Schlerf J, Hodge S, Haselgrove C, Albaugh M, Seidman L, Rauch S, Harris G, Biederman J, Caviness V, Kennedy D, Schmahmann J. MRI-based surface-assisted parcellation of human cerebellar cortex: an anatomically specified method with estimate of reliability. *NeuroImage* 25: 1146–1160, 2005.

[79] Marr D. A theory of cerebellar cortex. *J Physiol* 202: 437–470, 1969.

[80] Martin T, Keating J, Goodkin H, Bastian A, Thach W. Throwing while looking through prisms. I. Focal olivocerebellar lesions impair adaptation. *Brain* 119: 1183–1198, 1996.

[81] Maschke M, Gomez C, Ebner T, Konczak J. Hereditary Cerebellar Ataxia Progressively Impairs Force Adaptation During Goal-Directed Arm Movements. *J Neurophysiol* 91: 230–238, 2004.

[82] Mathiesen C, Caesar K, Lauritzen M. Temporal coupling between neuronal activity and blood flow in rat cerebellar cortex as indicated by field potential analysis. *J Physiol* 523: 235–246, 2000.

[83] Miall RC, Reckess GZ, Imamizu H. The cerebellum coordinates eye and hand tracking movements. *Nat Neurosci* 4: 638–644, 2001.

[84] Miller MJ, Chen N, Li L, Tom B, Weiss C, Disterhoft JF, Wyrwicz AM. fMRI of the Conscious Rabbit during Unilateral Classical Eyeblink Conditioning Reveals Bilateral Cerebellar Activation. *J Neurosci* 23: 11753 –11758, 2003.

[85] Molinari M, Leggio M, Solida A, Ciorra R, Misciagna S, Silveri M, Petrosini L. Cerebellum and procedural learning: evidence from focal cerebellar lesions. *Brain* 120: 1753–1762, 1997.

[86] Morton S, Bastian A. Cerebellar Contributions to Locomotor Adaptations during Splitbelt Treadmill Walking. *J Neurosci* 26: 9107–9116, 2006.

[87] Nissen MJ, Bullemer P. Attentional requirements of learning: Evidence from performance measures. *Cogn Psych* 19: 1–32, 1987.

[88] Petersen SE, Fox PT, Posner MI, Mintun M, Raichle ME. Positron Emission Tomographic Studies of the Processing of Singe Words. *J Cogn Neurosci* 1: 153–170, 1989.

[89] Pisella L, Rossetti Y, Michel C, Rode G, Boisson D, Pélisson D, Tilikete C. Ipsidirectional impairment of prism adaptation after unilateral lesion of anterior cerebellum. *Neurology* 65: 150–152, 2005.

[90] Ramnani N, Toni I, Josephs O, Ashburner J, Passingham RE. Learning- and expectation-related changes in the human brain during motor learning. *J Neurophysiol* 84: 3026–3035, 2000.

[91] Rancz EA, Ishikawa T, Duguid I, Chadderton P, Mahon S, Hausser M. High-fidelity transmission of sensory information by single cerebellar mossy fibre boutons. *Nature* 450: 1245–1248, 2007.

[92] Rao S, Mayer A, Harrington D. The evolution of brain activation during temporal processing. *Nat Neurosci* 4: 317–323, 2001.

[93] Ravizza S, Mccormick C, Schlerf J, Justus T, Ivry R, Fiez J. Cerebellar damage produces selective deficits in verbal working memory. *Brain* 129: 306–320, 2006.

[94] Richter S, Kaiser O, Hein-Kropp C, Dimitrova A, Gizewski E, Beck A, Aurich V, Ziegler W, Timmann D. Preserved verb generation in patients with cerebellar atrophy. *Neuropsychologia* 42: 1235–1246, 2004.

[95] Rijntjes M, Buechel C, Kiebel S, Weiller C. Multiple somatotopic representations in the human cerebellum. *Neuroreport* 10: 3653–3658, 1999.

[96] Schlerf J, Ivry RB, Diedrichsen J. Encoding of Sensory Prediction Errors in the Human Cerebellum. *J Neurosci* 32: 4913–4922, 2012.

[97] Schlerf JE, Verstynen TD, Ivry RB, Spencer RMC. Evidence of a Novel Somatopic Map in the Human Neocerebellum During Complex Actions. *J Neurophysiol* 103: 3330–3336, 2010.

[98] Schmahmann JD, Doyon J, McDonald D, Holmes C, Lavoie K, Hurwitz AS, Kabani N, Toga A, Evans A, Petrides M. Three-Dimensional MRI Atlas of the Human Cerebellum in Proportional Stereotaxic Space. *NeuroImage* 10: 233–260, 1999.

[99] Schmahmann JD. Disorders of the cerebellum: ataxia, dysmetria of thought, and the cerebellar cognitive affective syndrome. *J Neuropsychiatry Clin Neurosci* 16: 367–378, 2004.

[100] Seger CA, Desmond JE, Glover GH, Gabrieli JD. Functional magnetic resonance imaging evidence for right-hemisphere involvement in processing unusual semantic relationships. *Neuropsychology* 14: 361–369, 2000.

[101] Seidler R, Purushotham A, Kim S, Uğurbil K, Willingham D, Ashe J. Cerebellum activation associated with performance change but not motor learning. *Science* 296: 2043–2046, 2002.

[102] Shambes GM, Gibson JM, Welker W. Fractured Somatotopy in Granule Cell Tactile Areas of Rat Cerebellar Hemispheres Revealed by Micromapping; pp. 116– 140. *Brain Behav Evol* 15: 116–140, 1978.

[103] Shin JC, Ivry RB. Spatial and Temporal Sequence Learning in Patients with Parkinson's Disease or Cerebellar Lesions. *J Cogn Neurosci* 15: 1232–1243, 2003.

[104] Smith M, Shadmehr R. Intact Ability to Learn Internal Models of Arm Dynamics in Huntington's Disease But Not Cerebellar Degeneration. *J Neurophysiol* 93: 2809–2821, 2005.

[105] Snider R, Eldred E. Cerebrocerebellar relationships in the monkey. *J Neurophysiol* 15: 27–40, 1952.

[106] Spencer RMC, Verstynen T, Brett M, Ivry R. Cerebellar activation during discrete and not continuous timed movements: an fMRI study. *Neuroimage* 36: 378–387, 2007.

[107] Steinmetz JE, Rosen DJ, Chapman PF, Lavond DG, Thompson RF. Classical conditioning of the rabbit eyelid response with a mossy-fiber stimulation CS: I. Pontine nuclei and middle cerebellar peduncle stimulation. *Behav Neurosci* 100: 878–887, 1986.

[108] Sternberg S. High-speed scanning in human memory. *Science* 153: 652–654, 1966.

[109] Stoodley CJ, Schmahmann JD. Functional topography in the human cerebellum: A meta-analysis of neuroimaging studies. *NeuroImage* 44: 489–501, 2009.

[110] Straube A, Deubel H, Ditterich J, Eggert T. Cerebellar lesions impair rapid saccade amplitude adaptation. *Neurology* 57: 2105 –2108, 2001.

[111] Strick P, Dum R, Fiez J. Cerebellum and Nonmotor Function. *Annu Rev Neurosci* 32: 413–434, 2009.

[112] Swisher JD, Gatenby JC, Gore JC, Wolfe BA, Moon C-H, Kim S-G, Tong F. Multiscale Pattern Analysis of Orientation-Selective Activity in the Primary Visual Cortex. *J Neurosci* 30: 325 –330, 2010.

[113] Thach W. A role for the cerebellum in learning movement coordination. *Neurobiol Learn Mem* 70: 177–188, 1998.

[114] Thach WT, Goodkin HP, Keating JG. The Cerebellum and the Adaptive Coordination of Movement. *Annu Rev Neurosci* 15: 403–442, 1992.

[115] Thickbroom G, Byrnes M, Mastaglia F. Dual representation of the hand in the cerebellum: activation with voluntary and passive finger movement. *NeuroImage* 18: 670–674, 2003.

[116] Thomsen K, Offenhauser N, Lauritzen M. Principal neuron spiking: neither necessary nor sufficient for cerebral blood flow in rat cerebellum. *J Physiol* 560: 181–189, 2004.

[117] Thomsen K, Piilgaard H, Gjedde A, Bonvento G, Lauritzen M. Principal Cell Spiking, Postsynaptic Excitation, and Oxygen Consumption in the Rat Cerebellar Cortex. *J Neurophysiol* 102: 1503–1512, 2009.

[118] Tseng Y-W, Diedrichsen J, Krakauer JW, Shadmehr R, Bastian AJ. Sensory prediction errors drive cerebellum-dependent adaptation of reaching. *J Neurophysiol* 98: 54–62, 2007.

[119] Wiestler T, McGonigle DJ, Diedrichsen J. Integration of sensory and motor representations of single fingers in the human cerebellum. *J Neu*rophysiol 105: 3042–3053, 2011.

[120] Zhang Y, Forster C, Milner T, Iadecola C. Attenuation of activity-induced increases in cerebellar blood flow by lesion of the inferior olive. Am J Physiol Heart Circ Physiol 285: H1177–H1182, 2003.

5

A Practical Guide to an fMRI Experiment

Nasser H Kashou

1. Introduction

Functional Magnetic Resonance Imaging (fMRI) has been around for two decades now and research in this field has been exponentially rising. Many of this research has been dominated by basic science. Recent trends have brought the clinical realm into play in which valuable contribution can still be made. Allowing the clinician to understand the basic concepts behind an fMRI experiment is crucial to further developing and evaluating functional paradigms and research. Part of designing an fMRI experiment is understanding the physics and how fine tuning scanning parameters affect the image quality which in turn affect the findings of an fMRI study. The other part is understanding the physiology behind the acquired signal as well as the anatomy of the brain. To appreciate the complexity of the fMRI process see [1, 2].

In this chapter we present a practical guide to the novice on what important aspects needed to perform an efficient fMRI experiment from idea formulation to understanding the possible limitations of the results. In doing so, the basic concepts of fMRI beginning with image resolution and physics will be discussed along with advice on possible pearls and pitfalls of this process. Points covered will include paradigm design, scanning protocol, and limitations.

2. Basics physics

How is an image acquired in MRI? In this section a brief overview of the physics and steps needed is introduced. The main components to acquire an image in MRI are a magnet, three gradients and a radio frequency (RF) coil. In contrast to other imaging modalities, the magnet is always on, very strong and can range anywhere from 1.5 to 8 Tesla (higher for animal systems). Currently 1.5 and 3 Tesla are the standard magnets for clinical MRI. To get a grasp on the strength of the magnet, consider that the earth's magnetic field is equal to 0.5 Gauss where 10,000 Gauss is equal to 1 Tesla. This means if working with a 1.5 or 3 Tesla system then the magnet is 30,000 and 60,000 times stronger than the earth's magnetic field. This fact is probably the most important thing to know about MRI scanners, namely because of safety. Any ferrous material should never be brought near the scanner room. The magnet itself cannot provide images without having the two other components; the RF coil and three gradients (in x, y, and x planes). The RF coil is used to send a pulse at the same precessing frequency of the hydrogen nuclei (see below). In some systems the RF coil both transmits and receives. The gradients are turned on and off to cause a slight gradient increase in the magnetic field. All together these components initiate the process of acquiring viewable images. They also form the physical basis of scanning sequences.

But what is being measured? The interaction of protons in the magnetic field,i.e. nuclear magnetic resonance (NMR). Specifically, the hydrogen nuclei from water molecules. In general they have spins, like tops with orientation and a frequency ($\gamma = 42.56MHzT^{-1}$). γ is a proportionality constant called the gyromagnetic ratio. These protons are randomly pointing in different directions in our bodies, Fig. 1.

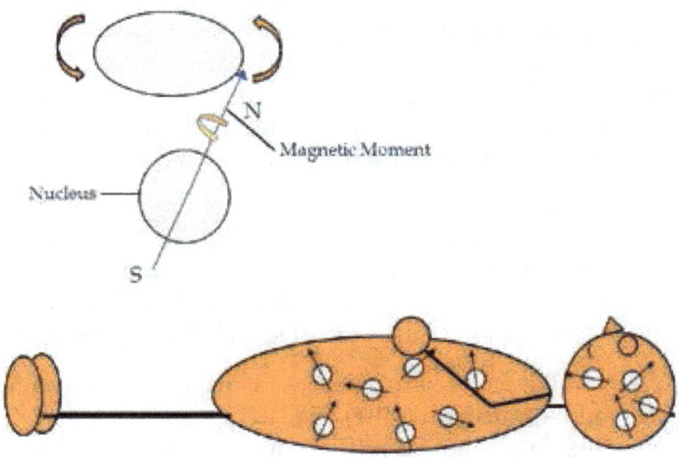

Figure 1. The human body is mainly water thus the hydrogen nuclei are exploited to extract an image in MRI. The nuclei (precess at 42.58 MHz/Tesla) have a spin with orientation and frequency and a magnetic moment, direction it points. These directions are random and thus no net magnetization.

Once we enter an MRI scanner there will be a net magnetization in the direction of the B_o field caused by the magnet. The larmor equation describes this interaction.

$$\omega_o = \gamma B_o \tag{1}$$

where ω_o is the angular frequency of precession of protons in an external magnetic field, and B_o is the strength of the external magnetic field.

The following steps illustrated in Figs. 2 and 3 are needed for the entire process. First the participant, after safety screening of any ferrous objects, is laid down and entered into the scanner. At this point there will be a net magnetization in the direction of the magnetic field (B_o) as a result of some protons aligning with the magnetic field. In a 1.5 Tesla scanner, 1 out of 100,000 hydrogen nuclei aligns itself with B_o [3]. Next some calibration and fine tuning is performed, called shimming. Then an RF pulse (typically 90°, known as flip angle, ϕ) is sent at the appropriate frequency based on the larmor equation. This knocks the particular protons of interest over by 90° as they absorb the energy however they will try to realign with the field and emit energy during this process. After turning off the RF pulse and as the protons return to their original orientations, they emit energy in the form of radio waves. Anytime between this process of realigning with B_0 the RF coil can measure the radio waves being emitted. This gives a signal from one location so the gradients are needed to encode space, Fig. 3. One gradient will phase encode while the second will frequency encode and the final one will slice encode. How this is done is dependent on the imaging parameters and pulse sequences (will not be discussed in this chapter) used. The use of different values of echo time (TE) and repetition time (TR) will determine the contrast or type of image acquired. Simply,TR is the time between transmitted RF pulses and TE is the time to listen to the signal. Varying these two parameters determines the contrast of an anatomical MRI allowing for a T1-weighted, T2-weighted or proton density (PD) image. In a T1-weighted image fat has a high signal (bright) and the cerebral spinal fluid (CSF) has a low signal (dark). In a T2-weighted image fat has low signal (dark) and CSF has high signal (bright). In a PD image the contrast is between that of T1 and T2. They are called T1 and T2 weighted because they are based on the T1 and T2 relaxation times. T1 relaxation is a measure of how quickly the protons realign with B_0 (returning to equilibrium) and T2 relaxation is a measure of how quickly the protons interact with each other (dephase).

Remember that radio waves have to be the right frequency to excite the protons. This frequency is proportional to the strength of the magnetic field. Turning on the gradients slightly increase the magnetic field allowing for manipulation of the frequencies that will affect protons in different parts of space. The slice encode process determines the slice thickness (ST) per user specification. This is repeated until the desired dataset is acquired.

The final step is to convert the acquired frequencies to image space/domain. This is done by using the inverse fast fourier transform (IFFT), Fig. 4. This is a quick overview of generating an image which is necessary to understand in order to properly design an efficient fMRI experiment.

3. Image quality

A key aspect and development in this field is the image quality. MRI image quality is dependent on many factors, some of which are TE, TR, the number of signal averages (NA), and resolution. There are tradeoffs among all these factors. Increasing TE allows for more T2 weighting, but decreases the signal to noise ratio (SNR). A long TR allows for more slices to be acquired, while decreasing T1 contrast and increasing scanning time. Thus, to decrease the scanning time, TR can be decreased which allows for more T1 contrast, but the SNR is lowered and fewer slices can be acquired. SNR increases as NA is increased, but only by a factor of $\sqrt{NA}$. Scan time, in turn, is directly proportional to NA. Resolution is a function of the number of phase encode (PE) steps, the number of frequency encode (FE) steps (matrix size), field of view (FOV), and slice thickness (ST). Thinner slices reduce partial volume effects (PVE) and increase resolution, but SNR and anatomic coverage are reduced proportionally. In-plane resolution is increased as FE steps and/or PE steps are increased, but SNR decreases. Scan time increases with the number of PE steps. However, changing the FOV or increasing the number of FE steps does not affect scan time. The smaller the FOV, the higher the resolution and the smaller the voxel size [4].

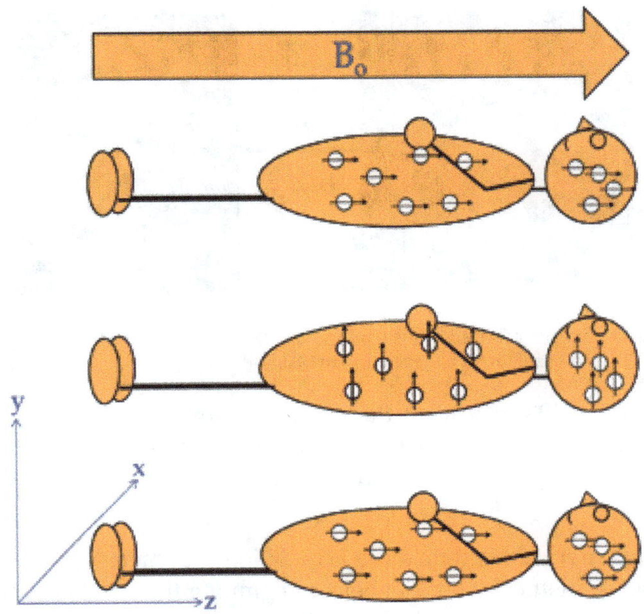

Figure 2. Illustration of the interaction between protons, the magnetic field and the RF pulse. In the magnet there is a magnetic field (B_o) 60,000 times stronger (for 3 Tesla) than the earth's magnetic field. When someone enters the bore of the magnet some of the hydrogen nuclei align with Bo causing a net magnetization (top). An RF pulse is sent at the same precessing frequency of the hydrogen nuclei. This tips the nuclei by 90°. (middle). The B_o field will force them to begin to realign, as this is happening the signal is being measured by the RF coil (bottom).

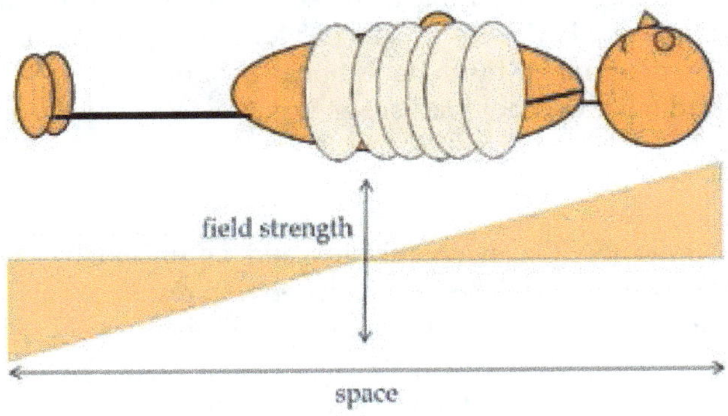

Figure 3. Using the gradient coils adds the ability to spatially encode the signals from previous process (see Fig. 2) by slightly modifying the magnetic field, thus a 2D/3D dataset in k-space can be mapped. The lower the magnetic field targets lower frequencies and higher field higher frequencies.

Note a common mistake is that displayed resolution is sometimes used interchangeably with nominal resolution. The nominal spatial resolution is the smallest tissue volume size that can be represented on an image. It is defined as the prescribed FOV in the frequency- and phase-encoding directions divided by the number of frequency- and phase-encoding points ($[\Delta x = FOV_x/N_x]$ and $[\Delta y = FOV_y/N_y]$), respectively [5]. For instance, on older scanner platforms this arises when a matrix of 96x96 is set. As a result the scanner automatically upsamples by zero padding the raw data to 128x128, and thus the displayed resolution

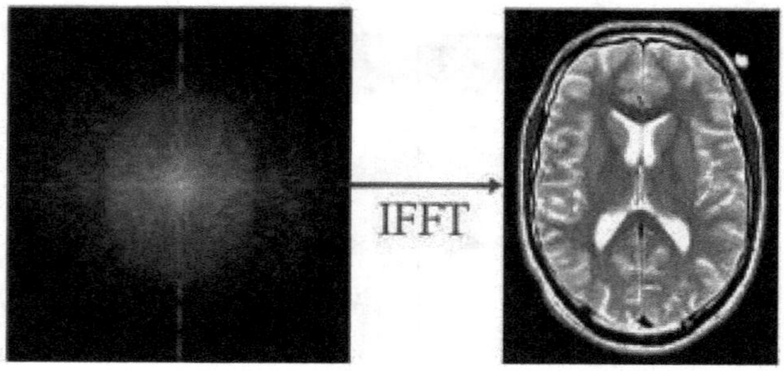

Figure 4. K-space data generated and collected by the gradients and RF coil is converted to the image domain via the inverse fast fourier transform (IFFT) as the final process to generating an MRI/fMRI image.

is $FOV_x/128$ and $FOV_y/128$ instead of the nominal (acquired) resolution of $FOV_x/96$ and $FOV_y/96$. This is because in the past these scanners interpolated anything that was not a factor of two from 64x64, e.g. 96x96 so the displayed resolution would not be the same as the nominal.

It is immediately apparent that from these acquisition parameters many things can either make for an efficient or inefficient dataset before beginning the fMRI task paradigm. In MRI, higher image resolution, i.e. smaller pixel/voxel sizes, is directly proportional to the magnet strength. Thus, going from 1.5 to 3 Tesla, the resolution can be doubled while using the same imaging parameters with the added advantage of shorter acquisition time. But with increase in resolution or signal there is also an increase in the noise. Note, for some applications (i.e. infant imaging) it may be advantageous to image at 1.5 Tesla.

In fMRI it is standard to achieve isotropic in plane resolution. For instance to attain a 3x3 pixel size then a matrix of 64x64 with a field of view (FOV) of 192mm can be set in the scanner. The voxel is determined by the additional parameter of slice thickness which is dependent on the third (slice encode) gradient as was previously alluded to, Fig. 5.

3.0.1. SNR

The signal to noise ratio (SNR) can be adjusted and optimized by choosing the proper imaging parameters. Note, there will be a tradeoff between resolution and SNR. For example if an increase from the 3x3x5 voxel resolution is desired then simply adjusting the matrix size to 128x128 while keeping all other parameters the same would yield a voxel of 1.5x1.5x5. Here the in plane resolution is doubled however the signal also suffers more noise. Similarly if a smaller slice thickness is chosen then SNR decreases and chances of partial volume effects increases. Next an explanation of the differences between MRI and fMRI is presented.

3.1. MRI vs fMRI

For both MRI and fMRI the process explained above applies. The difference is in the acquisition parameters and pulse sequences used. The most obvious difference is in the resolution, Fig. 6. MRI is denoted as the anatomical high resolution ($<$ 1 mm in-plane) image. In general this is one anatomical (T1) dataset with three spatial dimensions. Whereas fMRI is a set of low resolution (3 mm in plane) datasets with the addition of a time dimension, 4D. The difference in resolution is based on the imaging sequence used to acquire the data.

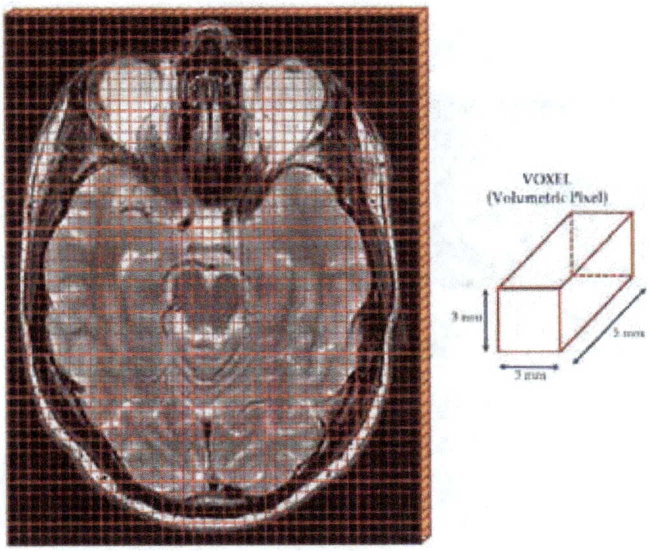

Figure 5. Image resolution is determined by the number of pixels in the x,y plane know as matrix size. This is dependent on how the gradients are phase and frequency encoded. In this case x=40, y=50. Assuming a field of view of 120 mm yields an in plane resolution of (120/40, 120/50) or (3, 2.4). Typically fMRI resolution at 3 Tesla is 3x3x5 with a FOV of 192 mm and matrix size of 64. The slice thickness is determined by a third gradient while performing the slice encoding phase.

In MRI about 5 minutes are used to scan the entire brain which allows for a very fine grid whereas in fMRI more than 100 volumes are acquired in the same amount of time. So, rather than 5 minutes to acquire one brain (MRI), only 2 seconds are allotted to acquire a brain (fMRI). When scanning for an anatomical image the participant simply lays in the scanner. But for an fMRI there is a specific task that needs to be repeated by the participant over the span of the 5 minutes. In doing so, the functional signal can be derived and analyzed. A description on preparing this task is given in Sections 5 and 6.

3.1.1. Artifacts

The main artifacts in fMRI are susceptibility due to structures such as the ear and nasal canals because of the air tissue interface. These artifacts cause a signal loss in the auditory and frontal regions respectively. If an experiment is interested in frontal lobe activation then the imaging parameters need to be optimized to minimize this. For a 3 Tesla system, being conservative and using 64x64 helps alleviate this.Other common artifacts are caused by retainers and braces which also cause a signal loss. This should be kept in mind when recruiting participants for a study. With a basic understanding of MR imaging an explanation of the origins of the functional signal can now follow.

4. BOLD

In the brain different regions are specialized to perform different sensory, motor and cognitive functions. Over the last two decades fMRI has been developed as a technique for mapping brain activation in these regions and has found widespread interest in basic and clinical research aimed at better understanding brain function. The fMRI technique is

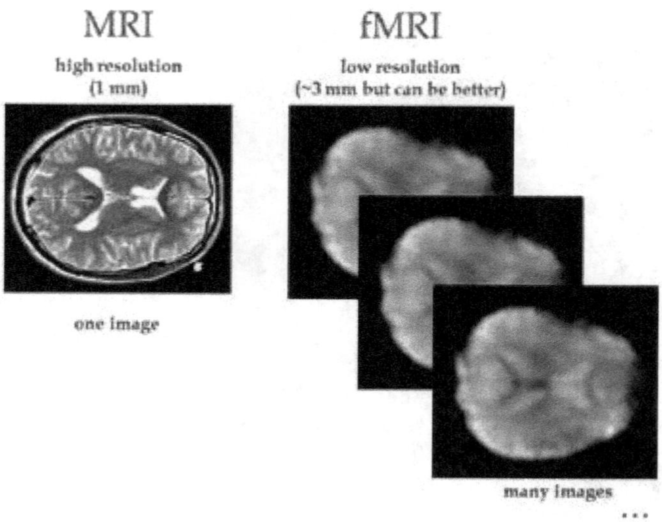

Figure 6. Illustrated is a visual comparison of the difference between MRI and fMRI. MRI is a set of high resolution slices that make up one 3D dataset while fMRI is a series of low resolution slices that make up many volumes, a 4D dataset (volumes + time). Note, images not to scale.

based on the detection of local perturbations of the deoxyhemoglobin concentration in the vicinity of neuronal activity. Neuronal activity at the synaptic level results in both an increase in oxygen consumption by the active cortex and an even greater increase of blood flow to the site. Because oxygen delivery exceeds oxygen utilization, the net effect is a local decrease in deoxyhemoglobin concentration near the activation site. The decrease in deoxyhemoglobin concentration at the site of neuronal activity causes a local increase the magnetic resonance signal, Fig. 7. This effect has been termed the Blood Oxygenation Level Dependent (BOLD) contrast mechanism [6]. This is possible because of the magnetic properties of hemoglobin which contains four Fe2+ ions. Specifically, deoxygenated blood is paramagnetic, meaning it has a small additive intrinsic magnetic field and oxygenated blood is diamagnetic meaning it tends to oppose external magnetic field. The ratio of deoxygenated to oxygenated blood changes when a particular task is performed as a result of the neurons firing which cause an increase in both blood flow into the neurons and oxygen consumption level to increase in that particular region of the brain. However, the blood flow increase is larger than proportional oxygen consumption. The result of this brief stimulus and in turn neural activation is the hemodynamic response function (HRF). The HRF has a characteristic shape with an initial dip immediately following the stimulus then an increase and finally an undershoot but can vary between participants [7]. Understanding the behavior of the HRF can help in designing an efficient fMRI paradigm. In summary BOLD fMRI capitalizes on the difference between two conditions; an active condition in which stimulus related neural activity is generated and a passive condition in which stimulus related neural activity is absent or kept to a minimum, Fig. 8.

5. Paradigms

There are several types of fMRI design paradigms: block, event-related (widely spaced and rapid) and mixed (block and event related). The development of the event related studies

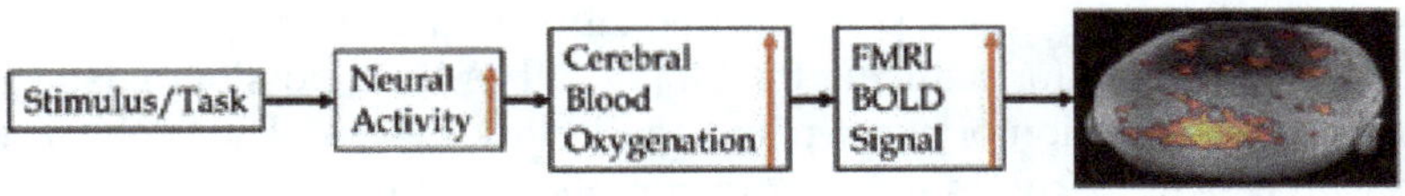

Figure 7. A simplified flow of events that lead to the BOLD fMRI signal. A specific stimulus/task causes an increase in neural activity which triggers a complex chain of changes to cause an increase in cerebral blood oxygenation. This complex series of events includes an increase in cerebral blood flow (CBF), an increase in cerebral metabolic rate for oxygen which in turn causes the cerebral blood volume (CBV) to increase. These events cause a decrease the local deoxyhemoglobin (HHb) content. This then allows for the detection of the signal which after post processing can be overlaid on an anatomical MRI.

[8–19] came several years after the advent of BOLD fMRI. Choosing the proper TR, TE FOV and matrix size values are all important and are dependent on the problem or question that is being investigated as will be discussed in section 6, but of equal importance is the type of of paradigm used. This in fact is intertwined with the imaging parameters. The importance of choosing a suitable TR to and interstimulus interval (ISI) ratio has been known early on, namely because BOLD is not necessarily steady-state rather transient signal [20]. For block designs, this is fairly straight forward. If using an event related paradigm then caution should be taken in choosing the proper TR. Software such as optseq (http://surfer.nmr.mgh.harvard.edu/optseq/) allows for a good randomization of stimuli for rapid event related designs based on specific imaging parameter. This ensures a robust randomized design.

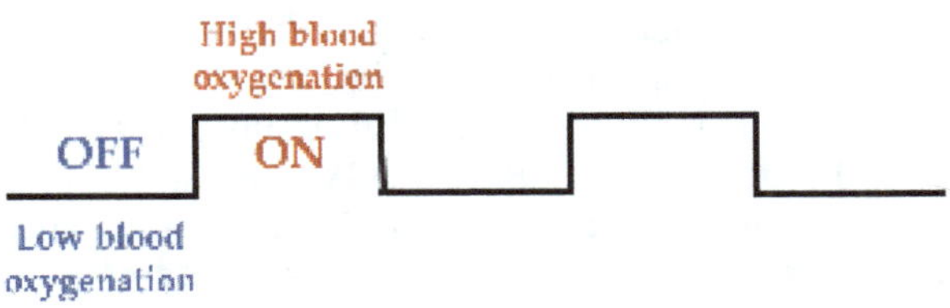

Figure 8. A typical block design should consist of two states, OFF (no task) and ON (task). The ratio of blood oxygenation is measured to determine the pixel with the fMRI BOLD signal change.

Block designs commonly consist of two states, Fig. 8, A (rest) and B (task), however in some situations where time or a factor like budget is an issue and a third or even a fourth state is added. Having four states complicates the design and strategies should be taken to design efficiently. The minimum block time and ISI can be around 20 seconds with an absolute minimum of 6 seconds and the maximum at 60 seconds. In two states the conditions would alternate a suggested minimum of three times, e.g. ABABABA. It is good practice to always end on a rest state. For three conditions there are several combinations for presentation, e.g. CACBCACBC; CABABABAC; CABCABCABC where C can be the rest condition and A and B are task 1 and task 2 respectively. The disadavantage of this paradigm is that the participant may start to predict or anticipate the task. In contrast event related can be more easily randomized because of the small stimulus duration. But how long should the stimulus last? Several groups have noted different durations that can still be detected by fMRI such as 2 seconds [21], 0.5 seconds [22] and 34 milliseconds [23]. This temporal resolution is a clear advantage in event related over block designs, however there is a tradeoff of SNR in the fMRI signal. It has been shown that going from a block to a widely spaced event related design decreases the SNR by approximately 33% [24] and about 17% [25] from a widely spaced to a rapid event related pardigm. In general block designs have larger BOLD signal change

[26, 27] and better statistical power [28]. An optimal ISI for a fixed stimulus duration of less than 2 seconds is about 12 seconds [24]. Additionally by randomizing the ISI the statistical power increases and allows for reducing the ISI [24, 29]. A third possibility is using a mixed design which is a combination of event-related and block design. The problem with this is the statistical processing becomes even more complicated and if not fully understood can lead to errors in data processing, analysis and interpretation. It is best to keep the paradigm as simple as possible. Note, for clinical use the majority if not all the fMRI scans will be block however this may change quickly as the experimental design aspects of fMRI continue to advance. Similar to choosing the imaging parameters, determining which paradigm to use will depend on the goal of the experiment.

6. Preparing an experiment

With the basics of MR physics and fMRI paradigms presented a more informed decision can be made on the experiment. In begining the journey into an fMRI experiment some basic questions need to be asked. Why are we doing this experiment, is generally our hypothesis. What are we looking for? For example, a specific behavior we are interested in. Where? This involves knowing the neuroanatomy. How? This is the type of fMRI design. The best way to explain this is to walk through an example. Why? We hypothesize that eye movements will cause activation. What? Moving the eyes. Where? In the cortex. How? Tell participant to move eyes. Initially this may look like a good set of answers but they are not. What is wrong with them? They are too general and leave room error, confounds, and reproducibility will be difficult as nothing was mentioned about the paradigm or scanning protocol. Several groups can follow the same logic and come up with different activation maps even if the scanning protocol was mentioned. For instance, full brain coverage axial scan with TR=3 seconds, TE=35ms, $\phi = 90^o$, matrix size=128x128, FOV=256mm ST=8mm. This would yield a voxel resolution of 2x2x8mm, SNR=75%, and allow for about 45 slices to be acquired. If full brain coverage was necessary then these parameters would be good, however from the vague answers this can not be determined. Also, note scanning time is still missing and no mention of the number of volumes to be acquired.

Let us now try to reword the answers to come up with a better starting point. Why? We hypothesize that eye movements will activate the visual cortex. What? Specifically moving the eyes to from left to right in a saccadic fashion. Where? Want to see activation differences between V1 and V2 in visual cortex. How? Will have a block paradigm of 30 seconds fixation followed by 30 seconds of guided saccadic eye movements. A backprojection system will be used to display the visual stimulus that will cue the participant to fixate on a white dot in the center of the screen. The dot will then automatically proceed to alternate back and forth between the center and the left side of the screen, note this is flipped because participant is looking through a mirror. A common mistake made by novice users. In regards to any stimulus that involves the visual cortex, it is good practice to either turn the lights off or keep on for all participants. Again, the number of variables and confounds should be at a minimum. It is always recommended to test the paradigm in the scanner before recruiting participants in order to debug and pick out issues like this. For statistical power want to repeat this on-off cycle six times. Using the same imaging protocol just mentioned allows for 120 volumes to be acquired in 6 minutes and 21 seconds. The 21 seconds are used for dummy scans to allow the scanner to warm up. For a particular participant whole brain coverage may only require 20 slices thus total slices acquired would be 120*20=2400. By providing a more informed set of answers and paradigm the study can be changed from an inefficient fishing expedition to an efficient specific study. Is this the most optimized design? Probably not but it is a better starting point. Since the interest is in the known regions of the visual cortex then whole brain coverage may not be necessary. That can buy more time, SNR, statistical power and/or image resolution.

Answering the questions differently will affect the way we want to scan the brain. If the following questions are asked then options from Fig. 9 will change. What brain areas are active during visual imagery? This is a very general question and may require an axial full brain coverage scan. Is the primary visual cortex (area 17) active during visual imagery? This is more specfic and allows for a more localized scan in the visual cortex. What areas of the brain are active during working memory? Again, this is very general. Is the prefrontal cortex active during working memory? Here the frontal cortex is targeted hence no need to scan the visual cortex.

The conventional scanning plane has been the axial however there is no rule against scanning in other planes or at an oblique angle. In fact, there are situations where going away from convention is advantageous. Depending on the answers given to the list of questions a very specific orientation and slices desired can be determined.

For example in Fig.9 it can be seen that it may not be necessary or the most efficient use of time and resolution to choose the axial or coronal planes even for visual cortex activation. The oblique plane scan at the visual cortex may be the best choice. Also if the other scans were chosen it would not have been necessary to acquire slices from the entire brain rather enough to cover the visual cortex. This saves acquisition time which can be invested in acquiring more volumes and increasing the resolution. A priori knowledge of the problem to be studied can go a long way in optimizing the fMRI experiment. Indeed it is advantageous to do full brain coverage if that is what the problem entails however it is not a good idea to go on a fishing expedition for activation sites. These are some aspects of several questions to ask before preparing an experiment. If thought out thoroughly they would minimize errors and confounding variables and in turn optimize the fMRI design and experience.

7. Collecting data

Once the questions to the problem are answered, the parameters are entered into the console of the MR scanner. This will then give the time required, number of slices, number of volumes, etc. to be acquired based on the matrix size, resolution and FOV chosen. It is recommended that the participant is made familiar with the task outside the scanner to minimize confusion and error. After entering the scanner the anatomical high resolution MR images are acquired followed by the fMRI scan. The latter is where the participant is instructed to simulataneously perform a task. This process can take an average of an hour. It is not recommended to go over this time too much mainly because of the attention and fatigue factor on the participant's end. If prepared and thought out properly the hour should be sufficient to collect the MRI and two or three fMRI sessions. At the end of the scanning session the images can be copied onto a DVD in DICOM (http://medical.nema.org/) format and taken to a local workstation for analysis. In the case of strictly clinical fMRI, for example, presurgical planning support, the scanners have a built in analysis tool that can output the results of activation on the console itself and these results can be pushed onto a PACS system. In this case the paradigm timing and design need to be entered into the console before the scanning begins. For research purposes using the built in system is not recommended. One reason being that the console can only process a single participant meaning no group analysis

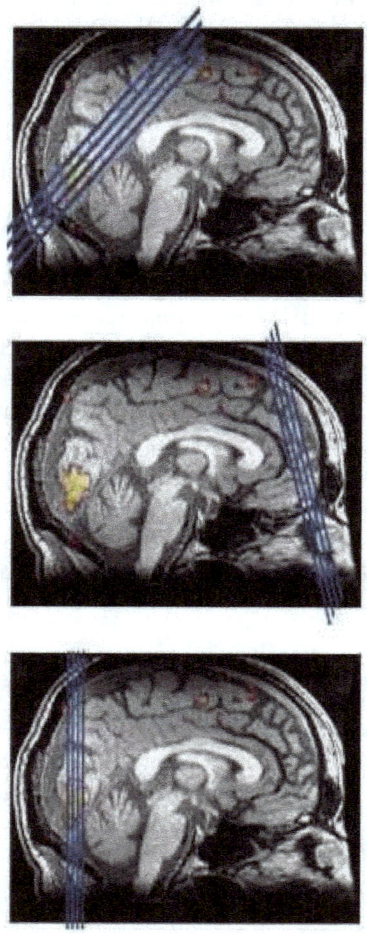

Figure 9. Illustration of four possible orientations overlaid on top fMRI results from an oculomotor paradigm coregistered withan anatomical MRI. In this case, all orientations except the third from top (oblique orientation at frontal cortex) would havecaptured the visual cortex activation.

can be performed. To date vendors have not added the option to do group analysis. This could be because the main users are clinicians whose priamry focus is treat one patient at a time. Section 8.2 lists possible software packages that can be used instead. For clinicians, it is also suggested that they use these packages for a more robust analysis especially for case studies and for confirming the results in situations of more critical care such as surgical resections.

8. Preparing data

After fMRI data is acquired, motion correction and filtering may be required. Each slice has to be aligned with the next within the volume and then registration is performed between volumes using the first as the fixed (stationary). From the saccadic eye movement example this means 19 slices need to be aligned to the first. The 2D slice alignment is repeated for all 120 volumes independently. Afterwards the slice aligned volumes are registered to each other in 3D. So 119 volumes are registered to this first (fixed volume). This is repeated for each participant dataset. For group comparisons the processed 4D datasets then have to be registered to a common space.

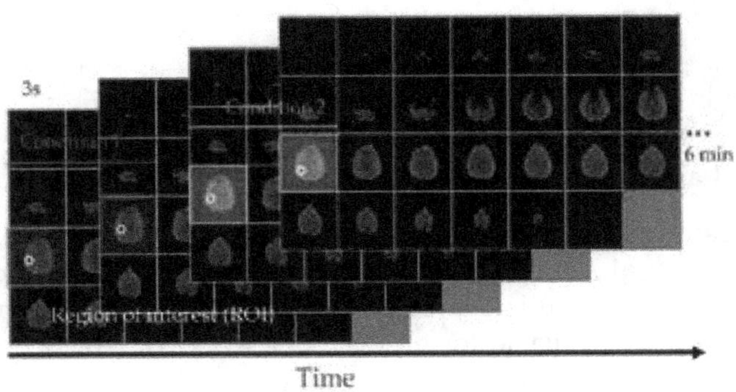

Figure 10. The signal intensity of a spatial region of interest (ROI) or a voxel can be traced over time, in this case every 3 secs for 6 minutes between two conditions. This intensity is fitted to the ON-OFF paradigm design (see Fig. 8) by using a general linear model regression analysis to determine if there is significant activation.

8.1. Statistics

Once all the data sets are aligned, time courses can be plotted for each voxel, Fig. 10. In the case of a block paradigm during condition 1 (fixation), it is expected that signal is low from a particular pixel and high for condition 2 (visually guided saccades). Regression analysis is performed on the voxels and the ones that follow this trend or fit the boxcar (from Fig. 8) can be identified as significantly activated regions of the brain responsible for the associated task or stimulus chosen. The statistics get more complicated for event related designs. If each block last 30 seconds with TR=3 seconds that means the intensity of one voxel from each volume will give result in a time series of 120 points with time as the x-axis and fMRI signal as the y-axis, again with a total time of 6 minutes (3*120=360 seconds). The mean and standard deviations for the duration between the two conditions is then calculated Fig. 11. The voxels that significantly follow this trend are then denoted by an orange color map and overlaid onto the original fMRI dataset. Depending on the resolution of the dataset this can be performed on more than 100,000 voxels, 128x128x20 = 327,680 voxels from the above example. Because of this number many voxels will be activated by chance (for $P<0.01$, 0.01*327,680 = 3,276) so bonferroni corrections are used. Rather than use $P<0.01$, $P<0.0000001$ is used (0.01/100,000 = 0.0000001). An alternative analysis that is commonly used is cluster grouping rather than individual voxels. In this way if a neighborhood of voxels are all following the paradigm then the chances of random activation can be eliminated.

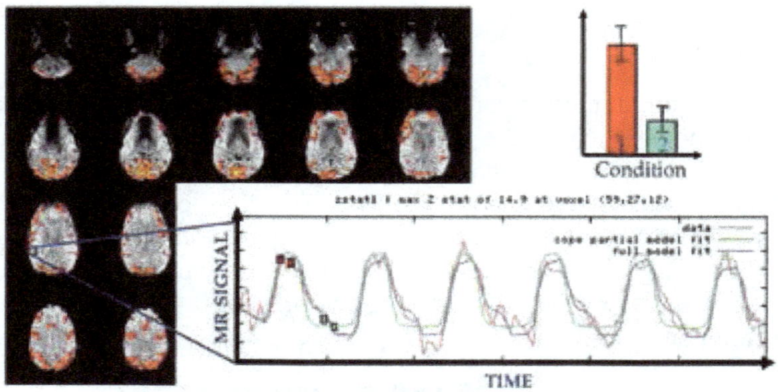

Figure 11. The orange pixels are the significant activation results of the general linear model (GLM) overlaid on top of the fMRIs. Looking at the ROI the raw signal is found to fit the model well for the two conditions.

8.2. Software packages

There are several software packages available for fMRI analysis. FSL (http://www.fmrib.ox.ac.uk/fsl/), AFNI (afni.nimh.nih.gov/afni), and SPM are all free with the exception that the latter requires a Matlab (http://www.mathworks.com/) license. FSL and SPM are available for all operating systems. AFNI is not available for Windows. More groups seem to be using a combination of these packages. For instance, using FSL for pre processing and SPM for post processing while others like to use AFNI for evaluating the susceptibility effects on the data to test efficacy of scanning protocol before beginning the experiment. The packages are all good in their own way and it comes down to user preference.

9. Pitfalls and limitations

Throughout the entire process of an fMRI experiment we need to be aware of our limitations. Are we using a 1.5, 3, or 7 Tesla magnet? The same exact design and protocol can be run on all three magnet strengths and give different results. All of these have their individual pearls and pitfalls and we should be able to identify them. The stimulus can easily be confounded if not designed efficiently. If interested in visual perception and using a visual stimulus then care needs to be taken to ensure that the lighting in the room, the stimulus size, contrast, duration, spatial and temporal frequency and distance to the participant stays fixed. If eye movements are of primary concern then investing in an MR compatible eye tracker would be necessary in order to confirm that indeed the participants are performing the task. In addition fMRI is susceptible to motion thus the head has to be held still and padding used. If motion is present then post processing algorithms can be utilized to correct them however only if they are minor. Otherwise the data will not be useful. It is crucial that the participants understand all the instructions. In an eye movement study, using the same visual stimulus but changing the instruction slightly found that significantly different regions were activated and recorded [30]. Participant comfort is a factor; if they are in pain then that will reflect on the results. At the same time if they are too comfortable then they will fall asleep. In designing the task paradigm things to consider are the timings, e.g. 15 vs 30 seconds. The latter may be to taxing on the eyes. It may advantageous to use a two state block design over a three state to alleviate participant confusion and simplfying the statistical analysis process. Reducing the time to 15 seconds and using only two states allow for more cycles to be repeated and give more power for statistical averaging. Alternatively, 15 seconds can be used to add a third state yet keep the total scan time of 6 minutes and introducing pseudo randomized cycles, however that would increase the complexity. Other limitations include both anatomical and physiological components. The size and location of the neuroanatomical site can limit what can be derived also the vascular response time may vary from approximately 2 ms to 6 s. The time of day certainly makes a difference on the fMRI signal so this should be kept in mind. Also, the amount of familiarity the participant has with the task will affect the intensity of the signal. Switching coils, or scanners in a middle of a study will definitely confound the data. This is of a bigger issue for multicenter trials, even if the same MR vendor is being used. All these factors can be minimized before the study begins and the data is collected.

After the data is collected, other issues arise. What is the minimum signficance level that will be accepted, p=0.05 vs p=0.01? What about gaussian smoothing the data, none, 5mm, 10mm? This depends on the SNR of the dataset. By smoothing the data activation clusters will spread and localization limited. Also, more regions will be activated. If fMRI voxel resolution is 2x2x2 mm and a smoothing kernel of 10mm is used then that decreased the resolution by a factor of five (10x10x10 mm). That in way defeats the purpose of sacrificing other parameters to achieve the $2mm^3$ voxel size. The degrees of freedom in the registration process need to be understood as well. Simply choosing 3, 6, 7 or 12 can cause alignment errors and erroneous activation maps. This becomes a bigger issue if partial brain images were acquired for fMRI and now they are trying to be aligned with a whole brain high resolution MRI. Eventhough the software packages above have built in tools for these steps the user has to be cognizant of the potential pitfalls. Remember there is to magic button to push and everything will come out perfect. The registration algorithms vary and the types of interpolation will introduce more blurring on top of the gaussian smoothing chosen. Many users think that because the fMRI activation maps are overlaid ontop of a high resolution anatomical MRI, that they have the same accuracy and resolution and do not appreciate the amount of approximations involved in the process. Overall an fMRI study needs much thought. There are many variables and confounds involved in setting up an fMRI design and this section touched on the importance of being aware of the limitations and keeping these variables as constant as possible when clinical, longitudinal or group studies are performed.

10. Conclusion

In designing an fMRI experiment there has to be a realization of the fact that there is no real (one) gold standard or solution. So rather than asking what is the solution? We should be asking, what can we control? Here are some concluding tips in answering this question. Before beginning anything we need to fully understand the experimental goals. Inevitably tweaking the fMRI imaging parameters need to performed. As a result the paradigm will also be adjusted accordingly, especially in the case of event related designs. Here are some design questions to answer: Design type? Blocked, Event-Related, Mixed? How many subjects? How much data to collect for each subject? How many stimulus conditions? How many repetitions for each condition? When should each stimulus be presented? TR? Number of slices? Getting in the habit of asking many questions before starting a study is key. Overall, the best solution is experience.

Author details

Nasser H Kashou

The Children's Radiological Institute, Nationwide Children's Hospital, USA

References

[1] Robert L Savoy. Experimental design in brain activation mri: cautionary tales. *Brain Res Bull*, 67(5):361–367, Nov 2005.

[2] Edson Amaro and Gareth J Barker. Study design in fmri: basic principles. *Brain Cogn*, 60(3):220–232, Apr 2006.

[3] R. L. Savoy. History and future directions of human brain mapping and functional neuroimaging. *Acta Psychol (Amst)*, 107(1-3):9–42, Apr 2001.

[4] V. D. KÃűchli D. Weishaupt and B. Marincek. *How Does MRI Work? An Introduction to the Physics and Function of Magnetic Resonance Imaging*. Springer, 2006.

[5] G. S. Slavin. Spatial and temporal resolution in cardiovascular mr imaging: Review and recommendations. *Radiology*, 234:330–338, 2005.

[6] S. Ogawa, T. M. Lee, A. R. Kay, and D. W. Tank. Brain magnetic resonance imaging with contrast dependent on blood oxygenation. *Proc Natl Acad Sci U S A*, 87(24):9868–9872, Dec 1990.

[7] G. K. Aguirre, E. Zarahn, and M. D'esposito. The variability of human, bold hemodynamic responses. *Neuroimage*, 8(4):360–369, Nov 1998.

[8] R. L. Buckner, P. A. Bandettini, K. M. O'Craven, R. L. Savoy, S. E. Petersen, M. E. Raichle, and B. R. Rosen. Detection of cortical activation during averaged single trials of a cognitive task using functional magnetic resonance imaging. *Proc Natl Acad Sci U S A*, 93(25):14878–14883, Dec 1996.

[9] R. L. Buckner, J. Goodman, M. Burock, M. Rotte, W. Koutstaal, D. Schacter, B. Rosen, and A. M. Dale. Functional-anatomic correlates of object priming in humans revealed by rapid presentation event-related fmri. *Neuron*, 20(2):285–296, Feb 1998.

[10] M. A. Burock, R. L. Buckner, M. G. Woldorff, B. R. Rosen, and A. M. Dale. Randomized event-related experimental designs allow for extremely rapid presentation rates using functional mri. *Neuroreport*, 9(16):3735–3739, Nov 1998.

[11] V. P. Clark, J. M. Maisog, and J. V. Haxby. fmri study of face perception and memory using random stimulus sequences. *J Neurophysiol*, 79(6):3257–3265, Jun 1998.

[12] A. M. Dale and R. L. Buckner. Selective averaging of rapidly presented individual trials using fmri. *Hum Brain Mapp*, 5(5):329–340, 1997.

[13] M. D'Esposito, E. Zarahn, and G. K. Aguirre. Event-related functional mri: implications for cognitive psychology. *Psychol Bull*, 125(1):155–164, Jan 1999.

[14] K. J. Friston, P. Fletcher, O. Josephs, A. Holmes, M. D. Rugg, and R. Turner. Event-related fmri: characterizing differential responses. *Neuroimage*, 7(1):30–40, Jan 1998.

[15] O. Josephs, R. Turner, and K. Friston. Event-related f mri. *Hum Brain Mapp*, 5(4):243–248, 1997.

[16] B. R. Rosen, R. L. Buckner, and A. M. Dale. Event-related functional mri: past, present, and future. *Proc Natl Acad Sci U S A*, 95(3):773–780, Feb 1998.

[17] A. D. Wagner, D. L. Schacter, M. Rotte, W. Koutstaal, A. Maril, A. M. Dale, B. R. Rosen, and R. L. Buckner. Building memories: remembering and forgetting of verbal experiences as predicted by brain activity. *Science*, 281(5380):1188–1191, Aug 1998.

[18] E. Wiener, L. R. Schad, K. T. Baudendistel, M. Essig, E. MÃijller, and W. J. Lorenz. Functional mr imaging of visual and motor cortex stimulation at high temporal resolution using a flash technique on a standard 1.5 tesla scanner. *Magn Reson Imaging*, 14(5):477–483, 1996.

[19] E. Zarahn, G. Aguirre, and M. D'Esposito. A trial-based experimental design for fmri. *Neuroimage*, 6(2):122–138, Aug 1997.

[20] C. J. Price, D. J. Veltman, J. Ashburner, O. Josephs, and K. J. Friston. The critical relationship between the timing of stimulus presentation and data acquisition in blocked designs with fmri. *Neuroimage*, 10(1):36–44, Jul 1999.

[21] A. M. Blamire, S. Ogawa, K. Ugurbil, D. Rothman, G. McCarthy, J. M. Ellermann, F. Hyder, Z. Rattner, and R. G. Shulman. Dynamic mapping of the human visual cortex by high-speed magnetic resonance imaging. *Proc Natl Acad Sci U S A*, 89(22):11069–11073, Nov 1992.

[22] P. A. Bandettini, A. Jesmanowicz, E. C. Wong, and J. S. Hyde. Processing strategies for time-course data sets in functional mri of the human brain. *Magn Reson Med*, 30(2):161–173, Aug 1993.

[23] R. L. Savoy, P. A. Bandettini, K. M. OâĂŹCraven, K. K. Kwong, T. L. Davis, J. R. Baker, R. M. Weisskoff, and B. R. Rosen. Pushing the temporal resolution of fmri: Studies of very brief visual stimuli, onset variability and asynchrony, and stimulus correlated changes in noise. In *Proc. Soc. Magn. Reson. Med. Third Sci. Meeting Exhib.*, volume 2, page 450, 1995.

[24] P. A. Bandettini and R. W. Cox. Event-related fmri contrast when using constant interstimulus interval: theory and experiment. *Magn Reson Med*, 43(4):540–548, Apr 2000.

[25] F. M. Miezin, L. Maccotta, J. M. Ollinger, S. E. Petersen, and R. L. Buckner. Characterizing the hemodynamic response: effects of presentation rate, sampling procedure, and the possibility of ordering brain activity based on relative timing. *Neuroimage*, 11(6 Pt 1):735–759, Jun 2000.

[26] G. H. Glover. Deconvolution of impulse response in event-related bold fmri. *Neuroimage*, 9(4):416–429, Apr 1999.

[27] R. B. Buxton, E. C. Wong, and L. R. Frank. Dynamics of blood flow and oxygenation changes during brain activation: the balloon model. *Magn Reson Med*, 39(6):855–864, Jun 1998.

[28] K. J. Friston, A. P. Holmes, C. J. Price, C. BÃijchel, and K. J. Worsley. Multisubject fmri studies and conjunction analyses. *Neuroimage*, 10(4):385–396, Oct 1999.

[29] A. M. Dale. Optimal experimental design for event-related fmri. *Hum Brain Mapp*, 8(2-3):109–114, 1999.

[30] Nasser H Kashou, Lawrence E Leguire, Cynthia J Roberts, Nick Fogt, Mark A Smith, and Gary L Rogers. Instruction dependent activation during optokinetic nystagmus (okn) stimulation: An fmri study at 3t. *Brain Res*, 1336:10–21, Jun 2010.

6

A Probabilistic Atlas of Human Visual Areas and Information-Theoretic Analysis of Individual Variability in their Loci

Hiroki Yamamoto

1. Introduction

The human visual cortex consists of multiple functionally distinct visual areas that have been individually localized on the cortical surface by brain imaging of their associated retinotopic activity. Thus, their locations can be quantitatively compared across individuals once they are expressed in a common coordinate space. In several studies (Dougherty et al. 2003, Fischl et al. 1999b, Hasnain et al. 1998), such comparisons have been performed using the Talairach stereotactic coordinate system (Talairach et al. 1967, Talairach & Tournoux 1988) as the common anatomical space. Because the Talairach system has been commonly used as a standard to describe the loci of brain activation or lesions, and to normalize the functional data between individual brains, evaluation of the interindividual variability within the Talairach space is essential for reliably interpreting a broad range of brain function data.

The Talairach system considers interindividual variations in overall brain size and shape but not the variations of smaller scale structures, such as the cortical sulci and gyri, which differ substantially and heterogeneously between individuals (Ono et al. 1990). Consequently, interindividual variability within the Talairach space is not only extensive, but also complex in morphology. Analysis of this variability is therefore not straightforward and requires conceptual and practical simplification.

Recently, we have proposed that inconsistency and uncertainty are fundamental concepts characterizing the interindividual variability within the visual areas (Yamamoto et al. 2011). This inconsistency refers to the disparity between the individuals regarding the location of a particular visual area. The inconsistency in the Talairach space has been assessed in several studies by calculating the variance of the position of a representative point within a visual area

(Dougherty et al. 2003, Hasnain et al. 1998) or by constructing a probabilistic map in which each point is associated with a probability that the visual area resides there (Amunts et al. 2000, Fischl et al. 1999b). Although the inconsistency provides a good basis for analyzing a single, isolated area, it is inherently insufficient for regulating multiple visual areas with pairwise adjacency. When transforming multiple areas together into Talairach space, their adjacency causes overlaps between the neighboring areas of different individuals. Therefore, in evaluating the interindividual variability in multiple visual areas, we must address another variable, uncertainty.

This uncertainty relates to the difficulty of knowing which visual areas reside at a given position where the greater the number of overlaps between the different areas, the greater the degree of uncertainty. We should emphasize that uncertainty is conceptually dissociated from inconsistency. Even if there is no area that has a high probability of being present at an anatomical point, the uncertainty at the point is zero if only a single area has a non-zero probability of being present. Conversely, even if an area has a high probability of being present, the uncertainty is large if other areas also have a high probability of being present. When brain activation is observed at a region described as having a high probability but also has a high uncertainty area, we cannot confidently attribute this region to a specific anatomical and functional area. In addition, when the individual brain activations are pooled in Talairach space, caution is warranted regarding the source of activation at such points because the activations of different areas are probably highly confounded. These considerations suggest that quantification of the uncertainty is crucial for reliable interpretation of the functional data in Talairach space. However, this issue has not been investigated.

In the present study, we applied a probabilistic and information theoretical framework to quantify the uncertainty and the inconsistency of multiple human visual areas that were localized based on functional MRI (fMRI) retinotopy measurements. Inconsistency was estimated by generating a probability map based on 10 hemispheres of five subjects, where each point was associated with a probability that it belonged to each retinotopic area. We used the Shannon entropy (Shannon 1948) as an uncertainty measure and generated a novel map we called an entropy map, where each point is associated with a Shannon entropy computed from the probability that the point belongs to each of the visual areas (Eq. (1) in the section 2.3). Generally, the Shannon entropy serves as a useful measure to quantify the uncertainty of a situation (Cencov 1982). In our study, the relevance is when one wants to predict or judge a visual area at a given Talairach point in clinical practice or scientific research, where higher entropy equates to a higher probability of incorrect classification. Using the probability and entropy maps, we analyzed the inconsistency and uncertainty of the locations of retinotopic areas registered in Talairach space.

Although Talairach registration was originally described as piecewise linear transformations, there are a number of methods used, where these include two main types; namely volume-based methods using linear, piecewise-linear, or nonlinear transformations and surface-based methods, allowing for a more precise alignment of the sulcal and gyral patterns (see Gholipour et al. 2007 for a recent comprehensive review). The choice of the transformation method is an important consideration that influences the results of our analysis. In our recent study

(Yamamoto et al. 2011), we employed a sophisticated surface-based method (Fischl et al. 1999b). In the present study, we used a single linear transformation (nine parameters, three each for translation, rotation, and orthogonal scaling) for the entire brain (Desmond & Lim 1997). Many more sophisticated, methods such as nonlinear volume methods (Ashburner 2007, Woods et al. 1998) and surface-based methods (Drury et al. 1996, Fischl et al. 1999b, Thompson et al. 1997) subsume and therefore outperform this method. Thus, the probability and entropy maps created using a single linear transformation can provide a baseline for the evaluation of the inconsistency and uncertainty in Talairach space. Understanding the limits of the transformation is important for performing reliable group analysis and interpreting the published Talairach coordinates of the activation foci because the linear transformation is still commonly used in both basic and clinical neuroscience.

2. Methods

2.1. Imaging

We studied ten hemispheres from five normal subjects (one female, four males; mean 33 years). The subjects were in good health with no past history of psychiatric or neurological disease. The study protocols were approved by the ethical committees of our institutions. All subjects provided written, informed consent prior to study enrollment. The structural and functional MRI measurements were performed using a standard clinical 1.5 Tesla scanner (GE, Signa NV/i). Prior to the experimental scans, high-contrast T1-weighted three-dimensional (3D) SPGR structural images (echo time (TE) = 3.0 ms, repetition time (TR) = 56 ms, flip angle (FA) = 55°; excitations (NEX) = 1, voxel size (VS) = 0.781 × 0.781 × 1.4 or 0.938 × 0.938 × 1.4 mm) of the whole brain were recorded for each subject, which was used for reconstructing the individual brain surface. For each subject, three types of images were obtained on each scan day, with a standard flexible surface coil placed at the occipital pole. First, T1-weighted Inversion Recovery 3D Fast SPGR structural images (TE = 2.7 ms, TR = 6.0 ms, inversion time (TI) = 600 ms, FA = 15°; NEX = 1, VS = 0.781 × 0.781 × 1.4 mm) were acquired for anatomical registration. Second, a set of 16 (three subjects) or 17 (two subjects) adjacent high-resolution T1-weighted spin echo anatomical slices (TE = 9 ms, TR = 420 ms, NEX = 2, VS = 0.781 × 0.781 × 4 mm) was obtained. Finally, multiple functional scans (6 – 8) were obtained in the same slice positions as the anatomical slices while the subject viewed visual stimuli (e.g., a flickering checkerboard ring), using a T2*-weighted two-dimensional gradient echo, echo planar imaging (TE = 50 ms, TR = 2000 ms, FA = 90°, VS = 1.563 × 1.563 × 4 mm).

2.2. Localization of retinotopic areas

After reconstructing each individual's cortical surface, locations of the retinotopic visual areas were identified with fMRI and standard retinotopic mapping procedures (Table 1). The surface was reconstructed to lie approximately in the middle of the gray matter, using a method that was a hybrid of volume segmentation (Drury et al. 1999) and surface deformation (Dale & Sereno 1993). We used mrGray software (Teo et al. 1997) for volume segmentation and a custom software for surface generation. The software generated an initial surface at the border of the white and gray matter using a marching cube algorithm (Lorensen & Cline 1987) and then deformed it to lie in the middle of the gray matter using the deformable template algorithm (Dale & Sereno 1993).

Technique	Method	Software
Cortical surface reconstruction	Step 1. Anatomical volume segmentation (cerebrospinal fluid, gray matter, white matter)	mrGray (Teo et al., 1997)
	Step 2. Triangular tessellation with the marching cube algorithm (Lorensen & Clein, 1987)	in-house software called BrainFactory (Yamamoto et al., 2002, 2008, 2011) written in C++ & Tcl/Tk using Visualization Toolkit (Kitware inc.)
	Step 3. Deformation of the tessellated surface with the deformable template algorithm (Dale & Sereno, 1993)	BrainFactory
Localization of retinotopic areas	Phase-encoding mapping with fMRI (Engel et al., 1994) Visual stimuli: a rotating wedge for visual field angular mapping and a expanding (fovea-16 deg eccentricity) annulus for eccentricity mapping, 60s /rotation(expansion) × 6 cycles Parcellation of visual areas: visual inspection of the retinotopy and the visual filed sign maps (Sereno et al., 1995)	BrainFactory
Brain registration	A linear rigid volume-based method (Desmond & Lim, 1997) Parameters: 9 parameters (3 scalings, 3 rotations, 3 translations) determined by visual inspection of anatomical landmarks Target brain:10 hemispheres from 5 subjects	BrainFactory

Table 1. Summary of key techniques

The surface regions delimiting areas V1d, V2d, V3d, V3B, V3A, V7, LOc, MT+, V1v, V2v, V3v, V4v, and V8 were determined by phase-encoded retinotopic mapping methods (DeYoe et al. 1994, Engel et al. 1997, Sereno et al. 1995), allowing visualization of the polar angle (Fig. 1A, upper panel) and eccentricity (Fig. 1A, lower panel) components of the retinotopic map. The retinotopic map was constructed using a phase-encoding technique where the receptive field centers were temporally coded using polar coordinates (Engel et al. 1994). The polar angle component of the map was measured by performing the fMRI while the subject viewed a wedge-shaped checkered pattern (24° center angle) that rotated counter-clockwise around the fixation point, making one rotation in 60 s. The eccentricity component was measured while the subject viewed a checkered annulus (2° width) that expanded from the fovea to 16° peripherally over 50 s and then disappeared for 10 s. Each stimulus underwent color (black/white, red/green, or blue/yellow) pattern reversal (1 Hz) and was presented in six cycles, evoking a periodic response at a given point on the retinotopy map, where the corresponding position in the visual field was encoded in the phase of the response. The response phase for each of the polar angles or eccentricity components was computed using Fourier analysis and mapped onto the cortical surface (Fig. 1A). More details of the surface reconstruction, the retinotopy mapping, and the parcellation schema have been described elsewhere (H. Yamamoto et al. 2008, Yamamoto et al. 2011).

2.3. Generation of the probability and entropy maps

Quantification of the inconsistency and uncertainty of the locations of the human retinotopic areas in the Talairach space comprised three basic steps: 1) construction of volumetric models of the retinotopic areas, 2) generation of the probability map, and 3) generation of the entropy map, as schematized in Fig. 1. In the first step, volumetric models of the retinotopic areas were constructed for each of the 10 hemispheres by first localizing them on the cortical surface (Fig. 1B) and then converting each area's surface to a volumetric model of 3 mm thickness (Fig. 1C). This conversion began by computing the distance from the surface of each area to the points of an output volume. The distance data was then thresholded at 1.5 mm (half the distance of the assumed thickness) to produce a draft version of the volumetric model for each area. Finally, the draft models of the different areas in one hemisphere were compared to each other to detect where the dilation caused the overlap among them, and the overlapped voxels detected were removed from the models, producing a final volumetric model for each area. The volumetric model is a 3D binary array of voxels, with each voxel having a label indicating the presence or absence of the area. We confirmed that each model did not overlap with the others and had no topological defects, such as discontinuities and holes, by visual inspection of the 3D volume and surface rendered models.

In the second step, the inconsistency associated with each area was assessed as its occurrence probability; that is, in the form of the probability map. For each area, we transformed 10 volumetric models constructed from the 10 hemispheres into Talairach space (Fig. 1D, E) and then counted the number of overlapping models for each anatomic point. We used a single homogeneous transformation (Table 1), which consists of nine parameters, three translations, three rotations, and three scalings with respect to the axes of a Cartesian frame. The homogeneous transformation was determined using a standard method (Desmond & Lim 1997). First, the translation and rotation components of the matrix were computed from the locations of the anatomical landmarks (AC, PC, and mid-sagittal plane) identified by visual inspection of the structural volume. The alignment was checked and corrected by graphically comparing the X-, Y-, and Z-axes with the three orthogonal slices of the standard volume and the reconstructed surface. Next, the scale components were determined by measuring the size of the brain along each of the three axes as the bounding box dimensions of the surface and then computing the scaling factors to match the size to that of the 1988 Talairach atlas brain (X dimension: 136 mm; Y: 172 mm; Z: 118 mm). The scaling factor was determined separately for the left and right hemispheres. Because the Talairach atlas only contains a right hemisphere, the volumetric models for the left hemispheres were mirrored around the Y-axis and treated as though they were in right hemispheres. The occurrence probability of each area of Talairach space was computed by dividing the number of overlaps by the total number of hemispheres ($N = 10$). This computation was repeated every 1 mm in the Talairach space covering the visual cortex, yielding a 3D probability map for each retinotopic area (Fig. 1F). Furthermore, the probability maps for all the retinotopic areas were integrated into a maximum probability map (Fig. 1G) where each voxel was assigned a label indicating which area had the greatest probability of being present there and was given the maximum value.

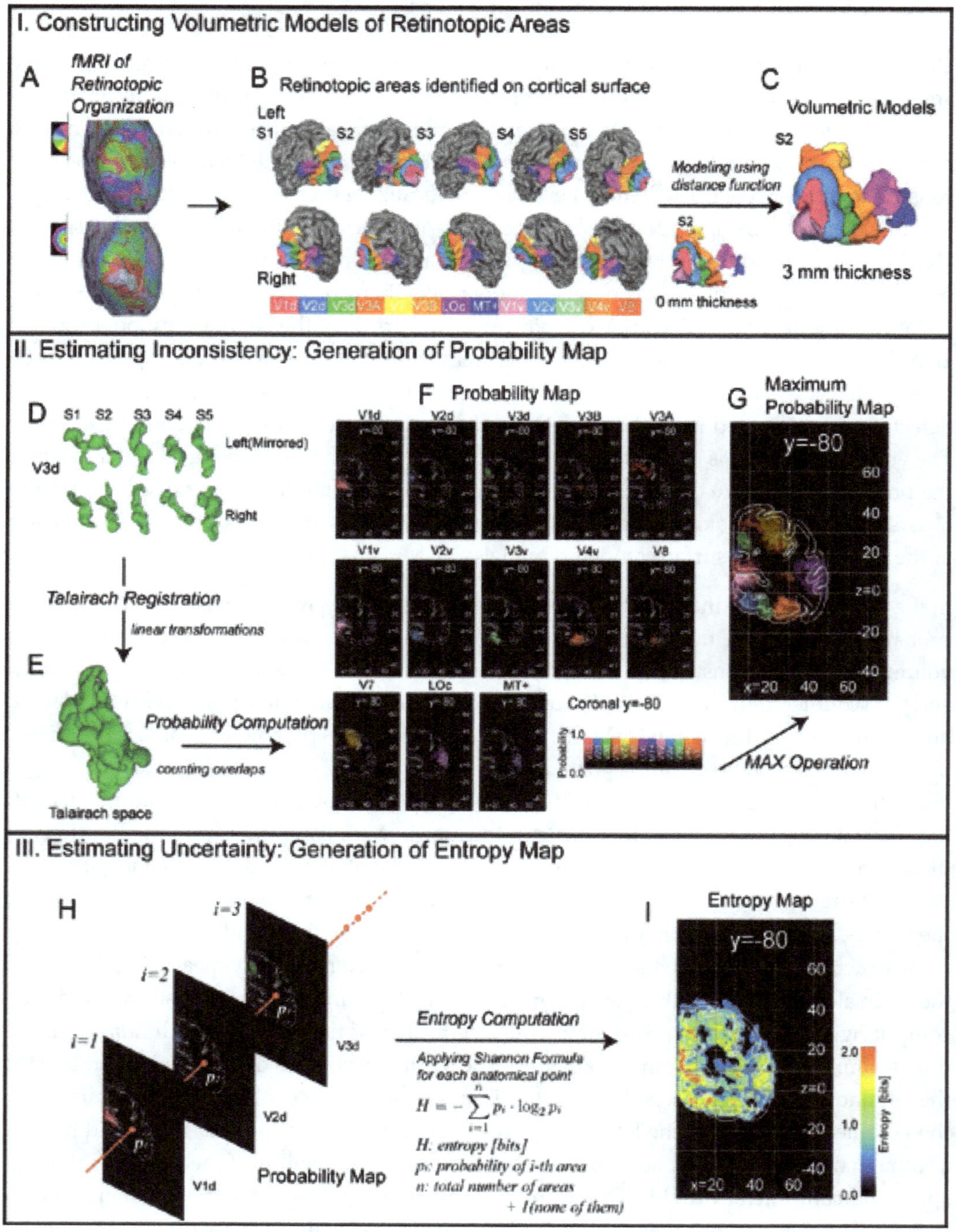

Figure 1. Overview of probabilistic atlas generation. See text for further explanation.

In the final step, the uncertainty associated with the retinotopic areas was assessed in the form of an entropy map (Fig. 1I) by calculating the Shannon entropy (Shannon 1948) from the occurrence probabilities of the different retinotopic areas (Fig. 1H), where this yields a quantitative measure of the uncertainty represented by a probability distribution. If no uncertainty exists in the distribution, the entropy equals zero, but if the entropy is greater than zero, it is maximal when all events are equally probable. The Shannon entropy (H) of the retinotopic areas can be expressed in terms of the occurrence probabilities (pi) of the different retinotopic areas and is given by

$$H = -\sum_{i=1}^{n} p_i \cdot \log_2 p_i \left[\text{bits}\right], \quad (1)$$

where n is the total number of candidate areas. By applying this equation to the probability maps of the retinotopic areas, we calculated the entropy for each point in the Talairach space covering the visual cortex (Fig. 1H, I). In the present analysis, $n = 14$; each of the 13 retinotopic areas = p_1, p_2,...p_{13} ; plus none of them, p_{14}. Thus, the maximum theoretical value for entropy is

$$-\sum_{i=1}^{14} \frac{1}{14} \log_2 \frac{1}{14} = \log_2 14 \cong 3.8 \left[\text{bits}\right], \quad (2)$$

2.4. Estimating two sources of uncertainty

We estimated two other kinds of entropies underlying the entropy about 14 possible states (retinotopic areas, and non-retinotopic area,) as computed above. The first was the entropy of two possible states, whether a voxel is located anywhere in the retinotopic areas (pr) or located outside of the areas (pnr), which was computed as follows:

$$H_r = -p_r \cdot \log_2 p_r - p_{nr} \cdot \log_2 p_{nr} \left[\text{bits}\right], \quad (3)$$

where

$$p_r = \sum_{i=1}^{13} p_i = 1 - p_{14} \text{ and } p_{nr} = p_{14}. \quad (4)$$

Because H_r is binomial, its maximum theoretical value is 1 bits. This binomial entropy would account for the uncertainty about whether a voxel is located within the visual cortex or is in the white matter, outside the brain or in the non-retinotopic cortex.

The second entropy type was the entropy of retinotopic areas computed on the probability distribution conditioned on a voxel being anywhere in the retinotopic areas, and was computed as follows:

$$H_c = -\sum_{i=1}^{13} p_{i/r} \cdot \log_2 p_{i/r} \left[\text{bits}\right], \tag{5}$$

where the conditional probability $p_{i/r} = p_i \, p_r$ and H_c was computed for voxels with $p_r \geq 0.2$, that is, for voxels that fell within any retinotopic area at least in two of ten hemispheres because it is impossible for areal overlap to occur for a voxel with $p_r = 0.1$. As the conditional entropy H_c has 13 possible states, its maximum theoretical value is

$$-\sum_{i=1}^{13} \frac{1}{13} \log_2 \frac{1}{13} = \log_2 13 \cong 3.7 \left[\text{bits}\right], \tag{6}$$

Please note, unlike the unconditional entropy H, H_c was computed on the probability distribution that did not comprise the event of "a voxel being in non-retinotopic area" and was rather conditional on the event of "a voxel being in retinotopic area". This conditional entropy would thus not be affected by the misalignment of cortical surfaces across hemispheres, and thereby reflect the uncertainty due to variability in the cortical locations of the areas in Talairach space.

2.5. Analysis and visualization software

The analyses were performed and visualized using BrainFactory software (Yamamoto 2011, H. Yamamoto et al. 2008, Yamamoto et al. 2002) written in VTK (Kitware, Clifton Park, NY) and MATLAB (Mathworks, Natick, MA), which has been successfully applied to cortical surface-based analysis of fMRI data (Ban et al. 2006, Ejima et al. 2007, Maeda et al. 2010, Yamamoto et al. 2011, T. Yamamoto et al. 2008) and cortico-cortical evoked potentials (Matsumoto et al. in press).

3. Results

To analyze the interindividual variability in the locations of the visual areas, we created a 3D probability map of the visual areas (e.g., for a coronal slice, see Fig. 1F) where each voxel was associated with the occurrence probabilities (N = 10) for each of the areas. It is difficult to display all such multivariate volume data in only two dimensions, so only the essence of the data is graphically presented in Fig. 2A in the form of a maximum probability map, where each point is color-coded according to the visual area with the greatest frequency (the maximum probability area), and the brightness represents the probability that the area resides at that voxel. The regions of maximal consistency are shown with maximal brightness, and the regions of minimal consistency are shown with minimal brightness. Figure 2A displays this information using the same coronal serial slices as the

1988 atlas of Talairach and Tournoux (1988), overlaid on the Talairach brain, the gray matter of which is outlined using white lines. The probability data in the horizontal and sagittal slices are also shown in Figs. 3A and 4A, respectively.

3.1. Inconsistency in the locations of visual areas: Probability map

The maximum probability area changes within the slices in the same hierarchical order as in the individual hemispheres. This topographic pattern is clearly illustrated in Fig. 5A, which shows the maximum probability map overlaid on the surface representation of the Talairach brain. The topographic preservation can be confirmed, except for the island-like V3 regions within V3B. In contrast to the near complete preservation of the topographic relations of the maximum probability areas, the probability maps of the corresponding areas (e.g., for a coronal slice, see Fig. 1F) revealed substantial inconsistency. As can be partially seen in Figs. 1F, 2A, 3A, and 4A, the probabilistic volume for a corresponding area (voxels having non-zero probabilities) is blurred so strongly that its extent is much wider than the thickness of the cortical gray matter. The strength of this tendency seems to vary among the visual areas, being strongest for area V7/IPS-0, which is located anterior to V3A (Tootell et al. 1998).

Positional inconsistency was quantitatively analyzed, and the results are shown in Fig. 6. Figure 6A illustrates the overall positional inconsistency, showing the distribution of maximum probability values within the voxels containing a non-zero probability. Most of the voxels were associated with small probabilities, with approximately half (47.3%) of them being associated with a value of 0.1 (only a single case representing a visual area) and 96.5% being associated with values less than 0.5 (0.2: 27.0%; 0.3: 15.1%; 0.4: 7.1%). The remaining 3.5% of the voxels were associated with probabilities equal to or larger than 0.5, with the maximum value being not 1.0 but 0.8 (0.5: 2.7%; 0.6: 0.67 %; 0.7: 0.14%; 0.8: 0.007%).

Separate analyses for the individual visual areas were also performed by spatially averaging all of the probability values within each area's probabilistic volume. The average probability is compared among the visual areas in Fig. 6B. The differences were not large, but the average probabilities were slightly lower for the dorsal areas (V3d, V7, and LOc), indicating a higher alignment inconsistency. Area V7 had the lowest values, as expected from the maximum probability map. The overall average of the average probabilities of the areas was 0.166 (SD: 0.013). The coefficient of variance (the SD divided by the mean) was 7.6%.

The analogous alignment inconsistency was evident when using another measure, percent blurring (Fischl et al. 1999b), which is defined as the percentage increase in the probabilistic volume of an area as compared with the mean volume of the individual areas. The percent blurring, which is compared among the visual areas in Fig. 6C, shows a pattern that is nearly reversed compared with the average probability (Fig. 6B), indicating a similar relative inconsistency among the visual areas. The average percent blurring for the group of areas was 460%.

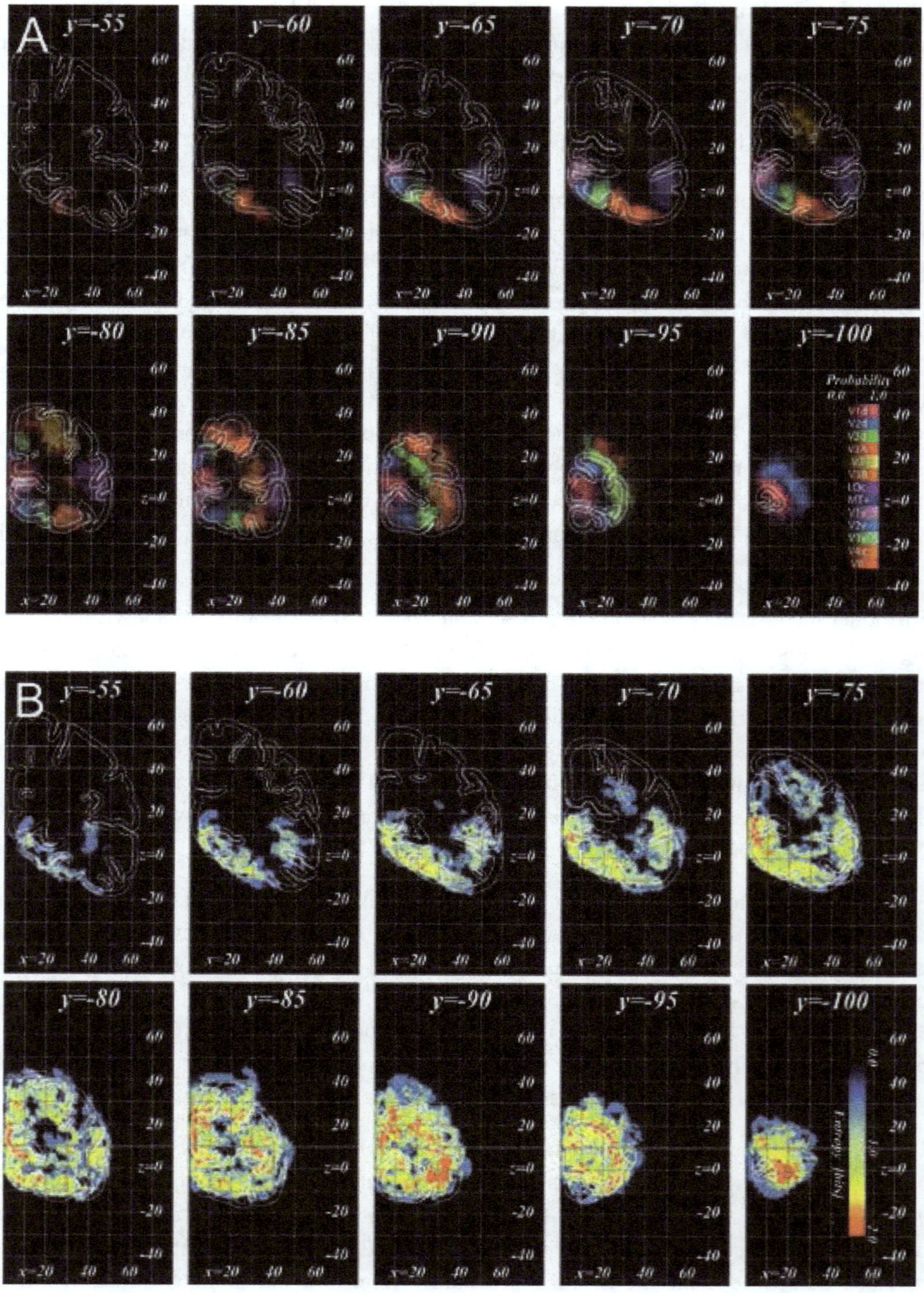

Figure 2. Maximum probability map (A) and entropy map (B) on serial coronal sections.

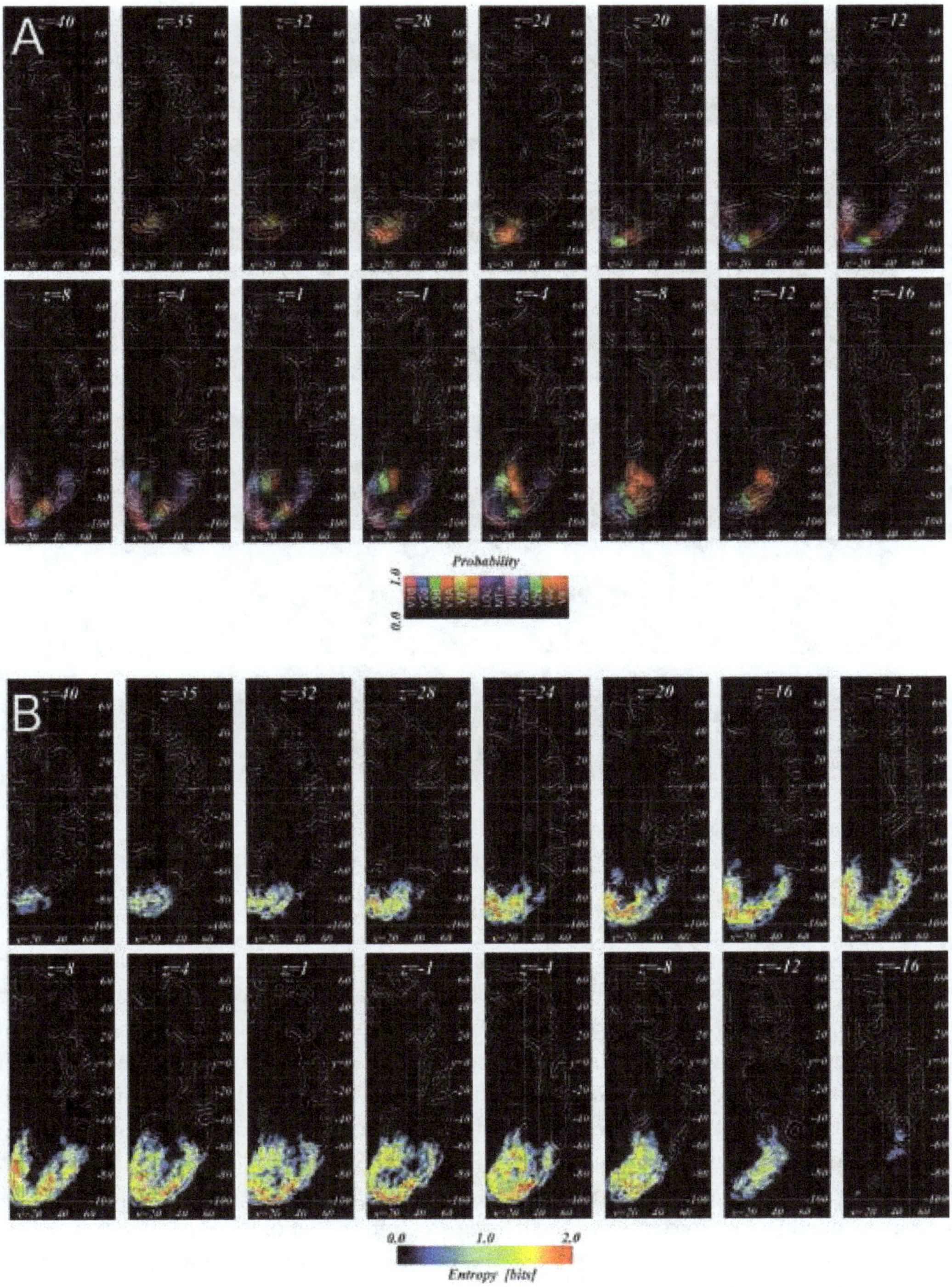

Figure 3. Maximum probability map (A) and entropy map (B) on serial horizontal sections.

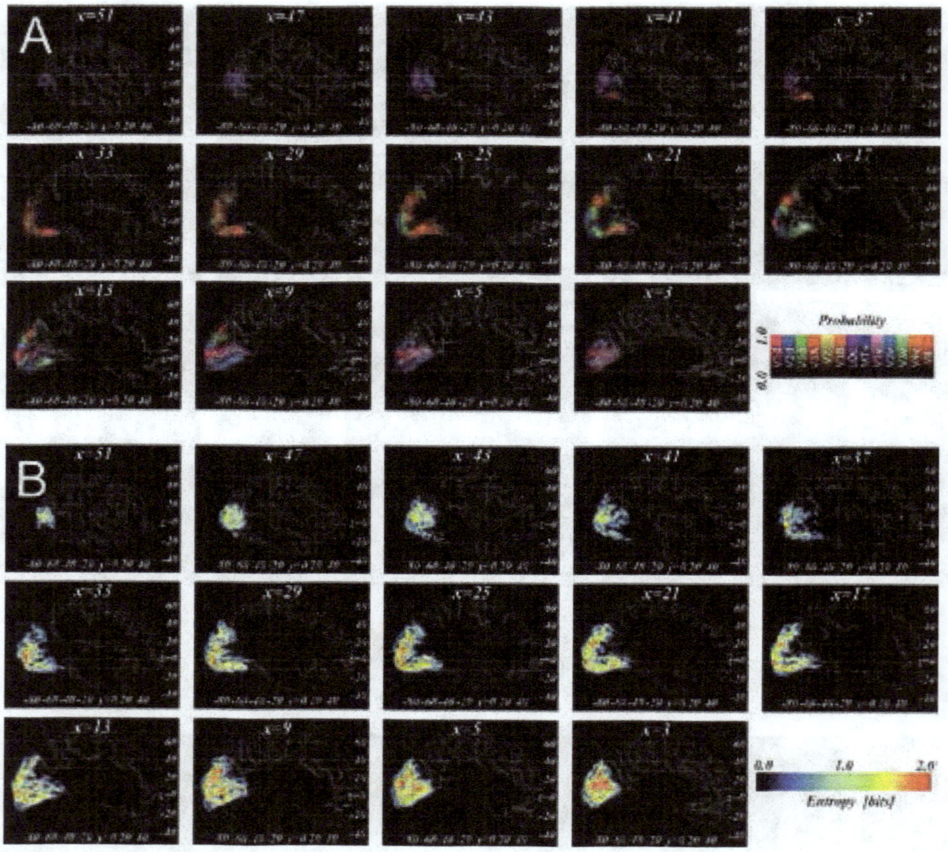

Figure 4. Maximum probability map (A) and entropy map (B) on serial sagittal sections.

3.2. Uncertainty in the locations of visual areas: Entropy map

Next, we performed a series of quantitative analyses regarding the uncertainty about which visual area actually resides at each voxel in Talairach space. As expected, registration of the individual visual areas into the Talairach space led to substantial overlaps among different visual areas. Figure 7A demonstrates this by showing the distribution of the number of overlaps among the areas. When considering the overlaps for all voxels associated with a non-zero probability (71804 voxels), these occurred in nearly half (46.7%) of the voxels and ranged from two to five overlapping areas per voxel (2: 35.4%; 3: 9.8%; 4: 1.5%; 5: 0.04%). Because it is impossible for overlap to occur in a voxel with a 0.1 probability (being in a visual area only for one hemisphere), we also computed the overlaps within the set of voxels with a probability greater than 0.1 (48116 voxels), finding the proportion of overlaps increased to occupy 69.6% of the voxels (2: 52.8%; 3: 14.6%; 4: 2.2%, 5: 0.05%).

To analyze the uncertainty resulting from the overlaps in an information theory framework (Shannon 1948), we introduced the Shannon entropy, a measure of the amount of uncertainty represented by a probability distribution. In our study, this distribution is the probability of occurrence of the 13 delineated areas plus the probability of occurrence of none of the areas at each voxel in Talairach space. If any of the probabilities is 1.0, such that there is no uncertainty, the Shannon entropy of the visual area is zero, but if not, the entropy is greater than zero. The entropy takes a maximum value of 3.8 bits when the probabilities of all events occurring are the same, such as when we are very uncertain of which of the 14 events has occurred. By applying Shannon's formula to the occurrence probabilities (Fig. 1H, I), we created a 3D map of the entropy of the visual areas within the same occipital region of Talairach space as the probability map.

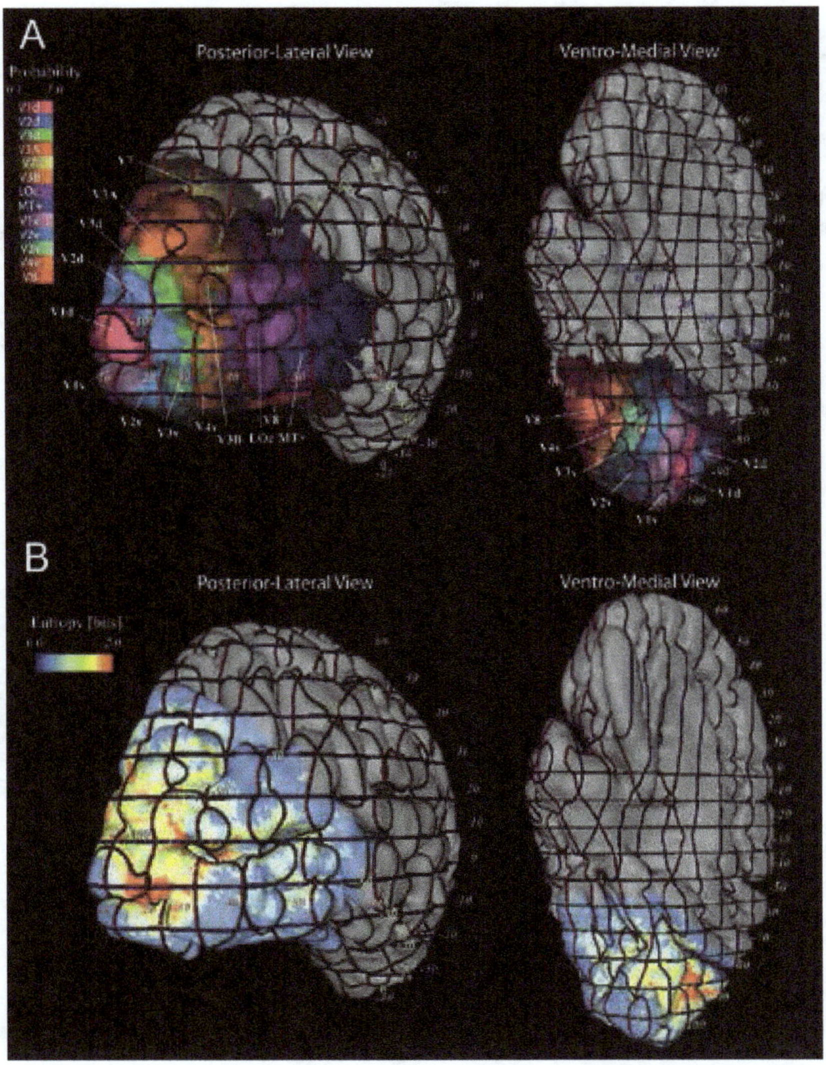

Figure 5. Surface representation of the maximum probability (A) and entropy map (B) of the areas.

Figure 2B/3B/4B shows the entropy map overlaid on the Talairach brain with the same coronal/horizontal/sagittal slice positions as the maximum probability map, where the entropy of the visual area at each voxel is color-coded from blue to red. Figure 5B also shows the entropy map overlaid on the surface representation of the Talairach brain in the same way as the maximum probability map (Fig. 5A). The entropy was less than 2 bits for most voxels, as evidenced by the predominance of blue and yellow regions. As shown in Fig. 7B, the larger the entropy, the smaller the number of voxels. The entropy values ranged from 0.47 to 2.45 bits, with a median value of 0.92 bits.

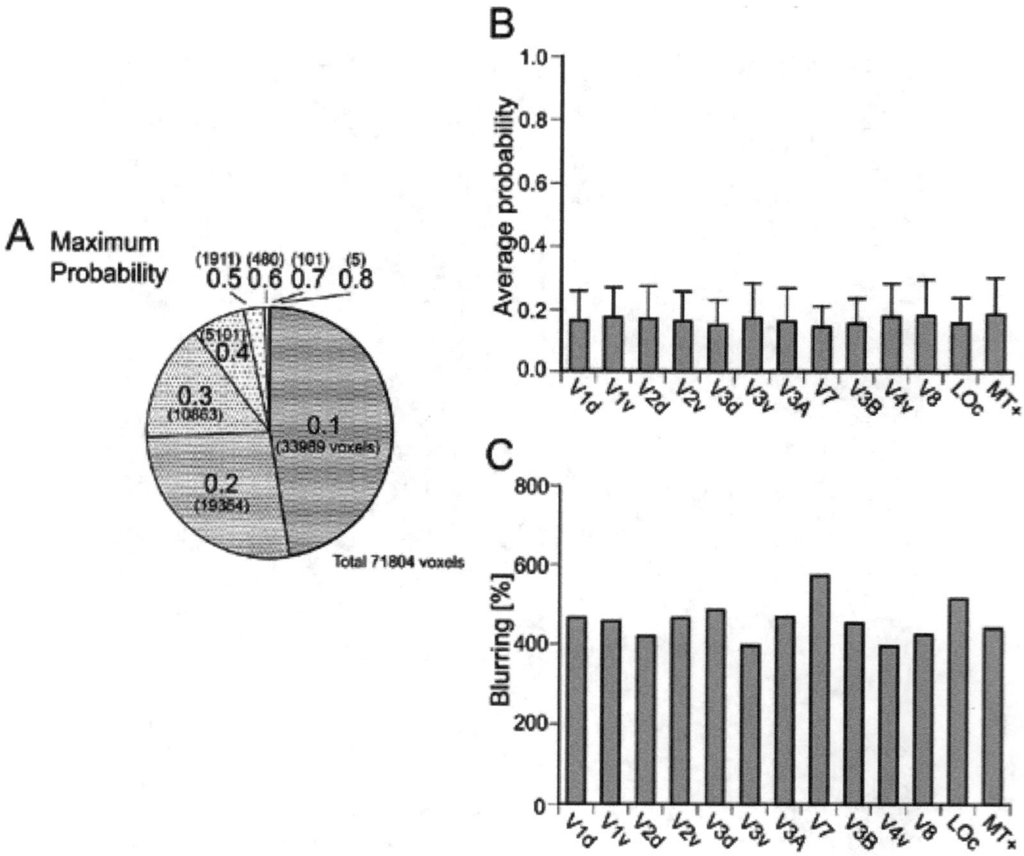

Figure 6. (A) Proportion of the maximum probabilities. The numbers of voxels are indicated in parentheses. (B) Average probability for each visual area across all the area voxels (probabilistic volume) in Talairach space, which is defined as the voxels being classified as an area for at least one hemisphere. Error bars denote SD. (C) Percent blurring of each visual area. This metric measures the amount of increase between the total volume of the area's voxels in its probability map and the mean volume of the area across hemispheres. If registration is perfect, the total volume in Talairach space will be equal to the mean volume, and percent blurring will be zero. For example, a value of 400% means that the total volume of the area's voxels is 5 times as big as the mean volume.

The comparison of the entropy map with the maximum probability map shows a topographical relationship between these. Regions with high entropy values (red) are generally located near places where multiple visual areas would be located in close proximity, such as the foveal confluence separating the dorsal and ventral region (e.g., [X,Y,Z]=[20,-100,0]) and the borders of areas (e.g., for V3d/V3A/V3B, [20,-90,20]). Conversely, the regions with low entropy values (blue) tend to lie outside of the crowded fields.

Entropy is conceptually and computationally distinct from maximum probability, such that its map has a unique importance. However, if these measures were empirically related to each other, the entropy map would become less important. For a potential relationship, one would expect that high entropy would generally be associated with a low probability of belonging to one area. Therefore, we examined the relationship between entropy and maximum probability on a voxel-by-voxel basis, but found no correlation consistent throughout their range (Fig. 8). Although the expected negative correlation was observed for the higher maximum probability levels (0.4—0.8), the number of voxels in the range occupied only 11% of all the area's voxels. The entropies of the voxels with lower probability levels, which occupied the remaining 89% of the voxels, dispersed widely and showed rather positive correlations with maximum probabilities. Consequently, the entropy provides information distinct from that conveyed by the maximum probability, which emphasizes the importance of the entropy map.

We also quantified the uncertainty at the level of the visual areas by averaging all of the entropy values within the probabilistic volume of each area. The average entropy is compared among the areas in Fig. 7C. The average entropy was smaller, less than 1 bit, for areas V7, V8, LOc and MT+, and was at a minimum for MT+. For other areas, the average entropy was greater than 1 bit and was at a maximum for V2d. The difference between the maximum and minimum was 0.47 bits. The average entropy for the group of areas was 1.07 bits (SD: 0.175). The coefficient of variance was 16.4%, which is about two-fold larger than the probability.

Comparison of the average entropy (Fig. 7C) with the average occurrence probability (Fig. 6B) and blurring (Fig. 6C) shows the dissociation between uncertainty and inconsistency at the cortical area level. For example, areas V7 and V8 display opposite patterns: V7 has the smallest average probability, the largest blurring, and the second smallest entropy value, whereas V8 has a relatively large average probability, small blurring, and comparable entropy with V7; thus, V7 exhibits relatively strong inconsistency with relatively small uncertainty, whereas V8 exhibits relatively weak inconsistency with relatively small uncertainty. As complementary examples, V3d exhibits relatively strong inconsistency with relatively large uncertainty, whereas V2d exhibits relatively small inconsistency with relatively large uncertainty.

3.3. Two sources of uncertainty in the locations of visual areas

Finally, we analyzed the potential sources of the areal uncertainty. There are at least two sources of entropy when computed over the probability distribution of 14 possible states (13 areas plus none of them), as stated above. The first is the uncertainty as to whether a voxel is located within the visual cortex or lies within the white matter, outside the brain, or in non-retinotopic areas. We estimated this cortical registration factor by computing the entropy over the probability distribution of two events of the "voxel being in any of retinotopic areas" or not. Figure 9A compares the estimated entropy (theoretical maximum, 1 bit) among the retinotopic areas. Although the binomial entropy was a little smaller for area V7, it was nearly

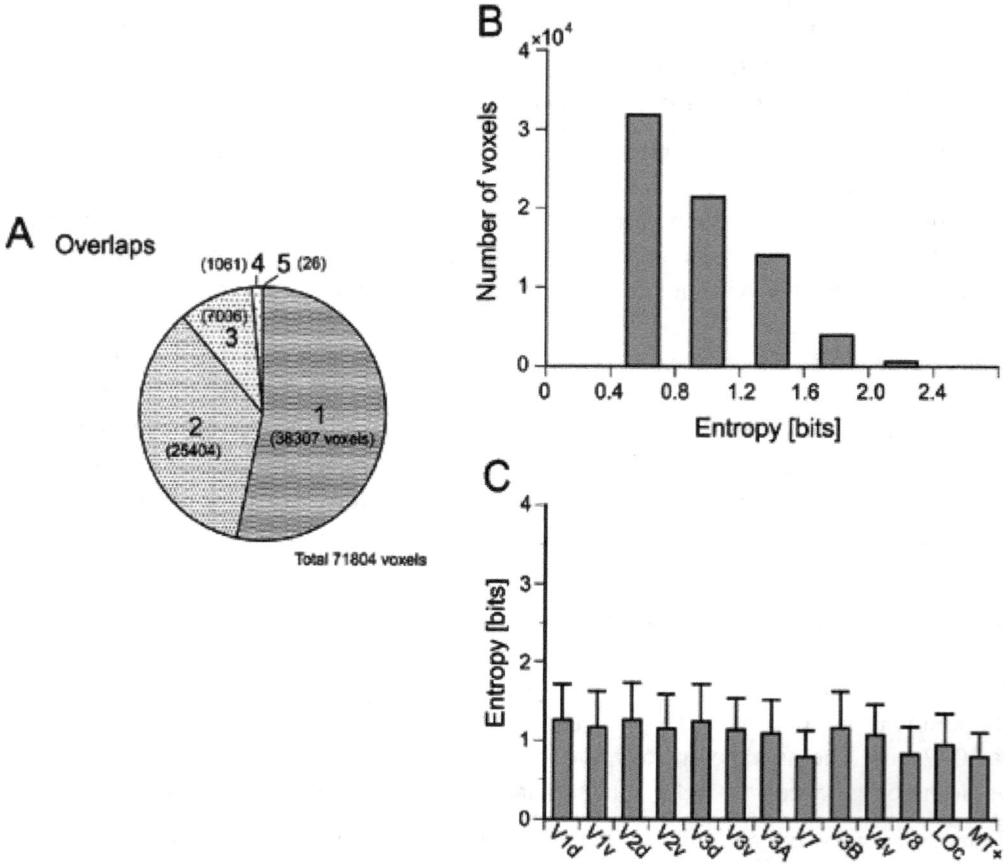

Figure 7. (A) Proportion of the number of overlaps among different visual areas in Talairach space. For example, an "overlap" of 1 means that these voxel correspond uniquely to a single area, whereas overlaps of 2 means that these voxel correspond two areas (one area for some hemispheres but another area for the other hemispheres). (B) Histogram of the entropy values. (C) Average entropy of each visual area across all the area's voxels (probabilistic volume). Error bars denote SD.

constant across the areas, as indicated by the fact that the standard deviation (0.022) was only 2.5% of the mean (0.87). The coefficient of variance was much smaller, by a factor of 6.4, compared with the result of the entropy over the full distribution of the 14 possible states (Fig. 5C). Therefore, this factor of uncertainty alone cannot explain the entropy difference among retinotopic areas.

The second factor was the uncertainty that remains even after the removal of the first uncertainty due to the registration, such as after knowing a voxel was being registered to some part of the retinotopic visual cortex. We estimated this by computing the entropy over the probability distribution of the retinotopic areas conditioned on a voxel belonging to any of the areas. This conditional entropy would reflect the underlying intersubject variability in the location on the cortical surface. Figure 9B compares the estimated conditional entropy (theoretical

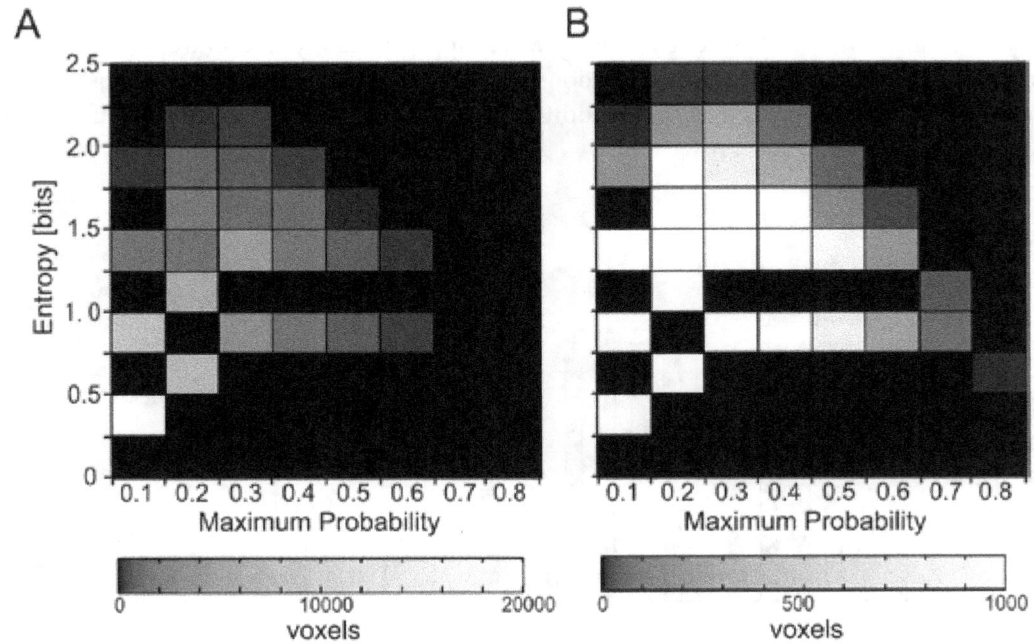

Figure 8. Two-dimensional histogram of entropy vs. maximum probability for all the area voxels. The histogram assigns a brightness value to each bin based on the number of voxels. The brighter the bin, the greater the number of voxels in that range. The brightness scale ranges from 0 to 20000 voxels. (B) Same histogram image as in A with a different, narrower scale to emphasize small differences in the number of voxels. The scale ranges from 0 to 1000 voxels.

maximum, 3.7 bits) among the retinotopic areas. Unlike the first binomial entropy due to cortical registration (Fig. 9A), the conditional entropy showed a substantial difference among the retinotopic areas, as indicated by a coefficient of variance of 27.6% (mean, 0.89; SD, 0.246), which was much larger, by a factor of 10.9, than the first entropy. The approximate ten-fold difference in the two entropy measures remained even when the comparison was limited to lower retinotopic areas, excluding the higher areas, V7, V8, LOc, and MT+, which are enclosed by more non-adjacent borders (coefficient of variance, 10.9% vs. 1.1%). Notably, the pattern of the difference among the areas (Fig. 9B) was similar to that found for the non-conditional entropy (Fig. 7C) but with more pronounced variability. The coefficient of variance and the difference between the maximum and minimum were larger, by factors of 1.7 and 1.6, respectively, than those obtained for the non-conditional entropy.

4. Discussion

The Talairach coordinate system has inherent limits in reducing the interindividual variability in the complex topography of the brain structure. The purpose of the present study was to apply a probabilistic and information theoretical framework for analyzing the residual interindividual variability of human visual area loci in Talairach space. The key feature of the framework is its ability to quantify the complementary aspects of the interindividual variability, inconsistency and uncertainty by constructing probability and entropy maps. The inconsistency and uncertainty of the locations of retinotopic areas found by analysis using this framework will be discussed below. In addition, we will discuss the applications of the maps and the framework.

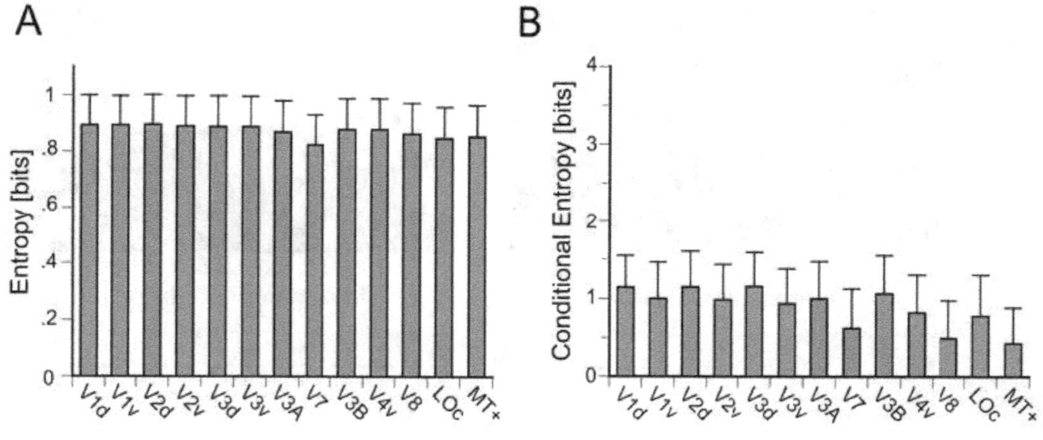

Figure 9. (A) Entropy computed on probability distribution whether a voxel is located in any retinotopic area or not. (B) Entropy computed on areal probability distribution *conditioned* on a voxel being in the visual cortex (retinotopic area). Error bars denote SD.

4.1. Inconsistency in the locations of visual areas: Probability map

In the present study, the alignment inconsistency of retinotopic areas (V1d/v, V2d/v, V3d/v, V4v, V8, V3A, V3B, V7, LOc, and MT+) was analyzed using a probabilistic approach (Mazziotta et al. 1995, Roland & Zilles 1994). The comprehensive application of this approach to visual areas was pioneered by Van Essen et al. (2001), who constructed probability maps of multiple areas (V1d/v, V2d/v, V3d/v, V3A, V4v, V8, MT+) identified using fMRI data from four hemispheres, using nonlinear surface warping in terms of the landmark coregistration rather than the standard linear Talairach transformation. Recently, we have also created probability maps using a similar surface based-method (Yamamoto et al. 2011). In this study, we generated probability maps of multiple retinotopic areas using standard linear Talairach transformation. Such maps have been made for the cytoarchitectonic definitions of areas V1 and V2 in five (Roland et al. 1997) and 10 brains (Amunts et al. 2000) and areas V3v and V4v in ten brains (Rottschy et al. 2007). Cytoarchitectonic studies of V1 and V2 have demonstrated that the probability volume of V2 surrounds that of V1 with substantial overlap, implying that the inconsistency was large, but not so large as to grossly violate the positional relationship. Our probability maps extend the observation to multiple functionally-defined visual areas.

Regarding the comparison across areas, it has been noted in cytoarchitectonic studies (Amunts et al. 2000) that the degree of inconsistency is smaller for V1 than for V2. However, such a pattern was not detected using the percent blurring measure in another study using fMRI

(Fischl et al. 1999b), where the comparison was made among V1d/v, V2d/v, and MT+. Consistent with this, the percent blurring measured in this study did not differ greatly among these areas. The discrepancy between anatomical and functional results may be resolved by examining them together using a common measure. One such integrated approach has been recently applied to areas V1 and V2 using probability maps, showing consistent results between the anatomical and functional probability maps (Wohlschlager et al. 2005). However, there appears to be a tendency for interindividual variability of the areas to increase in the anatomical map (see Fig. 5 in the study). Further studies are needed to elucidate the reason for this small discrepancy.

We also made a comparison across areas, introducing an intuitive measure of the average probability. Although the difference was not marked, we found slightly smaller average probabilities for areas V3d, V7, and LOc than for the other areas. A possible explanation is that as these areas are often buried in deep sulci, namely the intraparietal sulcus and lateral occipital sulcus, and that small differences in the courses of the sulci may prevent these areas from overlapping between the different subjects. The grand average across all areas was found to be only a little under 0.2, indicating substantial inconsistency.

4.2. Uncertainty in the locations of visual areas: Entropy map

Whereas the probability map allowed us to determine how probable it is that a particular visual area resides at a set of Talairach coordinates, the entropy map allowed us to quantify the uncertainty about the set of probability events. It should be stressed that even if events are highly probable, the entropy is large when the different events occur simultaneously, such as when the different areas overlap. The significance of the entropy map is in this dissociation. Indeed, our voxel-wise analysis of the relationship between the entropy and the maximum probability maps (Fig. 8) revealed that these statistics are largely unrelated, empirically supporting the dissociation of human visual areas in Talairach space. Although this dissociation has not been explicitly examined, the overlap between different structures has been noted previously in the context of the brain registration. Roland et al. (1997) identified areas V1 and V2 cytoarchitectonically and reported that the overlap between V1 and V2 is as large as the overlap between the different V1 areas. Van Essen (2005) analyzed the degree of overlap between the neighboring brain sulci using a probability map. Importantly, these studies all disregarded the occurrence probabilities of the overlapping structures, despite the uncertainty being maximal when each event is equiprobable. The present study extends these earlier analyses by relating the probabilities to the concept of uncertainty using entropy.

We found that the overall average of the entropy of retinotopic areas is approximately 1 bit in Talairach space, indicating that there are, on average, 1 bits of uncertainty about which retinotopic area is present at a point when its Talairach coordinates are specified. This means that there is an equal chance of each area being present for a point where two areas overlap. As for the spatial pattern of entropy distribution, the entropy map is not isotropic; it contains larger values around the borders of retinotopic areas and smaller values around their non-adjacent borders, which is expected given the possibility of overlaps between the different areas. In addition, we found that there is also a variation in entropy among retinotopic areas.

4.3. Two sources of uncertainty in the locations of visual areas

What causes the areal entropy and its variation in Talairach space? One possibility might be the poor alignment of the cortex under the simple Talairach volumetric registration because the probability distribution on which the entropy is computed contains information about whether a voxel belongs to the cortex. Indeed, the weakness of Talairach normalization is commonly agreed upon, and a prior probabilistic atlas of the human visual areas has been created using surface-based registration to partly overcome this problem (Van Essen et al. 2001, Yamamoto et al. 2011). The present study estimated the uncertainty caused by the inadequacy of Talairach registration by using the binomial entropy as either 'a voxel being in retinotopic area' or not and found that the measure is nearly constant among retinotopic areas. This suggests that the uncertainty due to registration is not a major factor underlying the uncertainty about retinotopic areas in Talairach space, thereby suggesting that the uncertainty due to intersubject variability in the relative size or cortical location of distinct areas (Dougherty et al. 2003, Ejima et al. 2003, Van Essen et al. 2001, Yamamoto et al. 2011) would be a significant factor.

This source of variability is, however, is not well understood. Therefore, we estimated this by computing the entropy for the probability distribution conditioned on a voxel in the cortex. Another approach could apply our non-conditional entropy measure to a surface-based group averaged brain, but this is beyond the scope of the present work. In addition, this method would lose some generality because the surface registration generally requires a set of anatomical or functional landmarks, and their selection would affect entropy. In contrast, our conditional entropy only assumes the association of a voxel to the cortex, such that it would constitute a baseline measure of the uncertainty remaining after surface-based normalization. The conditional entropy averaged across retinotopic areas was found to decrease by approximately 10%, supporting the general advantage of the surface-based normalization over Talairach normalization. This improvement would increase for the existing surface-based methods (Drury et al. 1996, Fischl et al. 1999b, Thompson et al. 1997) because they apply to the individual variability of gyral patterning. We also found that the difference in entropy across areas was amplified upon conditioning. This amplification underlines the fact that entropy provides information distinct from probability and confirms that the uncertainty due to intersubject variability in the layout of the cortical areas is a primary cause of the areal uncertainty in Talairach space. The much smaller observed conditional entropy of several higher areas confirms this idea because they are enclosed by many non-adjacent borders. However, with the exception of the apparent adjacency, we cannot specify the exact reason for the modest variations observed in lower retinotopic areas.

4.4. Preliminary comparison among registration methods

Three types of registration methods are commonly used, namely the linear volume-based, nonlinear volume-based, and surface-based methods. Among these, we evaluated a linear volume-based method for 5 subjects in the present study and a surface-based method for 16 subjects in a recent study (Yamamoto et al. 2011). Extending these studies, we initiated a comparison study among the three types of methods. Table 2 shows a preliminary summary of the results obtained for 16 subjects. As used in the present study, the linear volume-method is a single linear transformation; the nonlinear volume-based method used is an automated image registration (AIR) method (Woods et al. 1998) where a 12 parameter affine linear transformation was followed by a second-order 30 parameter, nonlinear polynomial model; the surface-based method used is an Automated Spherical Warping (Fischl et al. 1999b) of the FreeSurfer software package (Dale et al. 1999, Fischl et al. 1999a), which displaced the vertices of each labeled surface to match its folding pattern with that of the FreeSurfer average template surface. As expected, the surface-based method gave the best results for probability. However, surprisingly, the surface-based method lost its advantage for entropy (average entropy: ~ 1 bits). This suggests that the current technology is not perfect and should therefore be used with caution regarding the limits.

	Linear volume-based method	Nonlinear volume-based method	Surface-based method
Average probability	0.089 (0.016)	0.10 (0.013)	0.27 (0.074)
Average entropy [bits]	1.01 (0.18)	1.07 (0.20)	1.15 (0.23)

The average probability(entropy) over 12 areas (V1, V2d, V2v, V3d, V3v, V3A, V7, V3B, V4v, V8, LOc, MT+) was listed. Parenthesis indicates SD across the areas. 16 subjects' brain were coregistered with the three method (see text for description of the methods).

Table 2. Preliminary comparison among registration methods

4.5. Applications

The present probabilistic and information theoretical framework has a variety of applications related to interindividual variability in the human brain. Probability and entropy maps of retinotopic areas can readily benefit any application where it is necessary to predict which areas are present at an anatomical point with a high probability and to establish the uncertainty associated with the prediction given its Talairach coordinates. Using these maps, the researchers and clinicians can infer, with a known degree of uncertainty, the visual area that is most likely present at an activation site or a lesion site within a target brain for which any form of the direct identification is impossible. The non-conditional entropy is a useful measure of the uncertainty observed in a practical situation, such as to average functional activations for different subjects or regimens for stereotaxic surgical treatment, whereas the conditional entropy allows a more fundamental appreciation of uncertainty regarding the cortical location of visual areas when analyzing the layout and network of cortical areas. The other main application is in the field of brain registration and brain warping (Toga 1999). As demonstrated in this study, Talairach registration reduced the entropy of visual areas from approximately 4 bits to 1 bit. In this way, the performance of various registration methods can be compared quantitatively using the degree of reduction in the entropy of the structures to be coregistered. Finally, the present work on visual areas can be generalized to not only other functional structures, but also other anatomical structures. Thus, an important direction for future research is to extend the present framework to address brain structure-function relationships, which are the focus of an ongoing large-scale international project that aims to develop a probabilistic brain atlas representing many types of information on brain function and structure (Mazziotta et al. 2001). One such approach is quantifying relationships using the Shannon mutual information based on simultaneous probability maps of structural and functional areas (Yamamoto et al. 2003).

5. Conclusion

We made two kinds of multisubject maps (10 hemispheres from five subjects) to characterize interindividual variability in the positions of human visual areas (V1/2/3, V3A, V3B, V7, V4v, V8, LOc, and MT+), which were localized using fMRI and coregistered into standard Talairach space by a single linear transformation. The first is a probability map representing the amount of alignment inconsistency for each area, where each voxel in space is associated with a probability affiliated with a given area. The second, a novel map termed an entropy map where each voxel is associated with a Shannon entropy computed from the probabilities, represents the amount of uncertainty that exists regarding which area resides there and is maximal when all areas are equally probable. We demonstrate that the entropy map provides distinctly different information from the probability map, highlighting the significance of the entropy map. The overall average probability and entropy values were ~0.2 and ~1.0 bits, respectively, with some area differences. The difference increased when computing the entropy for the probability distribution conditioned on a voxel located anywhere in the visual cortex, suggesting that a major source of the observed uncertainty is not due to the poor alignment of the cortex, but to individual variability in the cortical locations of the visual areas. The probability and entropy maps generated in this study will readily benefit any application where it is necessary to predict the areas that are most likely present at an anatomical voxel and to establish the uncertainty associated with this prediction.

Acknowledgements

This work was supported by Grant-in-Aids for Global COE (Centers of Excellence) Program (D07), Scientific Research on Innovative Areas (No. 22135007), and Scientific Research (C) (No. 22530793) of Japan's Ministry of Education, Culture, Sports, Science and Technology.

Author details

Hiroki Yamamoto*

Graduate School of Human and Environmental Studies, Kyoto University, Japan

References

[1] Amunts K, Malikovic A, Mohlberg H, Schormann T & Zilles K. (2000). Brodmann's areas 17 and 18 brought into stereotaxic space-where and how variable? *NeuroImage,* Vol.11, No.1, pp. 66-84, ISSN 1053-8119

[2] Ashburner J. (2007). A fast diffeomorphic image registration algorithm. *NeuroImage,* Vol.38, No.1, pp. 95-113, ISSN 1053-8119

[3] Ban H, Yamamoto H, Fukunaga M, Nakagoshi A, Umeda M, Tanaka C & Ejima Y. (2006). Toward a common circle: interhemispheric contextual modulation in human early visual areas. *The Journal of neuroscience,* Vol.26, No.34, pp. 8804-9, ISSN 0270-6474

[4] Cencov NN. (1982). *Statistical decision rules and optimal inference,* American Mathematical Society, ISBN 0821845020, Providence, R.I.

[5] Dale AM, Fischl B & Sereno MI. (1999). Cortical surface-based analysis. I. Segmentation and surface reconstruction. *NeuroImage,* Vol.9, No.2, pp. 179, ISSN 1053-8119

[6] Dale AM & Sereno MI. (1993). Improved localization of cortical activity by combining EEG and MEG with MRI cortical surface reconstruction: A linear approach. *J Cogn Neurosci,* Vol.5, No.2, pp. 162-76, ISSN 1530-8898

[7] Desmond JE & Lim KO. (1997). On- and offline Talairach registration for structural and functional MRI studies. *Human Brain Mapp,* Vol.5, No.1, pp. 58-73, ISSN 1097-0193

[8] DeYoe EA, Bandettini P, Neitz J, Miller D & Winans P. (1994). Functional magnetic resonance imaging (FMRI) of the human brain. *J Neurosci Methods,* Vol.54, No.2, pp. 171-87, ISSN 0165-0270

[9] Dougherty RF, Koch VM, Brewer AA, Fischer B, Modersitzki J & Wandell BA. (2003). Visual field representations and locations of visual areas V1/2/3 in human visual cortex. *J Vis,* Vol.3, No.10, pp. 586-98, ISSN 1534-7362

[10] Drury HA, Van Essen DC, Anderson CH, Lee CW, Coogan TA & Lewis JW. (1996). Computerized mappings of the cerebral cortex: a multiresolution flattening method and a surface-based coordinate system. *Journal of Cognitive Neuroscience,* Vol.8, No.1, pp. 1-28, ISSN 1530-8898

[11] Drury HA, Van Essen DC, Corbetta M & Snyder AZ. (1999). Surface-based analyses of the human cerebral cortex., In: *Brain Warping* AW Toga, pp. 337-63, Academic Press, ISBN 0126925356, San Diego

[12] Ejima Y, Takahashi S, Yamamoto H, Fukunaga M, Tanaka C, Ebisu T & Umeda M. (2003). Interindividual and interspecies variations of the extrastriate visual cortex. *Neuroreport,* Vol.14, No.12, pp. 1579-83, ISSN 0959-4965

[13] Ejima Y, Takahashi S, Yamamoto H & Goda N. (2007). Visual Perception of Contextual Effect and Its Neural Correlates In: *Representation and Brain,* S Funahashi, pp. 3-20, Springer Verlag, ISBN 978-4-431-73020-0, Tokyo

[14] Engel SA, Glover GH & Wandell BA. (1997). Retinotopic organization in human visual cortex and the spatial precision of functional MRI. *Cereb Cortex,* Vol.7, No.2, pp. 181-92, ISSN 1047-3211

[15] Engel SA, Rumelhart DE, Wandell BA, Lee AT, Glover GH, Chichilnisky EJ & Shadlen MN. (1994). fMRI of human visual cortex. *Nature,* Vol.369, No.6481, pp. 525, ISSN 0028-0836

[16] Fischl B, Sereno MI & Dale AM. (1999a). Cortical surface-based analysis. II: Inflation, flattening, and a surface-based coordinate system. *NeuroImage,* Vol.9, No.2, pp. 195-207, ISSN 1053-8119

[17] Fischl B, Sereno MI, Tootell RB & Dale AM. (1999b). High-resolution intersubject averaging and a coordinate system for the cortical surface. *Hum Brain Mapp,* Vol.8, No.4, pp. 272-84, ISSN 1097-0193

[18] Gholipour A, Kehtarnavaz N, Briggs R, Devous M & Gopinath K. (2007). Brain Functional Localization: A Survey of Image Registration Techniques. *Medical Imaging, IEEE Transactions on,* Vol.26, No.4, pp. 427-51, ISSN 0278-0062

[19] Hasnain MK, Fox PT & Woldorff MG. (1998). Intersubject variability of functional areas in the human visual cortex. *Hum Brain Mapp,* Vol.6, No.4, pp. 301-15, ISSN 1097-0193

[20] Lorensen W, E. & Cline H, E. . (1987). *Marching cubes: A high resolution 3D surface construction algorithm.* Proceedings of the 14th annual conference on Computer graphics and interactive techniques, ISBN 0897912276, Anaheim, California, July 27-31, 1987

[21] Maeda K, Yamamoto H, Fukunaga M, Umeda M, Tanaka C & Ejima Y. (2010). Neural correlates of color-selective metacontrast in human early retinotopic areas. *Journal of Neurophysiology,* Vol.104, No.4, pp. 2291-301, ISSN 0022-3077

[22] Matsumoto R, Ikeda A, Fumuro T, Mikuni N, Miyamoto S, Fukuyama H, Takahashi R, Najm I, Shibasaki H & Luders H. (in press). Parieto-frontal network in humans studied by cortico-cortical evoked potential. *Human Brain Mapping,* ISSN 1097-0193

[23] Mazziotta J, Toga A, Evans A, Fox P, Lancaster J, Zilles K, Woods R, Paus T, Simpson G, Pike B, Holmes C, Collins L, Thompson P, MacDonald D, Iacoboni M, Schormann T, Amunts K, Palomero-Gallagher N, Geyer S, Parsons L, Narr K, Kabani N, Le Goualher G, Boomsma D, Cannon T, Kawashima R & Mazoyer B. (2001). A probabilistic atlas and reference system for the human brain: International Consortium for Brain Mapping (ICBM). *Philos Trans R Soc Lond B Biol Sci,* Vol.356, No.1412, pp. 1293-322, ISSN 0962-8436

[24] Mazziotta JC, Toga AW, Evans A, Fox P & Lancaster J. (1995). A probabilistic atlas of the human brain: theory and rationale for its development. The International Consortium for Brain Mapping (ICBM). *NeuroImage,* Vol.2, No.2, pp. 89-101, ISSN 1053-8119

[25] Ono M, Kubik S & Abernathey C. (1990). *Atlas of the Cerebral Sulci,* Thieme, ISBN 0865773629, Stuttgart, Germany

[26] Roland PE, Geyer S, Amunts K, Schormann T, Schleicher A, Malikovic A & Zilles K. (1997). Cytoarchitectural maps of the human brain in standard anatomical space. *Human Brain Mapping,* Vol.5, No.4, pp. 222-27, ISSN 1097-0193

[27] Roland PE & Zilles K. (1994). Brain atlases--a new research tool. *Trends Neurosci,* Vol. 17, No.11, pp. 458-67, ISSN 0166-2236

[28] Rottschy C, Eickhoff SB, Schleicher A, Mohlberg H, Kujovic M, Zilles K & Amunts K. (2007). Ventral visual cortex in humans: Cytoarchitectonic mapping of two extrastriate areas. *Hum Brain Mapp,* Vol.28, No.10, pp. 1045-1059, ISSN 1065-9471

[29] Sereno MI, Dale AM, Reppas JB, Kwong KK, Belliveau JW, Brady TJ, Rosen BR & Tootell RB. (1995). Borders of multiple visual areas in humans revealed by functional magnetic resonance imaging. *Science,* Vol.268, No.5212, pp. 889-93, ISSN 0036-8075

[30] Shannon CE. (1948). The mathematical theory of communication, I and II. *Bell System technical journal,* Vol.27, pp. 379-443

[31] Talairach J, Szikla G, Tournoux P, Prosalentis A, Bordas-Ferrier M, Covello L, Iacob M & Mempel E. (1967). *Atlas d'anatomie stereotaxique du telencephale.,* Masson, Paris

[32] Talairach J & Tournoux P. (1988). *Co-Planar Stereotactic Atlas of the Human Brain,* Thieme, ISBN 978-0865772939, Stuttgart/New York

[33] Teo PC, Sapiro G & Wandell BA. (1997). Creating connected representations of cortical gray matter for functional MRI visualization. *IEEE Transactions on Medical Imaging,* Vol.16, No.6, pp. 852-63, ISSN 0278-0062

[34] Thompson PM, MacDonald D, Mega MS, Holmes CJ, Evans AC & Toga AW. (1997). Detection and mapping of abnormal brain structure with a probabilistic atlas of cortical surfaces. *J Comput Assist Tomogr,* Vol.21, No.4, pp. 567-81, ISSN 0363-8715

[35] Toga AW. (1999). *Brain warping,* Academic Press, ISBN 0126925356, San Diego

[36] Tootell RB, Hadjikhani N, Hall EK, Marrett S, Vanduffel W, Vaughan JT & Dale AM. (1998). The retinotopy of visual spatial attention. *Neuron,* Vol.21, No.6, pp. 1409-22, ISSN 0896-6273

[37] Van Essen DC. (2005). A Population-Average, Landmark- and Surface-based (PALS) atlas of human cerebral cortex. *NeuroImage,* Vol.28, No.3, pp. 635-62, ISSN 1053-8119

[38] Van Essen DC, Lewis JW, Drury HA, Hadjikhani N, Tootell RB, Bakircioglu M & Miller MI. (2001). Mapping visual cortex in monkeys and humans using surface-based atlases. *Vision Res,* Vol.41, No.10-11, pp. 1359-78, ISSN 0042-6989

[39] Wohlschlager AM, Specht K, Lie C, Mohlberg H, Wohlschlager A, Bente K, Pietrzyk U, Stocker T, Zilles K, Amunts K & Fink GR. (2005). Linking retinotopic fMRI mapping and anatomical probability maps of human occipital areas V1 and V2. *NeuroImage,* Vol.26, No.1, pp. 73-82, ISSN 1053-8119

[40] Woods RP, Grafton ST, Watson JD, Sicotte NL & Mazziotta JC. (1998). Automated image registration: II. Intersubject validation of linear and nonlinear models. *J Comput Assist Tomogr,* Vol.22, No.1, pp. 153-165, ISSN 0363-8715

[41] Yamamoto H. (2011) BAVIEW: software for visualization and analysis of probabilistic atlases of human visual areas. *ESMRMB 2011,* Leipzig, DE, Oct. 6-8, 2011

[42] Yamamoto H, Ban H, Fukunaga M, Umeda M, Tanaka C & Ejima Y. (2008). Large- and Small-Scale Functional Organization of Visual Field Representation in the Human Visual Cortex., In: *Visual Cortex: New Research.,* TA Portocello, RB Velloti, pp. 195-226, Nova Science Publisher, ISBN 1604565306, New York

[43] Yamamoto H, Fukunaga M, Takahashi S, Mano H, Tanaka C, Umeda M & Ejima Y. (in press). Inconsistency and uncertainty of the human visual area loci following surface-based registration: Probability and Entropy Maps. *Human Brain Mapping,* doi: 10.1002/hbm.21200, ISSN 1065-9471

[44] Yamamoto H, Fukunaga M, Takahashi S, Tanaka C, Ebisu T, Umeda M & Ejima Y. (2002) BrainFactory: an integrated software system for surface-based analysis of fMRI data. *Human Brain Mapping 2002,* Sendai, Japan, June 2-6, 2002

[45] Yamamoto H, Fukunaga M, Tanaka C, Ebisu T, Umeda M & Ejima Y. (2003) A New Method for Quantifying Brain Structure-Function Relationships Based on Simultaneous Probability Map and Information Theory. *Society for Neuroscience 33rd Annual Meeting,* New Orleans, USA, Nov. 8-12, 2003

[46] Yamamoto T, Takahashi S, Hanakawa T, Urayama S, Aso T, Fukuyama H & Ejima Y. (2008). Neural correlates of the stereokinetic effect revealed by functional magnetic resonance imaging. *J Vis,* Vol.8, No.10, pp. 141-17, ISSN 1534-7362

7

Perfusion Based Functional MRI

Luis Hernandez-Garcia and Hesamoddin Jahanian

1. Introduction

In this chapter, we will discuss the perfusion imaging for functional MRI experiments as an alternative and complementary technique to the conventional Blood Oxygenation Level Dependent (BOLD) effect. We begin by discussing the motivation behind the development of perfusion based functional MRI techniques. In order to do so, we briefly review the underlying relationship between the brain's vasculature and neuronal activity. Increases in neuronal activity result in metabolic increases, which in turn elicit a local, complex, vasodilatory response. With this physiology in mind, we will discuss the advantages and disadvantages of perfusion MRI and BOLD imaging, and which situations are appropriate for each technique. We will discuss how the types of artifacts and noise characteristics present in each technique determine its applicability.

We will then survey a few examples of ASL based fMRI studies. These typically include clinical studies of pathological conditions, longitudinal studies of cognitive function and studies requiring sustained periods of the condition or state of interest (i.e., greater than 30 seconds).

We then proceed to survey the wide array of current techniques available to image cerebral perfusion, including non-MRI techniques. We will describe in broad strokes the basics of PET and SPECT imaging and the use of paramagnetic tracer injections in MRI to map cerebral perfusion. However, we will narrow our focus down to arterial spin labeling (ASL) techniques, which use the water in the arteries as a tracer by labeling it with radiofrequency pulses. Because of ASL's ability to image perfusion dynamically as well as quantitatively, this technique will be the main focus of this chapter.

We will discuss the technical aspects of ASL techniques by first describing the physics of the labeling process and the different labeling schemes available Here, we will discuss the advantages and disadvantages of each of these strategies in greater detail.

Next, we will discuss the requirements for image acquisition following the labeling period. We will give a brief survey of different image acquisition schemes that are typically used in the ASL literature. While slower non-echo planar techniques can be used for perfusion measurements at rest, functional imaging applications typically require faster, single-shot, echo-planar techniques. 3D acquisition techniques are also gaining prominence in ASL imaging because of signal-to-noise advantages, but they are often accompanied by blurring artifacts if not implemented properly.

We will then proceed to discuss the technical considerations for the analysis of ASL based functional MRI. We divide this section into the *detection* of perfusion changes due to brain activity and the *quantification* of perfusion from the ASL signal.

Linear regression techniques are typically used for detection of activation in ASL data, just as with BOLD data. However, ASL techniques typically rely on the subtraction of images acquired following a labeling pulse from control images that are free of label, in order to extract the perfusion information. As we will discuss in greater detail, there are several subtraction schemes that can be used to isolate the perfusion signal from the raw data. Each of these schemes has an effect on the content and properties of the resulting perfusion weighted signals. We will describe methods to leverage those statistical properties in order to maximize the statistical power of the analysis.

We then address the question of quantifying perfusion from the ASL images. We will discuss the tracer kinetics theory necessary for quantification, and we discuss strategies for quantifying perfusion from time-series data where the perfusion level is changing due to a known stimulation paradigm. In particular, we will discuss how the parameter estimates obtained in the same linear regression procedure used for signal detection can be used to obtain quantitative measures of perfusion both at baseline and perfusion increases due to neuronal activation.

2. Why perfusion FMRI?

Blood Oxygenation Level Dependent (BOLD) contrast fMRI is currently the dominant technique for functional imaging and has yielded a wealth of information about brain function. The observed BOLD contrast arises from a combination of several indirect phenomena that correlate with neuronal brain activation, such as increases in blood volume and perfusion and a decrease in the concentration of deoxy-hemoglobin, that causes the observed BOLD signal intensity to increase in the active area. However, this signal increase is a non-linear function of many physiological parameters as well as the scanner's own characteristics (Boynton, Engel et al. 1996; Buxton and Frank 1997; Buxton, Wong et al. 1998; Vazquez and Noll 1998). As a consequence, BOLD imaging results are typically reported as unitless statistical significance maps without a clear, quantitative, physiological interpretation.

One issue plaguing the BOLD effect technique is that, since the BOLD effect is based on sensitivity to local changes in magnetic susceptibility, artifacts due to susceptibility gradients are also greatly exacerbated. These artifacts are especially problematic in areas of the brain that lie near air spaces, such as the roof of the mouth, nose and ear canals, as well as the sinuses (Bandettini, Wong et al. 1992; Kwong, Belliveau et al. 1992).

The structure of the drift noise within a session has been shown to be autoregressive (Lund, Madsen et al. 2006) and difficult to remove or model. Furthermore, the height and shape of the BOLD response depend on the baseline perfusion and metabolic levels, and thus effects of interest can be confounded by the conditions of the experimental resting state (Cohen, Ugurbil et al. 2002; Mulderink, Gitelman et al. 2002). Thus, noise properties and drift of the BOLD signal make studies with long activation periods nearly impossible, as the effects of interest are confounded with the slow scanner drifts (Smith, Lewis et al. 1999). The same reasons prevent BOLD FMRI studies from answering questions about baseline conditions. For example, what is the effect of a given drug, therapy, or training regimen on the baseline activity of a brain structure of interest? How do the neural substrates of a specific cognitive function change with age?

Hence, there is a clear need for development of alternative and/or complementary *quantitative* methods to BOLD imaging for FMRI. As technology develops, we expect a paradigm shift toward quantitative methods that offer meaningful physiological interpretation and comparison across laboratories.

This is where perfusion comes in. Perfusion is a readily quantifiable physiological parameter, and is easier to relate to neuronal metabolism than the BOLD response. Furthermore, animal studies conducted at high field, and high spatial resolution have indicated that neuronal activity produces perfusion (Cerebral Blood Flow - CBF) changes that are more localized to the parenchyma than the BOLD effect, consistent with the notion that the BOLD effect is more weighted toward draining veins and away from the active tissue (Duong, Yacoub et al. 2002; Pfeuffer, Adriany et al. 2002; Nencka and Rowe 2007; Olafsson, Noll et al. 2008). Thus, a fast, repeatable technique to measure cerebral perfusion *directly* would be very desirable and complementary to BOLD imaging.

We note that recent blood volume imaging techniques, such as VASO (Lu, Law et al. 2005) and AVIS (Vazquez, Lee et al. 2006), hold promise for quantitative FMRI, but they are severely hampered in terms of signal to noise ration (SNR), temporal resolution, and multi-slice imaging capability in their present state. The corresponding models for quantification require many assumptions and/or multiple measurements per time point. (Gu, Lu et al. 2006; Changwei, Kai-Hsiang et al. 2008; Jin and Kim 2008 ; Christopher, Ronald et al. 2009). Other methods that indirectly measure the rate of oxygen consumption by the brain are also available, but they require ASL data and calibration studies involving hypercapnia experiments (Davis, Kwong et al. 1998; Hoge, Atkinson et al. 1999). Thus, at this stage, they are not practical for dynamic quantitative functional imaging and will not be the focus of this chapter.

3. A survey of quantitative perfusion imaging methods

Blood flow through any organ has been used as an important measure of its health and functionality for a long time (Kety and Schmidt 1945; Lassen and Perl 1979). As such, many techniques have been developed to measure blood flow based on tracer injections. The central idea behind these is always the same: some substance that can be detected easily (i.e. - radioactivity or fluorescence) gets injected somewhere upstream of the organ of interest, either an artery feeding of the tissue, a vein, or directly into the left ventricle of the heart. Then the concentration of the tracer is measured with the appropriate detector as it travels through the tissue of interest. Perfusion can then be calculated from the uptake curve of the tracer in the tissue.

With the advent of new imaging techniques, the detection process was incorporated into the imaging process, as in autoradiography, PET, or SPECT scanners. These imaging modalities use radioactive tracers to generate the raw signals from which the images are reconstructed. Hence, it was a straightforward leap to use the timing information in order to quantify perfusion through the existing tracer kinetic models.

In the case of MRI, perfusion can also be obtained by imaging the passage of a tracer through the tissue. Instead of being radioactive, though, MRI tracers are molecules that change the relaxation rates of blood and tissue – typically gadolinium compounds, such as Gd-DOTA or Gd-DTPA. MRI has the added benefit that it allows for fairly rapid imaging (1-2 seconds for a whole brain volume) so one can sample the wash-in and wash-out of the tracer through the tissue. One can also simultaneously measure the amount of dispersion of the bolus that occurs during the transit from the injection site to the region of interest. Knowledge of this dispersion provides a more accurate estimate of the tissue's perfusion rate. Unfortunately, one can only do one contrast injection at a time, as the tracer takes many hours to clear the body, so it is not a very useful technique for FMRI.

Thus, our focus is on arterial spin labeling (ASL) techniques. The principle behind ASL imaging is conceptually simple. As with other techniques, the measurement consists of measuring the concentration of a tracer as it passes through a tissue of interest. We will discuss the details in more depth later in this chapter, but for now, note that ASL deviates from the usual tracer strategy in two ways. First and foremost, no tracer is injected. Instead, the tracer is "created" inside the arteries feeding the organ by radio frequency (RF) electromagnetic pulses. These pulses are generated by standard MRI coils and invert the magnetization state of the water protons in the blood. After allowing a short period of time for inflow of the tracer into the tissue of interest, an image is collected. Just like in previous techniques, perfusion can be quantified by measuring the signal change due to the tracer – typically by subtracting the image with the tracer from a control image without the tracer. The second important difference is that the tracer used in ASL decays very quickly, since the longitudinal relaxation rate of arterial blood is in the order of 1600 ms. As a result, there is a significant penalty in the signal-to-noise ratio (SNR) but, on the bright side, the experiment can be repeated immediately and as many times as desired. One can think of ASL as a tracer (also referred to as "label" or "tag") that is completely non-toxic, rapidly decaying and it can be selectively injected into any artery (Detre, Leigh et al. 1992; Williams, Detre et al. 1992).

4. ASL and functional MRI

Although ASL is still limited by SNR and temporal resolution relative to BOLD imaging, some features of ASL make it a preferable option in many situations. The most important feature of ASL is the ability to quantify perfusion from the signal difference. This poses a significant advantage over BOLD contrast in that it allows the study of absolute baseline activity (i.e. – resting state) without comparison to an active state. This type of measurement is particularly desirable for studies concerned with pathological states, and/or testing the effects and specificity of different drugs. This ability to quantify perfusion is extremely useful in longitudinal studies over scanning sessions, whether involving activation or limited to the resting state. For example, we have used quantitative ASL to study the long-term effects of working memory training on brain activity, both at rest and during the performance of working memory tasks (Jaeggi, Studer et al. 2009).

Another interesting feature is that although the residual variance of an ASL time course within a single run is higher than with BOLD, it has been shown that the variance of non-quantitative ASL studies (i.e., relative CBF) across scanning sessions is dramatically less than that of BOLD, allowing studies that span days or even months (Aguirre, Detre et al. 2002; Wang, Aguirre et al. 2003; Wang, Aguirre et al. 2003). Furthermore, the variance across subjects is also lower in ASL than in BOLD, thus requiring fewer subjects to be scanned per experiment (Tjandra, Brooks et al. 2005).

Arterial spin labeling techniques allow greater flexibility in the image acquisition, especially when examining slow activation paradigms. Hence, they do not require T_2^* weighting and one can use standard Spin Echo imaging to collect the image data, dramatically reducing susceptibility artifacts. Functional imaging studies of the inferior brain structures, such as the basal ganglia, and the orbito-frontal cortex would benefit greatly from such techniques.

5. Some examples of ASL studies

Due to above mentioned properties of functional arterial spin labeling (FASL), it is particularly useful for the study of gradual changes in neural activity, longitudinal and multi-site studies. (N.B. in this chapter, we use the term FASL to indicate ASL time series used for FMRI purposes, but there is no technical difference between FASL and ASL). FASL has been used in several basic and cognitive neuroscience applications. It has been used in many studies to investigate visual, motor and language functions at 1.5T and 3T (Aguirre, Detre et al. 2002; Wang, Aguirre et al. 2003; Kemeny, Ye et al. 2005; Tjandra, Brooks et al. 2005; Leontiev and Buxton 2007; Ances, Leontiev et al. 2008; Chen, Wieckowska et al. 2008; Raoult, Petr et al. 2011) and has been compared to BOLD fMRI (Aguirre, Detre et al. 2002; Chen, Wieckowska et al. 2008; Raoult,

Petr et al. 2011) (Kemeny, Ye et al. 2005) (Tjandra, Brooks et al. 2005) (Hermes, Hagemann et al. 2007) indicating that the intra-individual reproducibility of FASL in terms of the area of activation and activation quantification is comparable to that of BOLD fMRI. FASL however, detects smaller activation volumes than BOLD fMRI but the areas had a high degree of co-localization between subjects. FASL also shows higher specificity compared to BOLD fMRI while maintaining high sensitivity in activation detection in the activated area (Raoult, Petr et al. 2011).

Due to the drift in the BOLD signal, study of slow changes in neural activity using BOLD is quit challenging. FASL is a suitable tool for these studies as well. Motor learning is an example of the gradual changes in the neural activity over time, which cannot be easily assessed using BOLD fMRI. In (Olson, Rao et al. 2006) Olson et al. used FASL to study continuous, gradual changes in neural activity during motor learning. Subjects were required to use four fingers to press keys as quickly and as accurately as possible in response to the presentation of visual cues. Olson et al. reported that subjects performing this task demonstrated a reduction of neural activity in response to motor execution after training as compared to the start of training. Because the change in performance is slow and continuous, it is assumed for this study that the neural correlate of performance improvement during training is a gradual reduction in regional activity. The authors used FASL to detect these neural changes and reported reliable correlations between performance improvements and decreases in blood flow in premotor cortex and the inferior parietal lobe. This study suggests that FASL is a suitable tool for the study of the slow changes in the neural activity resulting from different cognitive tasks.

FASL has also been used in higher level cognitive activation studies. There is an increasing body of evidence pointing to a neurobiological basis of personality. Characterizing the biological bases of personality dimensions is important to explaining individual differences in brain activity associated with more dynamic changes in experience (e.g., a psychotic episode) and cognition (e.g., activation paradigms in functional MRI) (O'Gorman, Kumari et al. 2006). In (O'Gorman, Kumari et al. 2006) O' Gorman et al. explored the biological bases of the major dimensions of models of personality using FASL. In this study, the correlation between personality factors with regional brain function was successfully investigated using FASL. The authors reported associations between perfusion in brain regions (including basal ganglia, thalamus, inferior frontal gyrus, cerebellum and cuneus) and different personality dimensions. These results suggest that variations in perfusion in certain brain regions correlated with variations in personality dimensions may reflect variations in brain function (O'Gorman, Kumari et al. 2006).

FASL provides reliable quantification of absolute cerebral blood flow (CBF) along with excellent reproducibility over long time periods, making ASL a sensitive technique for reliable visualization of brain function during the resting state as well as during task performance. This property allowed Rao et al. (Rao, Gillihan et al. 2007) to employ ASL to investigate the effect of genetic variation of the human serotonin transporter gene on resting brain function of healthy individuals. They studied the alteration of resting brain function in emotion-related regions (including the amygdala and ventromedial prefrontal cortex) in healthy individuals caused by the 5-HTTLPR genotype. Valid and reliable inferences of resting activity for applications such as this study could not be derived from BOLD fMRI because it only measures *relative* changes in neural activity, and the changes in signal intensity from scanner drift are much larger than the effects of interest.

Also, using ASL, authors (Rao, Gillihan et al. 2007) demonstrated an association of 5-HTTLPR genotype with resting amygdala and ventromedial prefrontal cortex function in the healthy human brain. Such alterations suggest a broad role of the 5-HTT gene in brain function that may be associated with the genetic susceptibility for mood disorders such as depression.

Neuronal modulations found using functional ASL (FASL), such as those reported in (O'Gorman, Kumari et al. 2006) and (Rao, Gillihan et al. 2007), may also be important in interpretation of the different manifestations of BOLD response (which typically rely on the modulation of cerebral hemodynamics for detection of task-induced activation) to a particular stimuli in different groups.

The presence of low frequency signal drift in the BOLD signal impedes using a long task block. This problem makes it difficult to investigate slow processes such as learning, emotion, sustained attention and behavioral states in healthy and clinical populations. Because of its efficacy in longitudinal designs and low frequency paradigms, FASL is a good candidate for these studies. Kim et al. (Kim, Whyte et al. 2006) successfully utilized FASL to study an uninterrupted 6-min continuous performance of the two high-level cognitive tasks (visual sustained attention and verbal working memory) which prior to FASL was only feasible for suboptimal short data acquisition blocks (40-90s). Understanding the neural correlates of these cognition function is very important because sustained attention is also implicated in various clinical disorders including attention deficit hyperactivity disorder, traumatic brain injury, and Alzheimer's disease (Kim, Whyte et al. 2006).

In another study, Rao et al. (Rao, Wang et al. 2007) used FASL and BOLD to measure brain activation patterns associated with natural vision while subjects were freely viewing a cartoon movie. Rao et al. reported that cerebral blood flow increases in multiple visual pathway areas and frontal areas, and decreases in ventromedial frontal cortex and superior temporal cortex during movie viewing compared to resting states. Concurrent BOLD contrast revealed similar but weaker activation and deactivation patterns. This study demonstrates the feasibility of using FASL for imaging both sustained and dynamic effects in neural activation during natural and ecologically valid situations (Rao, Wang et al. 2007).

With excellent reproducibility over long-term time periods, FASL is ideal for imaging a sustained behavioral state, such as stress. Wang et al (Wang, Rao et al. 2005) used FASL technique to measure perfusion changes associated with mild to moderate stress. The authors demonstrated that a positive correlation exists between the change in perfusion induced by the stress task and subjective stress rating in the ventral right prefrontal cortex and left insula/ putamen area. This study provides neuroimaging evidence that psychological stress induces negative emotion and vigilance and that the ventral right prefrontal cortex plays a key role in the central stress response.

Pharmacological functional (phMRI) studies are making a significant contribution to our understanding of drug effects on brain systems. Since noise spectrum of arterial spin labeling signal contains relatively less power at low frequencies, it is particularly useful for phMRI studies in which a change in brain activity is expected over the course of minutes, hours, or days to asses low frequency between- and within-session drug-induced changes (Wise and Tracey 2006) (16). As an example, Gollub et al. (Gollub, Breiter et al. 1998) used FASL to measure neuronal activation during visual stimulation before and after cocaine and saline infusions. The authors used FASL to determine whether acute intravenous cocaine use would change global cerebral blood flow and demonstrated that cortical gray matter cerebral blood flow was unchanged after saline infusion but decreased after cocaine infusion.

These studies demonstrate that FASL can be successfully utilized for the investigation of the cerebral blood flow changes associated with development of human brain, personality, high level cognitive operations, the behavioral states such as attention, natural vision, psychological stress and assessing low frequency drug effects. Increased applications of FASL to the investigation of cognitively impaired populations are expected to follow.

5. ASL methods

Now that we've seen the bigger picture, let's examine the details of carrying out the acquisition and analysis of ASL data. Any ASL sequence is basically made up of a labeling period, during which the inversion label is created, some delay time to allow the label to reach the tissue of interest, and then an imaging pulse sequence where the image is acquired. There may be additional pulses to shape the input function before the acquisition part, and there may be multiple coils involved in some variants, but in general, the structure remains the same. Thus, it is convenient to discuss labeling and imaging schemes independently, as they can be combined in multiple ways.

6. Labeling schemes

There are a number of MRI pulse sequence strategies that can be used to obtain ASL perfusion images. The first class of arterial spin labeling pulse sequences is "Continuous arterial spin labeling" (CASL). In the original continuous ASL formulation, low-power, long pulses (in the order of a second or two) are applied at a plane inferior to the brain. Typically this is below the circle of Willis where the arterial supply to the brain is perpendicular to the labeling plane. As usual, in order to achieve slice selection, the long RF pulses are applied at some frequency offset and in the presence of a slice-selective gradient. These pulses have very different effects on the stationary and the moving spins. While the stationary spins at the labeling plane become saturated and lose phase coherence (essentially destroying their magnetization), the spins that are moving through the labeling plane experience a gradual change of their resonant frequency (recall that the resonant frequency is directly proportional to the magnetic field). The difference between the resonance frequency of the protons and the transmission frequency changes from positive through negative as the spins move through the inversion plane and is zero at the center of it.

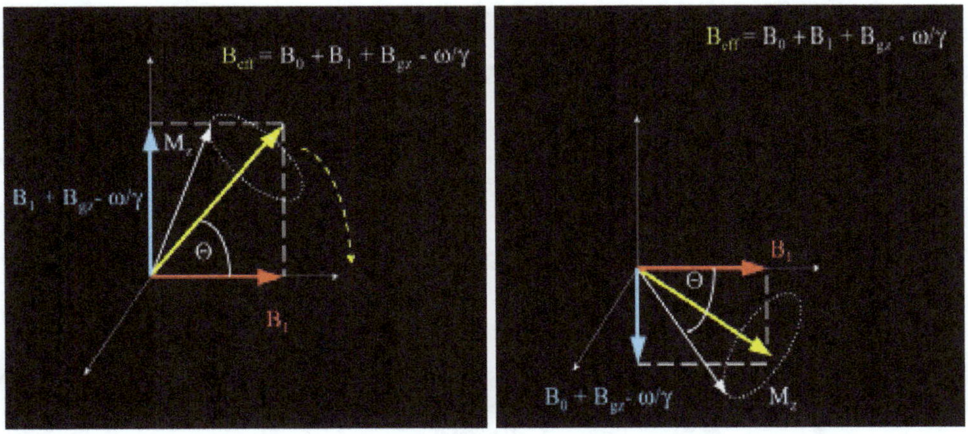

Figure 1. The Adiabatic Inversion Process - 1A – In the rotating frame of reference the magnetic fields due to the scanner's main magnetic field (B0), the RF coil's field (B1), the slice select gradient (Bz) and the opposing magnetization field add up to an "effective magnetic field" (Beff). The arterial water's magnetization vector precesses around Beff. 1B- As the spins move, the contribution from the slice select changes from positive to negative. As this happens, the magnetization vector continues to precess around the effective field, resulting in the inversion of the magnetization vector.

Because of this effective "frequency sweep", the net magnetic field generated by the combination of the main magnetic field (B0), the applied RF field (B1eff) and the magnetic field resulting from the spin's precession itself (ω/γ) experiences a rotation from pointing along the direction of the main magnetic field to pointing against it (see figure 1). If this rotation is slow relative to the precession frequency, the effect of the constant RF pulse on these moving spins is to create a "spin-locked" state. This means that the flowing proton's magnetization processes around the effective magnetic field and follows it as it rotated from pointing up to pointing down.

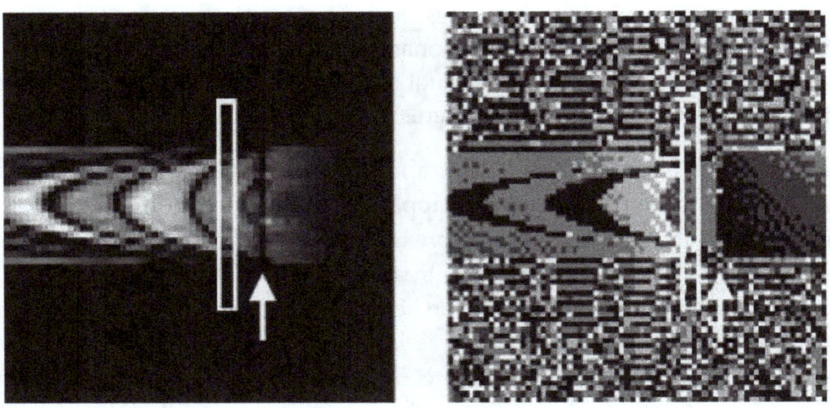

Figure 2. This image shows the magnitude (left) and phase (right) of an image of water flowing through a tube while experiencing adiabatic inversion. The banding pattern reflects periods where the pulses were turned on and off. Figure reproduced from (Hernandez-Garcia, Lewis et al. 2007).

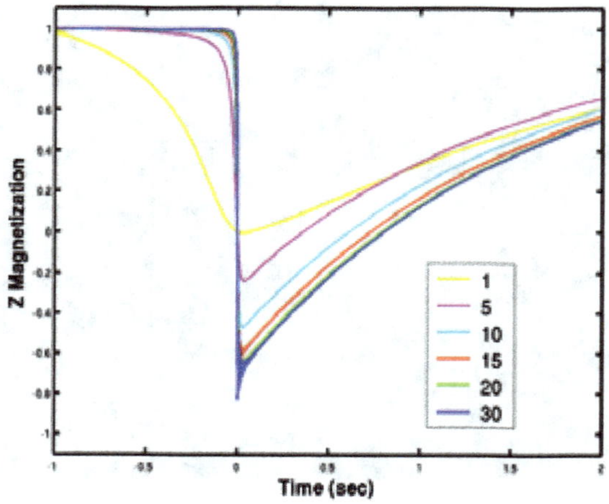

Figure 3. The longitudinal magnetization of the arterial water experiences adiabatic inversion at the labeling plane, then slowly decays back to its relaxed state. This phenomenon depends on a number of factors, such as the velocity of the spins, and the size of the slice select gradient and the RF fields used in the pulse sequence.

As the protons move through the inversion plane, the "effective" field (B_{eff}) to which they are locked rotates from pointing along the direction of the main magnetic field to pointing against it. The end result is that when the flowing spins leave the plane, their magnetization is inverted (figure 2 shows a practical demonstration of this phenomenon). This phenomenon is referred to as "flow driven adiabatic inversion" and is the basis for continuous arterial spin labeling techniques. It is important to note that immediately after inversion, the spins experience T1 relaxation and the label effectively decays in a matter of a couple of seconds, as depicted in figure 3.

The main caveat of continuous ASL is that the long inversion pulses applied at the neck for labeling purposes also produce a significant amount of magnetization transfer (MT) (Detre, Leigh et al. 1992; Williams, Detre et al. 1992) in the spins at the tissue of interest. Briefly, magnetization transfer consists of signal loss during acquisition when it is preceded by RF pulses, even if those are not applied on resonance. As a result of MT, subtracting a tagged image from a control image would indicate not only the perfusion effects but also the degree of magnetization transfer, which is of no interest to the investigator.

This would constitute a major obstacle, but a number of solutions have been devised. The original solution to this problem was to apply an MT preparation pulse with identical properties to those of the labeling pulse before collecting the control image. This preparation pulse was identical to labeling pulse but with a reversed slice select gradient such that the inversion pulse would be centered above the head. In that case, there is only magnetization transfer but no arterial spin labeling. While this works in principle, it is difficult to collect more than one slice at a time while appropriately compensated magnetization transfer symmetrically for all the slices. Another solution was to simply use a separate RF coil for labeling whose field pattern will not reach the brain (Zhang, Silva et al. 1995) (Talagala, Ye et al. 2004) (Hernandez-Garcia, Lee et al. 2004). While this approach works quite well and relatively simple to implement in principle, in practice it requires additional hardware that can be synchronized with the main MRI scanner's pulse sequence. It is also generally uncomfortable for the subjects to wear the additional neck coil and it can pose some logistical pulses.

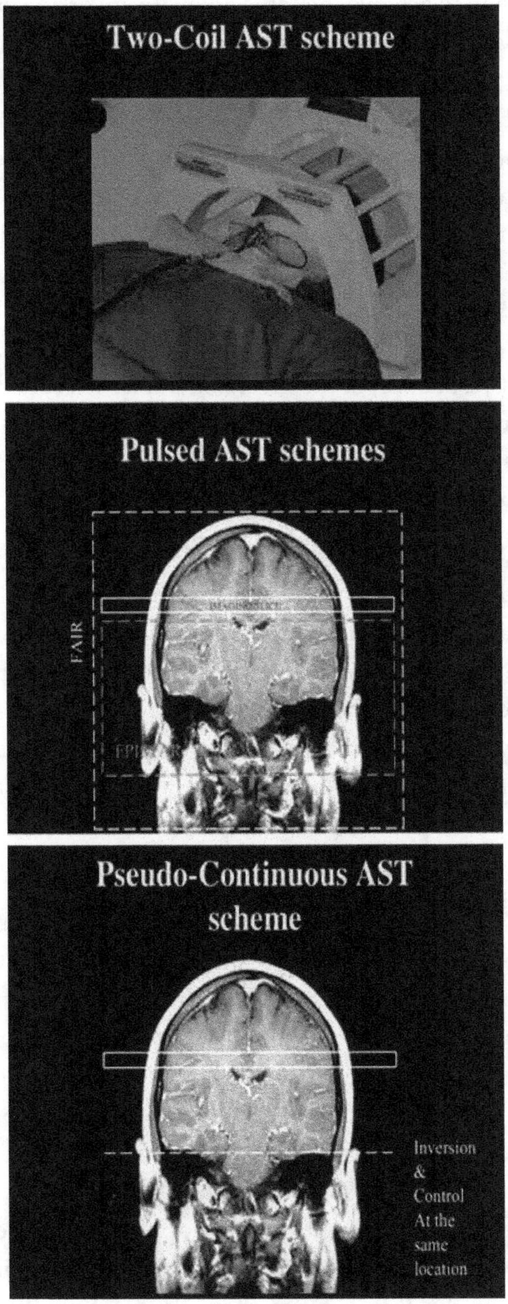

Figure 4. Labeling Schemes - Schematics indicating the relative locations of the inversion types of popular ASL schemes

Several other strategies to overcome the magnetization transfer problem have been tried to overcome this problem, such as amplitude modulated CASL (Wang, Zhang et al. 2005), but the most promising one is to break up the continuous labeling pulse into a train of pulses applied in rapid succession to achieve the same adiabatic inversion effect. In the control case, however, the same pulse train is applied but the phase of every other pulse is shifted by 180 degrees, such that every other pulse "un-does" the flip of the previous pulse. The end result is that both the control and the labeled image receive the same amount of magnetization transfer, the flowing blood's magnetization gets inverted prior to collecting the labeled image but it remains un-inverted during the collection of the control image. This technique, known as pseudo-continuous arterial spin labeling (PCASL) has greatly facilitated the use of continuous ASL because it addresses the magnetization transfer issue and is relatively easy to implement (Garcia, de Bazelaire et al. 2005; Wang, Zhang et al. 2005; Fernandez-Seara, Wang et al. 2007; Wu, Fernandez-Seara et al. 2007). The caveat is that PCASL is sensitive to magnetic field inhomogeneity (off-resonance) at the inversion plane. This effect can severely affect the efficiency of the labeling process, crippling the technique, and is exacerbated at higher magnetic fields. Fortunately, the loss of inversion efficiency can be recovered by adjusting the phase of the inversion pulses and introducing compensation gradients (Jahanian, Noll et al. 2011).

A second class of arterial spin labeling pulse sequences is "pulsed ASL" (PASL). This strategy is to label a slab containing the arterial supply to the organ of interest with a more standard, short RF inversion pulse and then allow the inverted spins to flow from that slab into the tissue of interest. The difference in signal intensity between the two images is provided by the un-inverted spins that flowed into the imaging slices during the inversion delay. This signal intensity difference can then be readily quantified and translated into perfusion images. This process mimics the injection of a bolus of tracer, rather than a constant infusion, as in the case of continuous ASL.

The simplest form of pulsed ASL is the EPISTAR technique (Edelman and Chen 1998), in which the inversion pulse (typically a hyperbolic secant) applied just below the region of interest followed by a delay to allow the inverted blood to flow into the tissue before collecting the image. Hyperbolic secant pulses are relatively short adiabatic pulses and exhibit no significant magnetization transfer effects, so there is no need for pre-compensation pulses before collecting the reference image. In the FAIR technique (the original pulsed ASL technique) the control image is preceded by an inversion pulse applied over the entire brain, followed by a short delay (Kim 1995; Kim and Tsekos 1997). The tagged image is collected following a similar hyperbolic secant inversion pulse, except that it is applied only over the slices of interest, followed again by the same short delay to allow for inflow of blood into the imaging region. There are many variants on this theme, but perhaps the most popular pulsed ASL technique is QUIPSS which uses additional pulses to saturate the trailing edges of the label, thus producing a clearly defined bolus (Wong, Buxton et al. 1997; Wong, Buxton et al. 1998).

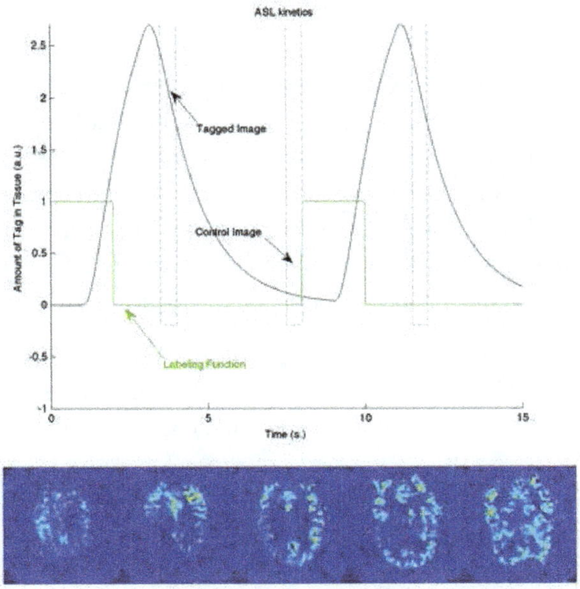

Figure 5. A - The uptake and release of the inversion label is relatively short, so there is only a limited amount of time to collect the images without a significant signal change. While including long post inversion delays reduce the sensitivity to the difference in slice timing, there is still only a limited amount of time to collect the images. If the process takes too long, different slices will have different SNR and sensitivity to perfusion changes from activation. B – This image, originally consisting of 24 slices, shows a noticeable change in SNR between the top and bottom slices. Here we only show slices 6, 9, 12, 15.

Whereas the pulsed approach only requires 1-2 seconds for the label to reach its maximum concentration in the tissue the continuous approach requires approximately 3 seconds before a steady state concentration of tag is reached. However, because of the longer inversion times of the continuous labeling scheme, the amount of tag to be detected is much larger and thus, the SNR of the method is also larger (Buxton, Frank et al. 1998; Wong, Buxton et al. 1998). Thus, the tradeoff between them is primarily one of speed versus SNR.

7. Image acquisition considerations in ASL

Image collection following the spin labeling process can be done in a number of ways, but it is important to take into account the goals of the specific application. As usual in MRI, there is a trade-off between acquisition speed, SNR and resolution.

In clinical and resting state applications, typical ASL scans use more standard image acquisition pulse sequences since the speed consideration is relaxed. Fast spin-echo acquisitions are a popular method because of their insensitivity to off-resonance artifacts and relatively high SNR and speed. For example (Fernandez-Seara, Wang et al. 2005; Fernandez-Seara, Wang et al. 2007) used a 3D GRASE acquisition sequence in conjunction with continuous ASL in order to boost the SNR of the acquired images in a functional imaging study of the medial temporal lobe.

Functional MRI requires image acquisition speed in order to capture the hemodynamic changes that take place during mental activity adequately. Fast imaging techniques that take advantage of echo-planar and echo-volumar acquisition and parallel imaging allow us to image the whole brain in a matter of a second or two with high spatial resolution. Consider the figure below, which indicates the concentration of tag in the tissue as it is taken up. Unfortunately, the rates at which the flows in and out of the tissue while decaying is such that we are constrained to roughly a half a second to acquire the whole volume.

If one slice is collected at the beginning of the uptake and another toward the end, the perfusion contrast will be vastly different. While one can account for it by including this delay in the quantification scheme, the SNR of the slices can still be significantly different.

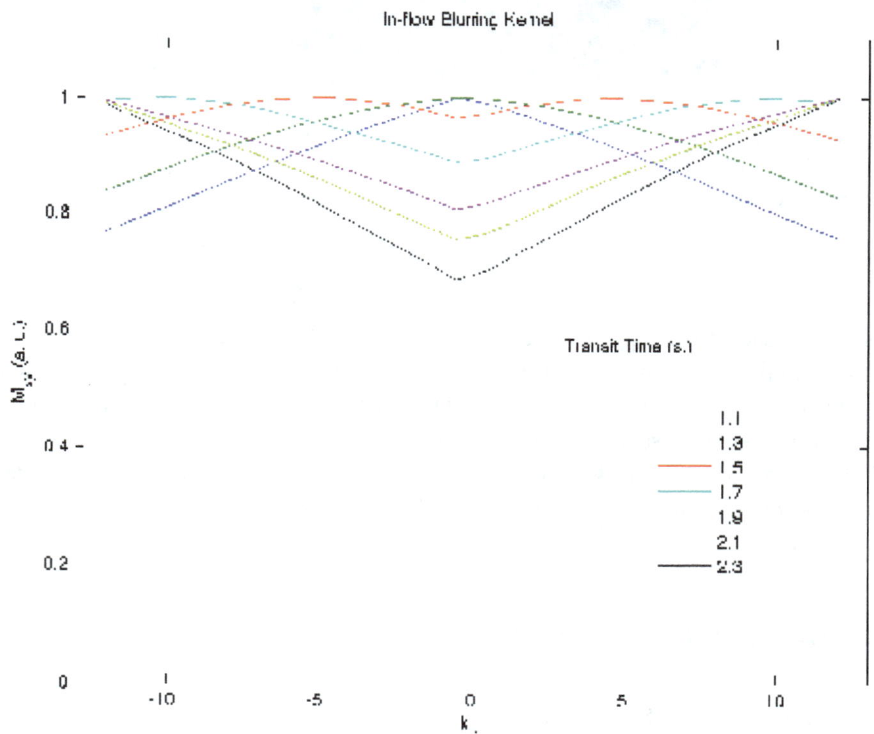

Figure 6. Depending on the transit time of the blood from the labeling plane to the imaging slab, the uptake of the label can induce a mild distortion along the slab-select location (or kz). Interestingly, this effect can be characterized by a point spread function that acts as either a high-pass or low-pass filter along the kz axis.

This acquisition time window means that there is a significant constraint in the number of slices that one can get after a single labeling period. For instance, using a fast spiral acquisition typically allows for acquisition of a single slice in at least 25 ms. At this rate one can acquire

20 slices in half a second, which is adequate but requires thick slices of about 6 mm thickness, assuming a 12 cm brain.

In this regard, there is recent interest in the development of 3D echo-planar and echo-volumar acquisition schemes. 3D imaging schemes can ensure the same acquisition delay for the entire imaging volume relative to the labeling period. The SNR of 3D imaging can be greater than 2D multislice because a larger volume contributes to each echo. For example, Gunther et al (Gunther, Oshio et al. 2005) proposed a multi-echo 3D acquisition that allows collection of a k-space plane at each echo. Unfortunately, this acquisition scheme imposes a T2 weighting on each plane of k-space depending on the acquisition order. The result is typically a severe blur of the volume along the z-direction. One can think of this as a blurring filter applied along the slice direction, and the shape of that filter's point spread function (PSF) is that of the T2 decay.

Another 3D alternative is to use multi-shot readouts as in (Talagala, Ye et al. 2004) but these typically require the use of low flip angles to preserve the magnetization throughout all the kz encoding steps. Low flip angles however result in reduction of the available signal. Gai et al (Gai, Talagala et al. 2011) have experimented with an increasing flip-angle schedule starting at 10 degrees that produces a constant signal along kz according to the Ernst formula. This approach produces a flat PSF, but at the cost of SNR. In recent investigation, we have found that a flip angle schedule that starts at 15 degrees and increases with a simple third order polynomial is a good compromise between SNR and blurring along the slice direction. The figure below illustrates this issue by calculating the PSF along the z-direction of different order polynomial flip angle schedules.

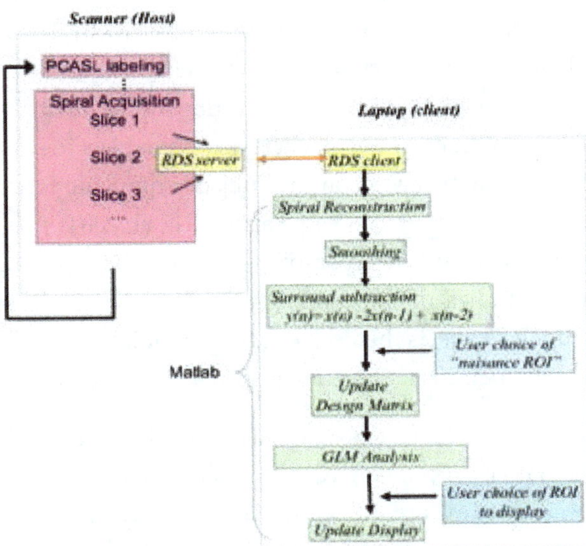

Figure 7. Real Time imaging with ASL requires coordination of the scanner's acquisition with an external computer that "catches" the data as it is generated by the scanner and carries out the analysis within the interval between two images. (Figure from (Hernandez-Garcia, Jahanian et al. 2011))

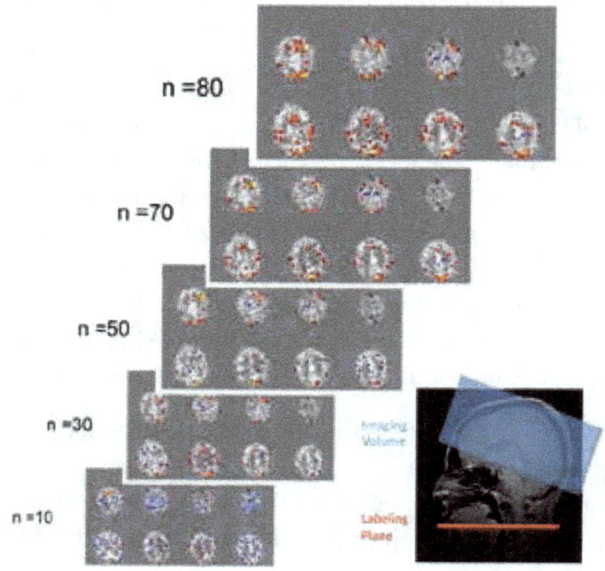

Figure 8. This figure shows an updated view of the real time FASL acquisition during a visuo-motor stimulation paradigm. As one can see, the activation maps evolve over time and become better defined as more data become available. (Figure from (Hernandez-Garcia, Jahanian et al. 2011))

Real-time functional magnetic resonance imaging (rtfMRI) is an exciting extension to conventional fMRI techniques that enables the user to analyze fMRI data as it is being collected. The requisite is that the reconstruction and analysis must be carried out before acquisition of the next image in the time series (about two seconds for standard FMRI). Thus, in rtfMRI the results are immediately available as the subject is being scanned, and can be used to reveal and/or guide the subject's cognitive processes. Thus, by collecting the data in real time, the investigator can fine tune the design's parameters to suit each specific subject (deCharms 2008). One can also design interactive paradigms based on the subject's dynamic functional activity (fMRI biofeedback or brain-computer interface (Yoo, Fairneny et al. 2004)). Furthermore, it allows the investigator to determine the subject's compliance during the experiment. Examples of real time FMRI also include studies of the modulation of motor-area cortical activation and emotional processing by the subjects themselves (Yoo and Jolesz 2002; Posse, Fitzgerald et al. 2003; deCharms, Christoff et al. 2004; Phan, Fitzgerald et al. 2004; Caria, Veit et al. 2007).

A number of processing strategies have been developed in order to carry out real time FMRI analysis, such as cumulative correlation (Cox, Jesmanowicz et al. 1995), sliding-window correlations with reference vector optimization (Gembris, Taylor et al. 2000), online general linear model [GLM] analysis (Nakai, Bagarinao et al. 2006). There are also a number of combined methods to collect behavioral, physiological and MRI data while performing near real-time statistical analysis (Voyvodic 1999). The recent advances in computational speed have made it relatively easy to implement any of these analysis methods.

8. Quantifying perfusion from the ASL signal

In the original implementation of continuous ASL, quantification was done by writing the well-known Bloch equations that describe the longitudinal magnetization with one modification: the authors included terms to account for the inflow of arterial blood and outflow of venous blood. (Recall that the Bloch equations describe the behavior of a magnetization vector in the presence of magnetic fields such as the ones present in an MRI pulse sequence Please see textbooks like Haacke's (Haacke 1999) or Bernstein (Bernstein, King et al. 2004) for an introduction). Like this $\frac{dM_{tissue}(t)}{dt} = f \cdot M_{art}(t) - \frac{f}{\lambda} \cdot M_{tissue}(t) - \frac{M_{tissue}(t)}{T1}$

Here, $M_{tissue}(t)$ would be the longitudinal magnetization of the tissue protons. $M_{art}(t)$ is the incoming arterial magnetization. In the control image it would be positive, but in the labeled image, it would be negative. Note that this must be adjusted to reflect the efficiency of the inversion efficiency (α) and its decay during transit time from the labeling plane to the tissue (Δ). Hence, $M_{art}(t) = (2\alpha e^{-(\Delta/T1art)} M_{art}(0))$.

T_{1art} and T_1 are the longitudinal relaxation rates of the arterial blood and the tissue. The parameter λ is blood brain partition coefficient and it relates the concentrations of label in blood and tissue at equilibrium. The key parameter is f, the perfusion rate that describes the rate at which water moves in and out of the tissue. By writing the steady state solutions for this equation in the case of control and tagged images, one can solve for f.

An equivalent but perhaps more generalizable approach was presented by Buxton et al (Buxton, Frank et al. 1998) in which they treated the ASL experiment as a standard tracer kinetics experiment. In this formulation, the concentration of "label" in the tissue, C_{tissue} is given by the subtraction of control and tagged images, and can be modeled as a linear system. In that case, the observed signal difference between control and tagged images is the convolution of an input function with a system function.

$$C_{tissue}(t) = f \cdot M_{art}(t) * [r(t)m(t)]$$

In this case, the input function is a fraction of the arterial blood (determined by the perfusion rate, f). The system function is a combination of the tissue "retention" function, e^{-ft}, which describes how the label clears away with an exponential decay, and also the T_1 decay function of the tag in the tissue, e^{-t/T_1}.

In subsequent work the pulse sequence's timing parameters, including the TR, duration of the tagging period (ω), post inversion delay (τ) and transit time (δ) were taken into account to yield the following equation relating the subtraction image (ΔM) to the perfusion rate. If the post inversion delay is longer than the transit time, the perfusion rate can be calculated by

$$f = \frac{\lambda \cdot \Delta M \cdot R_{1\,app}}{\left(\frac{M_{control}}{1 - e^{-TR \cdot R_1}}\right) \cdot 2 \cdot \alpha \cdot e^{-\delta \cdot R_{1a}} \left(e^{(\delta - \omega) \cdot R_{1app}} - e^{(\delta - \tau - \omega) \cdot R_{1app}}\right)}.$$

Note that R_1 is simply the reciprocal of the T_1 relaxation rate (or $1/T_1$) used for convenience. In keeping with the notation of the authors, R_{1a} refers to the relaxation of arterial blood and R_{1app} refers to the apparent relaxation rate of the tissue.

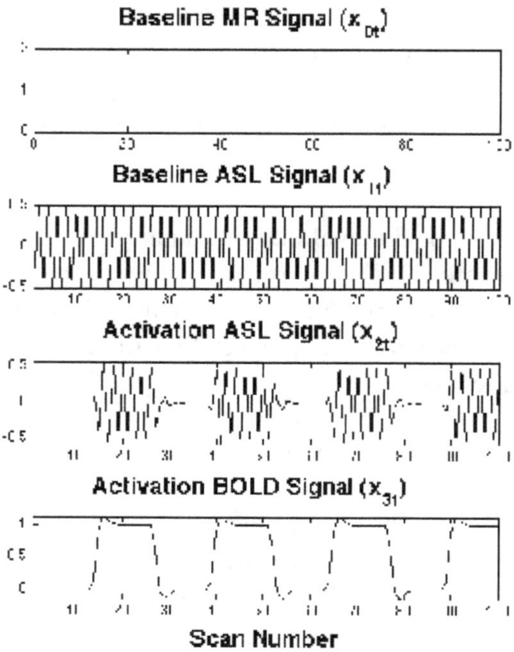

Figure 9. The regressors in a design matrix for a simple functional ASL experiment (only two conditions) include both the usual baseline and BOLD effects (regressors 0 and 2). In order to capture the variance due to resting and activation blood flow, we must include regressor 1 and 3, which are modulated by the presence of the arterial label. Reproduced from (Hernandez-Garcia, Jahanian et al. 2010)

On a practical note, R_{1a} and R_{1app} may vary from subject to subject when dealing with clinical populations or across age groups, so in those cases, it is important to make those measurements separately and use the measured values in the calculation. In the healthy subjects typically used for FMRI research, this is not so much of a factor and literature values are typically employed for the relaxation rates.

9. Quantification of perfusion in FASL data

While the above framework is useful for situations where perfusion is constant, it's more challenging to quantify dynamic perfusion changes as in the case of FMRI experiments. The very slow sampling rate of ASL makes it difficult to get perfusion values during the transitions between active and resting states, so investigators are often forced to settle for collecting only a few perfusion measurements obtained at the baseline and a few measurements at the plateau of the activation, and none from the transition. Unfortunately, this reduces the number of samples available for quantification, which can be fatal in a low SNR technique like ASL. Furthermore, it precludes event-related fMRI, where there is not much of a plateau of activation.

In order to overcome this problem, one can formulate a general linear model (GLM) that specifies BOLD and ASL effects. One can then estimate the coefficients of this model and translate them into meaningful, quantitative measures of perfusion by using standard tracer kinetic models. This concept is based on the simple realization that the difference images used in ASL quantitative models have a direct relationship to the coefficients (or amplitudes) of the regressors or the general linear model. Since estimation of a general linear model is the standard way of analyzing FMRI data by the bulk of the functional imaging community, this approach constitutes a natural next step in the analysis.

For example, let us consider an ASL FMRI experiment with a baseline condition and a single activation condition with tag and control ASL images acquired in each. One such experiment can be characterized by a linear model, as previously described (Mumford, Hernandez-Garcia et al. 2006). Let y_t be the time course (a vector) of image intensity at a particular voxel obtained from an ASL experiment. In Fig. 9 are the regressors of a simple ASL design matrix representing the linear model

$$y_t = \beta_0 + \beta_1 x_{1t} + \beta_2 x_{2t} + \beta_3 x_{3t} + \varepsilon_t$$

for time t=1, …, n. The first regressor, the baseline vector $x_{0t,}$ =1 and its coefficient parameter, the scalar β_0, indicate the baseline signal, and can be interpreted as a measure of spin density. The second regressor x_{1t} describes the baseline difference between control and tagged images ($\Delta\Delta M$) and thus its amplitude, β_1, is indicative of baseline perfusion. The third regressor x_{2t} with its regression coefficient β_2 describes differences between control and tagged images (ΔM) due to activation, and the fourth regressor x_{3t} with its regression coefficient β_3 describes the BOLD effect changes. By realizing that the amplitude of the oscillation (β_2) induced by the ASL scheme corresponds to the difference between control and tagged images, perfusion can be computed dynamically by translating the coefficient parameter estimates of the oscillations into the appropriate control-tag differences.

Quantification of perfusion effects in continuous ASL data without background suppression can be done directly by adapting the same kinetic model by Wang et al (Wang, Alsop et al. 2002) that we discussed in the previous section. The ΔM parameters are replaced with the GLM parameter estimates as follows

$$f_{effect,t} = \frac{\lambda \cdot R_{1app} \cdot \hat{\beta}_{effect}}{\left(\frac{\hat{\beta}_0}{1-e^{-TR/T_1}}\right) \cdot 2 \cdot \alpha \cdot e^{-\delta \cdot R_{1a}} \cdot \left(e^{(\delta-\omega) \cdot R_{1app}} - e^{(\delta-\tau-\omega) \cdot R_{1app}}\right)} \cdot x_{effect,t}$$

where $\hat{f}_{effect,t}$ is the estimated perfusion change due to the effect of interest, α is the inversion efficiency, $x_{effect,t}$ is the regressor for the effect at time t, $\hat{\beta}_{effect,t}$ is the coefficient parameter estimate of the regressor representing the effect of interest (for example, the amplitude of the perfusion changes due to activation in the above model are captured by β_2), $\hat{\beta}_0$ is the baseline state signal (T_1-weighted spin density), λ is the blood brain partition coefficient, R_1, R_{1a}, R_{1app}

are the longitudinal relaxation rates of arterial blood, tissue, and tissue in the presence of perfusion. The term δ is the arterial transit time, while *TR, w,* and τ are repetition time, post labeling delay, and labeling duration.

As previously noted (Wang, Alsop et al. 2002), when long post-inversion delays (w) are used, the equation becomes insensitive to changes in arterial transit time. Note also that the sign of $\hat{\beta}_{effect}$ can be positive or negative depending on the acquisition order of the control and tagged pairs.

But, what about the error on those parameter estimates? Both Ordinary and Generalized Least Squares estimation yield estimates of the linear model's parameters as well as their variances. Thus, the same relationship can be used to derive the standard deviation of the estimates in perfusion units. In order to calculate the variance of the estimated *perfusion* effects, we propagate the errors of the relevant coefficient parameter estimates through the kinetic model.

Propagation of error can be calculated in a straightforward way from the partial derivatives of the model relative to the coefficient parameters of interest (Bevington and Robinson 2003). We refer the readers to the article by Hernandez-Garcia et al (Hernandez-Garcia, Jahanian et al. 2010) for the derivation.

We have seen that instead of calculating a perfusion time series one image at a time, we can make a linear model of what that perfusion time series should be, and then estimate the corresponding coefficients and their variance. If the model is accurate, this yields much better estimates of the perfusion time series. To illustrate this point, figure 10 shows the perfusion time courses at a given voxel obtained from the traditional method versus the GLM method. Since the residual variance estimates are reduced, the activation maps and residual variances are greatly improved, as illustrated in figure 11.

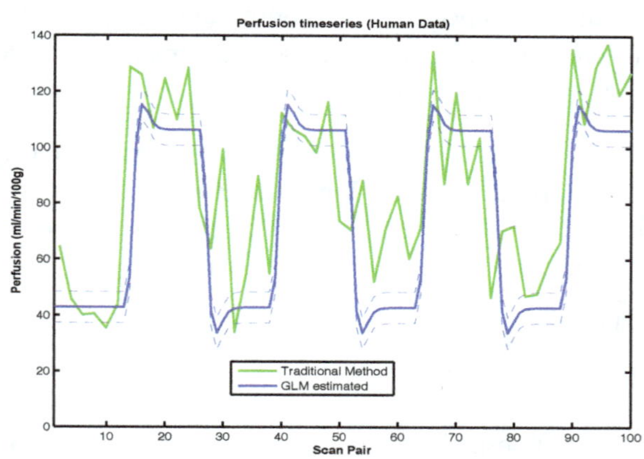

Figure 10. The green line shows the individual perfusion time series calculated at each individual time point. The propagation of errors through the equation makes the result noisy. However, by using all the data at once to estimate the coefficients of a linear model, one can also obtain such a time course if the activation paradigm is known. Reproduced from (Hernandez-Garcia, Jahanian et al. 2010)

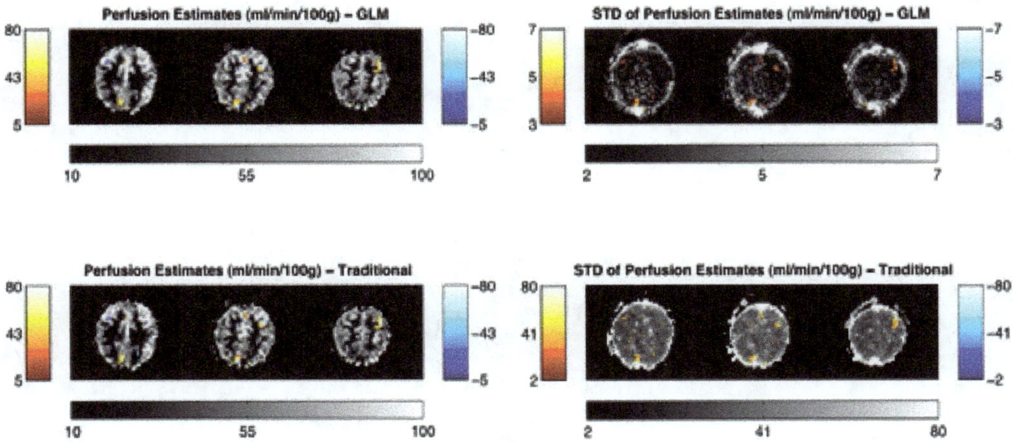

Figure 11. By translating the coefficients of a GLM into perfusion estimates, the residual variance is greatly reduced in comparison to calculating the perfusion time series first and then estimating a general linear model. The result is more accurate activation maps. As with all linear models, one must know the activation paradigm a priori. Reproduced from (Hernandez-Garcia, Jahanian et al. 2010)

10. About the subtraction of the ASL time series

As we have described earlier, the perfusion information in the ASL images is contained in the subtraction of tagged images from control images, which are previously acquired in an alternating order. While differencing the image time course reduces the degree of autocorrelation in ASL data (Aguirre, Detre et al. 2002 ; Liu and Wong 2005) and is widely used, this topic deserves some attention, as there are multiple options available with their corresponding side effects.

In its simplest form, subtraction is done by "pairwise differencing" in which every two images is used to obtain a single perfusion image. As a result, the raw data are no longer autocorrelated, but they are also sub-sampled severely and, consequently, aliasing can occur. By this sub-sampling one also gives up almost half of the degrees of freedom in the analysis, so it translates into a major loss of power. There are other ways to difference the data, however. For example, one can make a "running subtraction" in which one would subtract from every image the previous one, but reverse the sign of the subtraction at every image. Similarly, one would subtract from every control image the average of the two neighboring tagged images (i.e., "surround subtraction"). In this case, only two degrees of freedom are lost, and the data are still whitened. The caveat is that all these differencing processes have a smoothing effect on the time course so fast changes in perfusion are dampened, and we may not be able to observe them. The "sinc subtraction" scheme consists of interpolating the value of the control images at the time of acquisition of the tagged images and, likewise, interpolating the tagged images to obtain their value at the time of the control images. The two up-sampled time courses are then subtracted from each other.

pairwise

$$y_2[m]=y_c[m]-y_t[m] \Leftrightarrow D_2=\begin{pmatrix}1 & -1 & & & & 0\\ & & 1 & -1 & & \\ & & & & \ddots & \\ 0 & & & & 1 & -1\end{pmatrix}$$

running

$$y_3[n]=(-1)^n\cdot(y[n]-y[n+1]) \Leftrightarrow D_3=\begin{pmatrix}1 & -1 & & & 0\\ & -1 & 1 & & \\ & & 1 & -1 & \\ & & & \ddots & \ddots \\ 0 & & & -1 & 1\end{pmatrix}$$

surround

$$y_4[n]=(-1)^n\cdot(2y[n]-y[n+1]-y[n+2]) \Leftrightarrow \begin{pmatrix}1 & -2 & 1 & & & \\ & -1 & 2 & -1 & & \\ & & 1 & -2 & 1 & \\ & & & \ddots & \ddots & \ddots \\ & & & -1 & 2 & -1\end{pmatrix}$$

Figure 12. Examples of differencing matrices that can be used for functional ASL.Whether we use an ordinary least squares (OLS) approach on differenced data or a generalized least squares approach (GLS) on raw data can make a significant difference in the statistical power of the analysis. It's not important for blocked designs, but in the case of event related designs, whose frequency content is relatively higher, it makes a significant difference, whether the inter stimulus interval (ISI) is randomized or not. Reproduced from (Mumford et al. 2006)

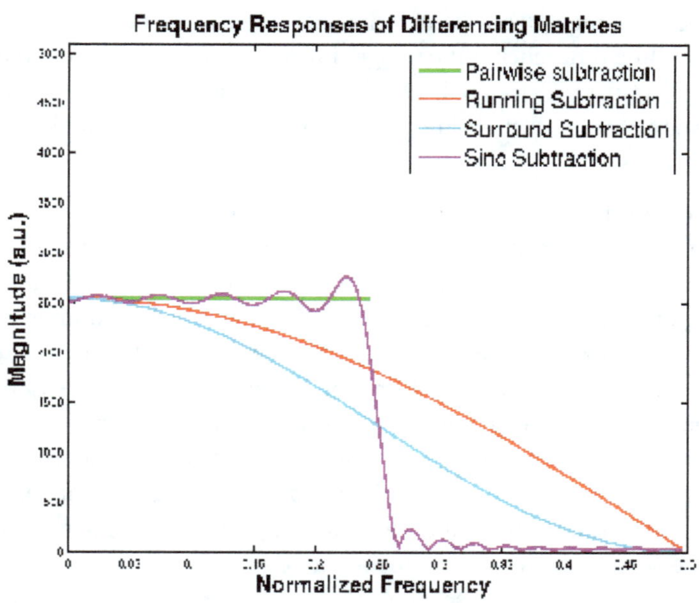

Figure 13. The effect of the differencing process on the frequency content of the ASL signal. Reproduced from (Mumford, Hernandez-Garcia et al. 2006).

From a signal processing point of view it is useful to note that the differencing schemes can be thought of as multiplying the time course by a "differencing matrix". Figure 12 shows some of the differencing matrices that are commonly used. This differencing process, in addition to isolating the perfusion weighting, also behaves like a filter applied to the data and frequency responses can be computed accordingly. For example, figure 13 shows the filtering effect on the frequency content by several differencing "filters".

Those frequency responses can be derived analytically for a given input y[n] whose discrete Fourier transform is given by $Y(e^{jw})$, yielding the equations in Table 1.

Note that pairwise subtraction and sinc subtraction do not have a straightforward linear response since they involve down-sampling the data. In both of those cases, the down-sampling process causes the top half of the frequency spectrum to alias into the bottom half before the filtering process. In terms of their frequency response, they are very similar except for the imperfections of the sinc kernel used in the implementation. In terms of detection and statistics, sinc subtraction preserves greater degrees of freedom than pairwise subtraction, which reduces the number of time points by half.

Type of Differencing		Fourier Domain Expression
D_1	No subtraction	$Y_1(e^{j\omega}) = Y(e^{j\omega})$
D_2	Pairwise subtraction	$Y_2(e^{j\omega}) = 0.5 \cdot [Y(e^{j\omega/2})(1 - e^{j\omega/2}) + Y(e^{j(\omega+2\pi)/2})(1 - e^{j(\omega+2\pi)/2})]$
D_3	Running subtraction	$Y_3(e^{j\omega}) = Y(e^{j(\omega+\pi)})(1 - e^{j(\omega+\pi)})$
D_4	Surround subtraction	$Y_4(e^{j\omega}) = Y(e^{j(\omega+\pi)})(-1 + 2e^{j(\omega+\pi)} - e^{2j(\omega+\pi)})$

Table 1. Frequency Responses of the differencing schemes

With that in mind, it is important to take the differencing matrix into account when constructing a general linear model for analysis. In the previous section we constructed a model that contained both BOLD effects and ASL effects (see figure 9). Let X represent the corresponding design matrix. We can then re-write the general linear model equation with an additional Differencing matrix, like this:

$$DY = DX\beta + D\varepsilon.$$

It is crucial to note that whatever we do to the data, we must also do to the model if that model is to be as accurate as possible. Hence we difference the data, we must also difference the model, including the noise term. If no differencing is applied, the matrix D can be the identity.

At this point, the objective is the same as in the standard GLM analysis: estimate the model's coefficients (β) and determine whether they are statistically significant. Our choices are to pick a differencing matrix, D, and solve by ordinary least squares (OLS), or do nothing to the data (use D = I) and solve be generalized least squares (GLS).

As it turns out, this decision largely depends on the type of experimental paradigm and on the design matrix. Figure 14 shows a comparison between the statistical power obtained from analyzing ASL data with different amount of noise the two strategies: differencing and not differencing. In one case the data are analyzed with a Generalized Least Squares (GLS) model and not differenced. In the other case, the data are pairwise differenced and analyzed with the usual ordinary least squares (OLS).

Specifically, it shows the statistical power for no differencing with GLS and that of pairwise differencing with OLS for the 3 study designs over SNR values ranging between 0.25 and 2. The dotted lines on the random event related figure indicate ± 2 standard deviations of the average power over the 100 simulations. As expected, the power is similar between the two methods for the block design, but the "no differencing GLS" model is shown to have larger power for the event related study designs. The random event related design can have up to 14% (s.d. 0.7%) lower power when OLS is used compared to GLS. (Mumford, Hernandez-Garcia et al. 2006). An added benefit is that the GLS approach also enables us to estimate both BOLD and ASL effects simultaneously, which may be desirable in some analyses.

A final note is that the above quantification method using the GLM can be used whether the data are differenced and undifferenced, as long as the design matrix is constructed carefully to reflect the differencing scheme.

11. Challenges facing ASL

So far, we have illustrated the utility of ASL in functional MRI, but we must reiterate that ASL is not a panacea, though. Arterial spin labeling techniques pose a number of challenges. These challenges must be overcome so that ASL techniques can take a more central role in the study of brain function.

ASL is challenged by low SNR, since less than 10% of the water in a given voxel is contributed by blood (Pawlik, Rackl et al. 1981; Weiss, Buchweitz et al. 1982) and the label decays quickly. This problem can be partially alleviated by continuous arterial spin labeling, which increases the amount of label that is introduced into the tissue. Gains in the SNR have also been made with the development of pulse sequences that employ background suppression pulses, as these dramatically reduce the noise contribution from stationary tissue (Garcia, Duhamel et al. 2005). However, these background suppression pulses interfere with the ability to quantify perfusion, so they limit the measurement to relative CBF measures (Shin, Liu et al. 2011).

Another major challenge to ASL techniques is low temporal resolution because ASL measurements take from 3 to 6 seconds depending on the amount of time spent labeling the arterial blood. Collecting multi-slice data can be challenging because the imaging RF pulses can interfere with the inversion label of the arterial water (Silva, Zhang et al. 1995). Lastly, all slices must be acquired within a short period of time in order to sample the label before it clears from

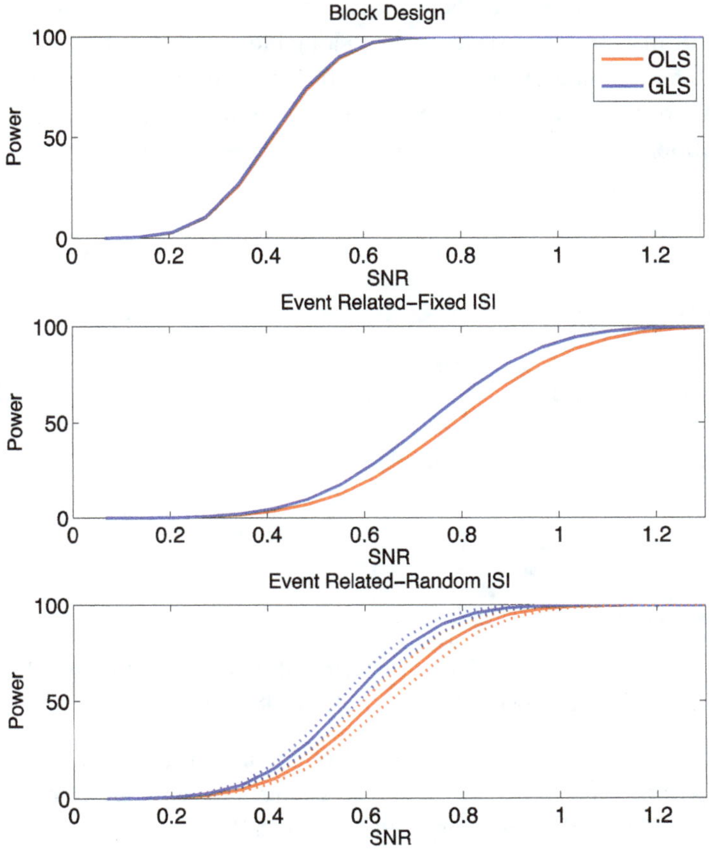

Figure 14. Whether we use an ordinary least squares (OLS) approach on differenced data or a generalized least squares approach (GLS) on raw data can make a significant difference in the statistical power of the analysis. It's not important for blocked designs, but in the case of event related designs, whose frequency content is relatively higher, it makes a significant difference. Reproduced from (Mumford, Hernandez-Garcia et al. 2006).

the tissue of interest. As we have discussed earlier, functional MRI experiments often require the ability to scan the whole brain at a rapid rate in order to localize and characterize brief, subtle changes in cerebral activity (i.e., event related experiments). Collecting multi-slice ASL images in a rapid manner is challenging, given the SNR and clearance rate of the label. While one can collect images at a rate roughly equivalent to the transit time of the subject (roughly 1.5 seconds) the number of slices at this rate is limited to less than five at the present time (Hernandez-Garcia, Lee et al. 2004; Hernandez-Garcia, Lee et al. 2005).

12. Conclusions

In this chapter we have examined arterial spin labeling as technique for functional MRI in depth. As we have seen, there are some clear advantages to collecting ASL data for functional studies in some circumstances, but other times it may not be beneficial at all. ASL is really well suited for longitudinal studies and studies with long blocks of activation, but it may not be so well suited for event related experiments. ASL offers quantitative measures of perfusion at rest and activation. On a per subject basis, the technique's limitations are low SNR and temporal resolution, but there are significant gains in terms of population variance and contrast between resting and active states.

Author details

Luis Hernandez-Garcia and Hesamoddin Jahanian

University of Michigan, FMRI Laboratory, USA

References

[1] Aguirre, G., J. Detre, et al. (2002). "Experimental design and the relative sensitivity of BOLD and perfusion fMRI." *Neuroimage* 15(3): 488-500.

[2] Ances, B. M., O. Leontiev, et al. (2008). "Regional differences in the coupling of cerebral blood flow and oxygen metabolism changes in response to activation: implications for BOLD-fMRI." *Neuroimage* 39(4): 1510-1521.

[3] Bagarinao, E., K. Matsuo, et al. (2003). "Estimation of general linear model coefficients for real-time application." *Neuroimage* 19(2): 422-429.

[4] Bandettini, P. A., E. C. Wong, et al. (1992). "Time course EPI of human brain function during task activation." *Magn Reson Med* 25(2): 390-397.

[5] Bernstein, M. A., K. F. King, et al. (2004). *Handbook of MRI pulse sequences*, Elsevier Academic Press.

[6] Bevington, P. R. and D. K. Robinson (2003). *Data reduction and error analysis for the physical sciences*. Boston, McGraw-Hill.

[7] Boynton, G., S. Engel, et al. (1996). "Linear systems analysis of functional magnetic resonance imaging in human V1." *J Neurosci* 16(13): 4207-4221.

[8] Buxton, R. and L. Frank (1997). "A model for the coupling between cerebral blood flow and oxygen metabolism during neural stimulation." *J Cereb Blood Flow Metab* 17(1): 64-72.

[9] Buxton, R., L. Frank, et al. (1998). "A general kinetic model for quantitative perfusion imaging with arterial spin labeling." *Magn Reson Med* 40(3): 383-396.

[10] Buxton, R., E. Wong, et al. (1998). "Dynamics of blood flow and oxygenation changes during brain activation: the balloon model." *Magn Reson Med* 39(6): 855-864.

[11] Caria, A., R. Veit, et al. (2007). "Regulation of anterior insular cortex activity using real-time fMRI." *Neuroimage* 35(3): 1238-1246.

[12] Changwei, W. W., C. Kai-Hsiang, et al. (2008). "Vascular space occupancy-dependent functional MRI by tissue suppression." *Journal of Magnetic Resonance Imaging* 28(1): 219-226.

[13] Chen, J. J., M. Wieckowska, et al. (2008). "Cerebral blood flow measurement using fMRI and PET: a cross-validation study." *International journal of biomedical imaging* 2008: 516359.

[14] Christopher, B. G., A. S. Ronald, et al. (2009). "Estimating cerebral blood volume with expanded vascular space occupancy slice coverage." *Magnetic Resonance in Medicine* 61(5): 1193-1200.

[15] Cohen, E. R., K. Ugurbil, et al. (2002). "Effect of basal conditions on the magnitude and dynamics of the blood oxygenation level-dependent fMRI response." *J Cereb Blood Flow Metab* 22(9): 1042-1053.

[16] Cox, R. W., A. Jesmanowicz, et al. (1995). "Real-time functional magnetic resonance imaging." *Magn Reson Med* 33(2): 230-236.

[17] Davis, T. L., K. K. Kwong, et al. (1998). "Calibrated functional MRI: mapping the dynamics of oxidative metabolism." *Proc Natl Acad Sci U S A* 95(4): 1834-1839.

[18] deCharms, R. C. (2008). "Applications of real-time fMRI." *Nat Rev Neurosci* 9(9): 720-729.

[19] deCharms, R. C., K. Christoff, et al. (2004). "Learned regulation of spatially localized brain activation using real-time fMRI." *Neuroimage* 21(1): 436-443.

[20] Detre, J., J. Leigh, et al. (1992). "Perfusion imaging." *Magn Reson Med* 23(1): 37-45.

[21] Duong, T., E. Yacoub, et al. (2002). "High-resolution, spin-echo BOLD, and CBF fMRI at 4 and 7 T." *Magn Reson Med* 48(4): 589-593.

[22] Edelman, R. and Q. Chen (1998). "EPISTAR MRI: multislice mapping of cerebral blood flow." *Magn Reson Med* 40(6): 800-805.

[23] Fernandez-Seara, M. A., J. Wang, et al. (2007). "Imaging mesial temporal lobe activation during scene encoding: comparison of fMRI using BOLD and arterial spin labeling." *Hum Brain Mapp* 28(12): 1391-1400.

[24] Fernandez-Seara, M. A., Z. Wang, et al. (2005). "Continuous arterial spin labeling perfusion measurements using single shot 3D GRASE at 3 T." *Magn Reson Med* 54(5): 1241-1247.

[25] Gai, N. D., S. L. Talagala, et al. (2011). "Whole-brain cerebral blood flow mapping using 3D echo planar imaging and pulsed arterial tagging." *J Magn Reson Imaging* 33(2): 287-295.

[26] Garcia, D., C. de Bazelaire, et al. (2005). *Pseudo-continuous Flow Driven Adiabatic Inversion for Arterial Spin Labeling*. Proceedings International Society for Magnetic Resonance in Medicine, Miami, FLA.

[27] Garcia, D. M., G. Duhamel, et al. (2005). "Efficiency of inversion pulses for background suppressed arterial spin labeling." *Magn Reson Med* 54(2): 366-372.

[28] Gembris, D., J. G. Taylor, et al. (2000). "Functional magnetic resonance imaging in real time (FIRE): sliding-window correlation analysis and reference-vector optimization." *Magn Reson Med* 43(2): 259-268.

[29] Gollub, R. L., H. C. Breiter, et al. (1998). "Cocaine decreases cortical cerebral blood flow but does not obscure regional activation in functional magnetic resonance imaging in human subjects." *Journal of cerebral blood flow and metabolism : official journal of the International Society of Cerebral Blood Flow and Metabolism* 18(7): 724-734.

[30] Gu, H., H. Lu, et al. (2006). "Noninvasive quantification of cerebral blood volume in humans during functional activation." *Neuroimage* 30(2): 377-387.

[31] Gunther, M., K. Oshio, et al. (2005). "Single-shot 3D imaging techniques improve arterial spin labeling perfusion measurements." *Magn Reson Med* 54(2): 491-498.

[32] Haacke, E. M. (1999). Magnetic resonance imaging : physical principles and sequence design. New York, Wiley.

[33] Hermes, M., D. Hagemann, et al. (2007). "Reproducibility of continuous arterial spin labeling perfusion MRI after 7 weeks." *Magma* 20(2): 103-115.

[34] Hernandez-Garcia, L., H. Jahanian, et al. (2011). "Real-time functional MRI using pseudo-continuous arterial spin labeling." Magnetic resonance in medicine : official journal of the Society of Magnetic Resonance in Medicine / Society of Magnetic Resonance in Medicine 65(6): 1570-1577.

[35] Hernandez-Garcia, L., H. Jahanian, et al. (2010). "Quantitative Analysis of Arterial Spin Labeling FMRI Data Using a General Linear Mode." *Mangetic Resonance Imaging* 28(7): 919-927.

[36] Hernandez-Garcia, L., G. R. Lee, et al. (2004). "Fast, pseudo-continuous arterial spin labeling for functional imaging using a two-coil system." *Magn Reson Med* 51(3): 577-585.

[37] Hernandez-Garcia, L., G. R. Lee, et al. (2005). "Quantification of perfusion fMRI using a numerical model of arterial spin labeling that accounts for dynamic transit time effects." *Magn Reson Med* 54(4): 955-964.

[38] Hernandez-Garcia, L., D. Lewis, et al. (2007). "Magnetization transfer effects on the efficiency of flow-driven adiabatic fast passage inversion of arterial blood." *NMR Biomed* 20: 733-742.

[39] Hoge, R. D., J. Atkinson, et al. (1999). "Linear coupling between cerebral blood flow and oxygen consumption in activated human cortex." *Proceedings of the National Academy of Sciences of the United States of America* 96(16): 9403-9408.

[40] Jaeggi, S. M., B. E. Studer, et al. (2009). *Improving Fluid Intelligence – Single N-back Is As Effective As Dual N-back.* Annual Meeting of the Psychonomic Society, Boston, MA.

[41] Jahanian, H., D. C. Noll, et al. (2011). "B0 field inhomogeneity considerations in pseudo-continuous arterial spin labeling (pCASL): effects on tagging efficiency and correction strategy." *NMR in Biomedicine*: n/a-n/a.

[42] Jin, T. and S.-G. Kim (2008). "Improved cortical-layer specificity of vascular space occupancy fMRI with slab inversion relative to spin-echo BOLD at 9.4+T." *Neuroimage* 40(1): 59-67.

[43] Kemeny, S., F. Q. Ye, et al. (2005). "Comparison of continuous overt speech fMRI using BOLD and arterial spin labeling." *Human Brain Mapping* 24(3): 173-183.

[44] Kety, S. S. and C. Schmidt (1945). "THE DETERMINATION OF CEREBRAL BLOOD FLOW IN MAN BY THE USE OF NITROUS OXIDE IN LOW CONCENTRATIONS." *American Journal of Physiology*(143): 53-66.

[45] Kim, J., J. Whyte, et al. (2006). "Continuous ASL perfusion fMRI investigation of higher cognition: quantification of tonic CBF changes during sustained attention and working memory tasks." *Neuroimage* 31(1): 376-385.

[46] Kim, S. (1995). "Quantification of relative cerebral blood flow change by flow-sensitive alternating inversion recovery (FAIR) technique: application to functional mapping." *Magn Reson Med* 34(3): 293-301.

[47] Kim, S. and N. Tsekos (1997). "Perfusion imaging by a flow-sensitive alternating inversion recovery (FAIR) technique: application to functional brain imaging." *Magn Reson Med* 37(3): 425-435.

[48] Kwong, K., J. Belliveau, et al. (1992). "Dynamic magnetic resonance imaging of human brain activity during primary sensory stimulation." *Proc Natl Acad Sci U S A* 89(12): 5675-5679.

[49] Lassen, N. A. and W. Perl (1979). *Tracer kinetic methods in medical physiology.* New York, Raven Press.

[50] Leontiev, O. and R. B. Buxton (2007). "Reproducibility of BOLD, perfusion, and CMRO2 measurements with calibrated-BOLD fMRI." *Neuroimage* 35(1): 175-184.

[51] Liu, T. and E. Wong (2005). "A signal processing model for arterial spin labeling functional MRI." *Neuroimage* 24(1): 207-215.

[52] Lu, H., M. Law, et al. (2005). "Novel approach to the measurement of absolute cerebral blood volume using vascular-space-occupancy magnetic resonance imaging." *Magn Reson Med* 54(6): 1403-1411.

[53] Lund, T., K. Madsen, et al. (2006). "Non-white noise in fMRI: does modelling have an impact?" *Neuroimage* 29(1): 54-66.

[54] Mulderink, T. A., D. R. Gitelman, et al. (2002). "On the use of caffeine as a contrast booster for BOLD fMRI studies." *Neuroimage* 15(1): 37-44.

[55] Mumford, J. A., L. Hernandez-Garcia, et al. (2006). "Estimation efficiency and statistical power in arterial spin labeling fMRI." *Neuroimage* 33(1): 103-114.

[56] Nakai, T., E. Bagarinao, et al. (2006). "Dynamic monitoring of brain activation under visual stimulation using fMRI--The advantage of real-time fMRI with sliding window GLM analysis." *Journal of Neuroscience Methods* 157(1): 158-167.

[57] Nencka, A. S. and D. B. Rowe (2007). "Reducing the unwanted draining vein BOLD contribution in fMRI with statistical post-processing methods." *Neuroimage* 37(1): 177-188.

[58] O'Gorman, R. L., V. Kumari, et al. (2006). "Personality factors correlate with regional cerebral perfusion." *Neuroimage* 31(2): 489-495.

[59] Olafsson, V. T., D. C. Noll, et al. (2008). "Fast Joint Reconstruction of Dynamic R2* and Field Maps in Functional MRI." *Medical Imaging, IEEE Transactions on* 27(9): 1177-1188.

[60] Olson, I. R., H. Rao, et al. (2006). "Using perfusion fMRI to measure continuous changes in neural activity with learning." *Brain and Cognition* 60(3): 262-271.

[61] Pawlik, G., A. Rackl, et al. (1981). "Quantitative capillary topography and blood flow in the cerebral cortex of cats: an in vivo microscopic study." *Brain Res* 208(1): 35-58.

[62] Pfeuffer, J., G. Adriany, et al. (2002). "Perfusion-based high-resolution functional imaging in the human brain at 7 Tesla." *Magn Reson Med* 47(5): 903-911.

[63] Phan, K. L., D. A. Fitzgerald, et al. (2004). "Real-time fMRI of cortico-limbic brain activity during emotional processing." *Neuroreport* 15(3): 527-532.

[64] Posse, S., D. Fitzgerald, et al. (2003). "Real-time fMRI of temporolimbic regions detects amygdala activation during single-trial self-induced sadness." *NeuroImage* 18: 760-768.

[65] Rao, H., S. J. Gillihan, et al. (2007). "Genetic variation in serotonin transporter alters resting brain function in healthy individuals." *Biological Psychiatry* 62(6): 600-606.

[66] Rao, H., J. Wang, et al. (2007). "Imaging brain activity during natural vision using CASL perfusion fMRI." *Human Brain Mapping* 28(7): 593-601.

[67] Raoult, H., J. Petr, et al. (2011). "Arterial spin labeling for motor activation mapping at 3T with a 32-channel coil: Reproducibility and spatial accuracy in comparison with BOLD fMRI." *Neuroimage* 58(1): 157-167.

[68] Shin, D., H. Liu, et al. (2011). *Effect of background suppression on CBF quantitation in pseudo continuous arterial spin labeling*. International Society for Magnetic Resonance in Medicine, Montreal, QC, Canada.

[69] Silva, A., W. Zhang, et al. (1995). "Multi-slice MRI of rat brain perfusion during amphetamine stimulation using arterial spin labeling." *Magn Reson Med* 33(2): 209-214.

[70] Smith, A. M., B. K. Lewis, et al. (1999). "Investigation of Low Frequency Drift in fMRI Signal." *Neuroimage* 9(5): 526-533.

[71] Talagala, S., F. Ye, et al. (2004). "Whole-brain 3D perfusion MRI at 3.0 T using CASL with a separate labeling coil." *Magn Reson Med* 52(1): 131-140.

[72] Tjandra, T., J. C. W. Brooks, et al. (2005). "Quantitative assessment of the reproducibility of functional activation measured with BOLD and MR perfusion imaging: Implications for clinical trial design." *Neuroimage* 27(2): 393-401.

[73] Vazquez, A. and D. Noll (1998). "Nonlinear aspects of the BOLD response in functional MRI." *Neuroimage* 7(2): 108-118.

[74] Vazquez, A. L., G. R. Lee, et al. (2006). "Application of selective saturation to image the dynamics of arterial blood flow during brain activation using magnetic resonance imaging." *Magn Reson Med* 55(4): 816-825.

[75] Voyvodic, J. T. (1999). "Real-time fMRI paradigm control, physiology, and behavior combined with near real-time statistical analysis." *Neuroimage* 10(2): 91-106.

[76] Wang, J., G. Aguirre, et al. (2003). "Empirical analyses of null-hypothesis perfusion FMRI data at 1.5 and 4 T." *Neuroimage* 19(4): 1449-1462.

[77] Wang, J., G. Aguirre, et al. (2003). "Arterial spin labeling perfusion fMRI with very low task frequency." *Magn Reson Med* 49(5): 796-802.

[78] Wang, J., G. K. Aguirre, et al. (2003). "Arterial spin labeling perfusion fMRI with very low task frequency." *Magn Reson Med* 49(5): 796-802.

[79] Wang, J., D. Alsop, et al. (2002). "Comparison of quantitative perfusion imaging using arterial spin labeling at 1.5 and 4.0 Tesla." *Magn Reson Med* 48(2): 242-254.

[80] Wang, J., H. Rao, et al. (2005). "Perfusion functional MRI reveals cerebral blood flow pattern under psychological stress." *Proceedings of the National Academy of Sciences of the United States of America* 102(49): 17804-17809.

[81] Wang, J., Y. Zhang, et al. (2005). "Amplitude-modulated Continuous Arterial Spin-labeling 3.0-T Perfusion MR Imaging with a Single Coil: Feasibility Study." *Radiology* 235(1): 218-228.

[82] Weiss, H., E. Buchweitz, et al. (1982). "Quantitative regional determination of morphometric indices of the total and perfused capillary network in the rat brain." *Circ Res* 51(4): 494-503.

[83] Williams, D., J. Detre, et al. (1992). "Magnetic resonance imaging of perfusion using spin inversion of arterial water." *Proc Natl Acad Sci U S A* 89(1): 212-216.

[84] Wise, R. G. and I. Tracey (2006). "The role of fMRI in drug discovery." *Journal of magnetic resonance imaging : JMRI* 23(6): 862-876.

[85] Wong, E., R. Buxton, et al. (1997). "Implementation of quantitative perfusion imaging techniques for functional brain mapping using pulsed arterial spin labeling." *NMR Biomed* 10(4-5): 237-249.

[86] Wong, E., R. Buxton, et al. (1998). "Quantitative imaging of perfusion using a single subtraction (QUIPSS and QUIPSS II)." *Magn Reson Med* 39(5): 702-708.

[87] Wong, E., R. Buxton, et al. (1998). "A theoretical and experimental comparison of continuous and pulsed arterial spin labeling techniques for quantitative perfusion imaging." *Magn Reson Med* 40(3): 348-355.

[88] Wu, W. C., M. Fernandez-Seara, et al. (2007). "A theoretical and experimental investigation of the tagging efficiency of pseudocontinuous arterial spin labeling." *Magn Reson Med* 58(5): 1020-1027.

[89] Yoo, S. S., T. Fairneny, et al. (2004). "Brain-computer interface using fMRI: spatial navigation by thoughts." *Neuroreport* 15(10): 1591-1595.

[90] Yoo, S. S. and F. A. Jolesz (2002). "Functional MRI for neurofeedback: feasibility study on a hand motor task." *Neuroreport* 13(11): 1377-1381.

[91] Zhang, W., A. Silva, et al. (1995). "NMR measurement of perfusion using arterial spin labeling without saturation of macromolecular spins." *Magn Reson Med* 33(3): 370-376.

8

The Neurometabolic Underpinnings of fMRI BOLD Dynamics

Christopher W. Tyler and Lora T. Likova

1. Introduction

The primary indicator of brain activity in the fMRI technique is known as the blood oxygenation level dependent (BOLD) signal, which derives from the hemodynamic response of the local blood vessels. Although much effort has gone into the analysis of the temporal dynamics of this signal as a reflection of the underlying neural activity that elicits it, the link between neural activity and the hemodynamic response is not direct, but involves a chain of metabolic processes mediated by the astrocytic glial cells in the cerebral cortex. This review focuses on the role of the metabolic pathways mediated by the glial cell in coupling the neural activity to the BOLD responses in the blood vessels, and the consequent implications for the processes governing the fMRI BOLD dynamics.

2. The chain of metabolic processing

In general terms, the stimulus impinging on the subject generates a sequence of neural responses starting with the transduction into a neural signal within the sensory receptors, which then propagates to the brain and activates various populations of neurons within the voxels being analyzed by the fMRI technique (Logothetis, 2003). For instance, the neural signals arriving from the visual pathway generate synaptic activation of the populations of neurons in the occipital cortex, which generates an energetic demand for the restoration of the neurotransmitter molecules carrying the activation signals across the synapses. The chain of cortical processing progresses from the neural events through the metabolic demand mediated by the glucose/lactate cycle in neighboring astrocyte glial cells to the processes of oxygen delivery by the adjacent arterioles and capillaries that is detected by the

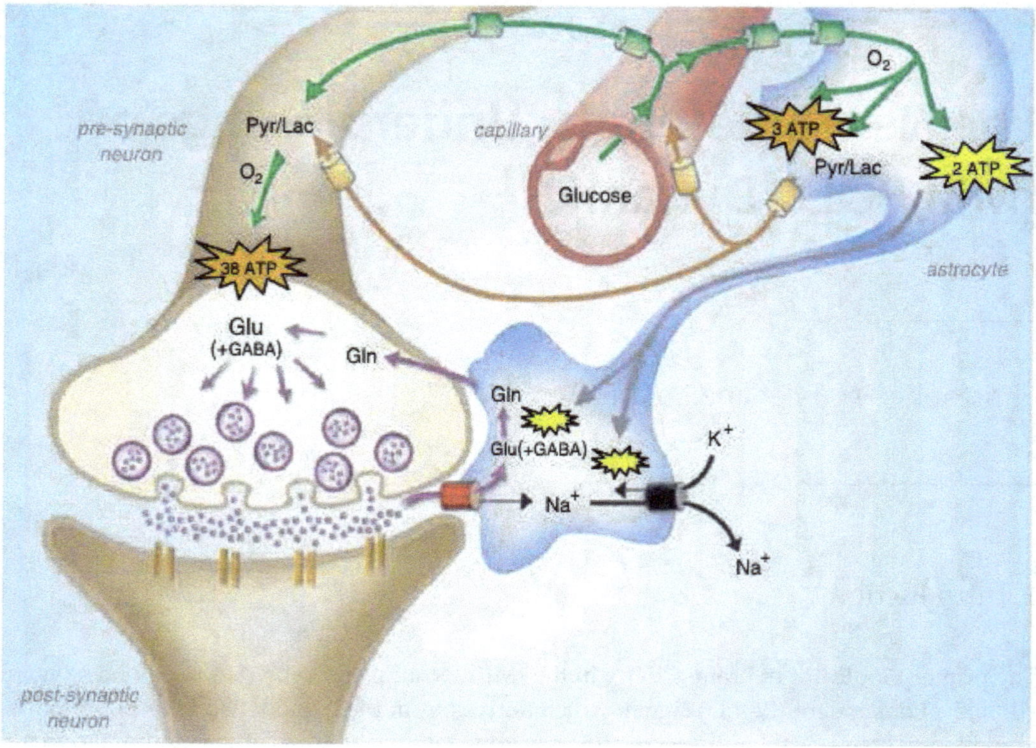

Figure 1. The astrocytes as the substrate for the neurovascular coupling of the neural metabolism. (From Hyder et al., 2006, with permission).

imaging methodology. The first element in this metabolic chain is the local astrocyte processes, which provide glucose to the neuron and replenish its supply by an ATP metabolism, which is fueled by oxygen diffusing through the astrocyte cytoplasm from their endfeet connections to neighboring blood vessels (Magistretti & Pellerin, 1999; Magistretti, 2009). The integrated metabolic demands are met primarily by the astrocytes, which integrate the required energy consumption over time and space and make a complementary metabolic demand on the adjacent vasculature.

In detail, the pathways are complex, involving lactate, glucose and glycogen metabolic mechanisms, mediated by both intracellular astrocyte and supplementary extracellular transport (Dienel & Cruz, 2008; Ghandi et al., 2009) but the connection between this local glucose metabolism close to the synapse and the oxygen-based hemodynamics in the blood vessel remains unclear. Three hypotheses for this neuro-hemodynamic coupling may be adduced, although all thee remain to be tested:

- aerobic glucose metabolism. This is the concept of a direct coupling between the neural glucose metabolism and the vascular oxygen supply, in which the neural metabolism is supported by oxygen transported from the blood vessels either within the encapsulating astrocytes or through the extracellular cytoplasm (having passed through the astrocytic sheath) to reach the site of the neural synapses and provide the oxidative metabolism of the glucose to reconstitute the ATP used in the neural response. Studies in rat cortex have demonstrated a linear relationship between neural activity, glutamatergic neurotransmitter flux and the cerebral rate of oxygen metabolism (Hyder et al., 2002; Smith et al., 2002). Since cells are predominantly linear summators of the excitatory and inhibitory transmitter release across their synaptic population, the energetic demand driving the BOLD signal is most closely coupled to the net transmitter signal impinging on the cells, and hence to intracellular potential in the cells. The problem with this hypotheses is that it evokes a process with a time constant of the order of minutes (Margaria et al., 1933), which is too slow to account for the 5 s time constant of the BOLD response, despite its high efficiency.

- anaerobic glucose metabolism. This is the concept that the entire neural metabolic process is based on anaerobic glucose delivery from the blood vessel, and that the variation in the oxygenation fraction of the hemoglobin is an epiphenomenon. On this hypothesis, the metabolic demand the site of the neural synapse generates a signal in the astrocytes to release nitric oxide in the filopodia (endfeet) wrapping the arterioles, stimulating an increase in the arteriolar volume with a consequent increase in the proportion of oxyhemoglobin in that region of tissue. The ~5 s time constant of decay of the nitric oxide in the presence of hemoglobin (Hakim et al., 1996) meshes well with that of the BOLD response dynamics. The nitric oxide release signal is presumably mediated by a calcium signal traveling 'antidromically' through the astrocyte (Bezzi et al., 1998; Koehler et al., 2006), accounting for the 1-2 s onset delay in the onset of the BOLD signal.
- anaerobic stimulation of the combined metabolic pathway. This is a mixed concept in which the anaerobic metabolic demand from the neural glucose metabolism stimulates the NO-mediated arteriolar dilation with the consequent increase in both glucose and oxygen transport into the astrocytes (and extracellular cytoplasm). On this concept, the slow diffusion of the oxygen and glucose molecules to the synaptic sites is irrelevant to the BOLD response time course. The critical factors is that the metabolic demand generated by the neural glycolysis is fast enough to elicit an NO signal to the arterioles that, together with its decay time constant, again generates an arteriolar volume time course compatible with the measured BOLD dynamics. On this interpretation, the question of how long the transported products take to reach their metabolic targets, to provide the needed aerobic recovery from the anaerobic depletion, is invisible to the BOLD signal probe.

Thus, the most likely basis of the metabolic demand driving the cortical BOLD signal is the energetic load deriving from the total conductance changes in the postsynaptic membrane generated by a range of processes consequent on transmitter release at the synaptic inputs to each neuron. The summed metabolic demand in the nexus of active cortical neurons adjacent to a capillary forms the drive for the metabolic response in that region of cortex. Thus, the transmitter release is tightly coupled to the activation of the post-synaptic receptors on the recipient cell membrane and consequently to the energetic demands of the membrane receptor activation and to a lesser extent to the subsequent recycling of the transmitter molecules. The majority of these energetic demands are met by the conversion of glutamate to glutamine in the neighboring astrocytes (Sibson et al., 1998, 2001; Rothman & Schulman,

1998). The glutamine is then taken up by the neurons for reconversion to glutamate for use as a transmitter, releasing energy within the neuron in the process.

3. The time course of astrocytic responses

The first element in this chain is the astrocytes surrounding the neuron, which provide glucose to the neuron and replenish its supply by ATP metabolism fueled by oxygen from neighboring blood vessels. It may be emphasized that the astrocyte metabolic processes are as slow, relative to the intracellular signal dynamics, as are the processes of hemodynamic oxygen supply. The time constant of the astrocyte responses at the cell body is known to be of the order of several seconds (Kelly & van Essen, 1974; Filosa, Bonev & Nelson, 2004; Metea & Newman, 2006), and it is clear that these slow responses must mediate the hemodynamic component.The hemodynamic processes provide the requisite oxygen exchange to replenish the energy depletion in the astrocytes and other intermediary processes. The hemodynamic response of the blood vessels to increase their oxygen supply in response to the neural metabolic demand G(t) is mediated by coupling with the astrocyte endfeet. The fMRI BOLD analysis provides an estimate of the ratio of oxygenated to deoxygenated hemoglobin in the blood complement of a given voxel. The post-neural processing stages are often modeled as a linear hemodynamic response kernel convolved with the presumed neural signal. However, this approach overlooks the key role of the pre-hemodynamic processes of the glial and other intermediaries. To reflect the contributions of these intermediary processes, we will term it a 'metabolic response kernel' (MRK) incorporating both the glial and hemodynamic components of the metabolic recovery processes. The metabolic demand has been shown to have a short time course, on the order of the membrane response to a single presynaptic spike. The time constant of the metabolite diffusion through the astrocyte cytoplasm is known to be of the order of several seconds (Filosa, Bonev and Nelson, 2004; Metea and Newman, 2006), so it is clear that there must be a substantial pre-hemodynamic component from these slow responses.

This analysis is borne out by an examination of the time courses of the astrocyte signals. These represent some of the shortest time courses that could be found in a search of the literature on astrocyte signals. These studies make it clear that the calcium signal represents the final control signal for the vasodilation that initiates the sequence of hemodynamic processes that generate the BOLD signal. This calcium signal again has the about the same time constant as the other processes, peaking at times of approximately 5 sec after the stimulus onset (Kelly & Van Essen, 1974; Filosa, Bonev & Nelson, 2004; Metea & Newman, 2006), which implies that the astrocyte response to the neural signal is a slow process with a time constant of the same order as that of the typical BOLD signal.

4. The form of the metabolic response kernel

The time domain approach of present analysis allows the extraction of the maximum possible information about the temporal evolution and processing nonlinearities of the neural signals underlying particular BOLD activation profiles. Our analysis reveals that much information about the neural response properties are reflected in the BOLD signals, even if the time-resolution is insufficient to reproduce the exact neural signal. Examples of such 'transparency' of response properties are particularly clear in the case that the full metabolic response kernel is monophasic.

This monophasic assumption was tested for rat cortex by both Martindale et al. (2003) and de Zwart et al. (2005), who showed that the empirical dispersion of the BOLD response generated increasing delay with distance from the activation site, but were always well-fit by a monophasic model of the BOLD impulse response. Similarly direct measurements of cerebral blood flow and the concentrations of oxygenated and deoxygenated hemoglobin in the human brain (Hoge et al., 2005) reveal only a monophasic temporal waveform for each of these contributors to the BOLD response. These results are all compatible with the inference of a dominant monophasic positive BOLD response in cat LGN and cortex reviewed above (Thompson et al., 2003, 2004, 2005). This form also seems to be a fair approximation in the case of human fMRI because the canonical response kernel (commonly known as the HRF) provided in the SPM-5 software package, although biphasic, has a negative lobe of less than 10% of the amplitude of the positive lobe. It is therefore only a minor modification of this standardized kernel to assume that it has no negative lobe, which is the assumption made for the following analysis. (As will be explained below, the residual biphasic component can be readily attributed to *neural* rather than hemodynamic rebound signals.) Armed with this assumption, we show how several properties of the neural signal are reflected in the recorded BOLD waveform.

5. Implications for the variety of BOLD response waveforms

Armed with this assumption, we show how several properties of the neural signal are reflected in the recorded BOLD waveform. This demonstration assumes a linear relationship between the neural response and the BOLD waveform, in order to make its properties clear before introducing the nonlinear aspects of the analysis.

- **Polarity**. The BOLD response polarity will be an accurate reflection of the polarity of the neural response for any monophasic neural response.
- **Latency**. Any delay in the neural response will also be reflected in the consequent BOLD response. Of course, the metabolic processing sequence may introduce additional delays, but neural delays such as response reaction times or perceptual ambiguity delays should be accurately reflected in the BOLD waveform once the inherent delays of the MRK are taken into account.

- **Transience.** It is an established property of the BOLD response that it is largely sustained for an appropriately sustained neural response (Birn, Saad & Bandettini, 2001; Boynton et al., 1996; Glover, 1999; Logothetis, 2002, 2003; Shmuel et al., 2006). Hence, transience of the BOLD response for a sustained stimulus implies a transience of the underlying neural response. For example, the onset of a sustained light is known to generate transient neural responses in most cortical neurons responding to it. Such stimulation will generate a transient BOLD response even though the stimulation and photoreceptor response are sustained.

- **Number of phases.** For a monophasic MRK (HRF), the BOLD waveform will have the same number of phases as the input stimulus, if the neural input is balanced for positive and negative lobes. Thus, the fact that the measured BOLD waveform is typically biphasic does not imply that the MRK is necessarily biphasic. The negative lobe may derive from a biphasic neural response to a stimulus rather than to blood dynamics.

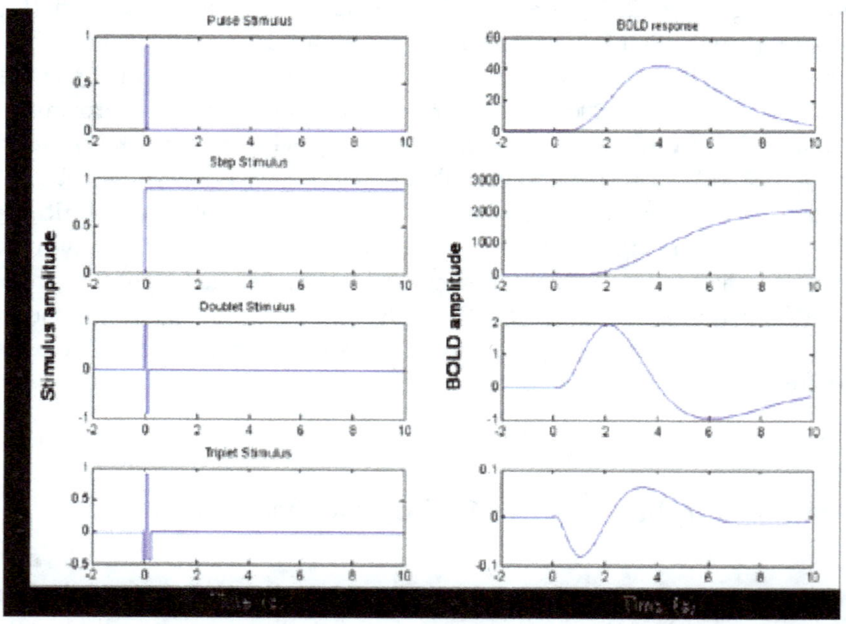

Figure 2. Left panels: (A) neural impulse response, (B) step response, (C) balanced doublet and (D) balanced triplet response. Right panels present convolution of each of these responces with the MRk shown at right. Note that differences in neural response characteristics (left panels) at the tim scale of 100 *ms* generate profound changes in the simulated BOLD waveforms (right panels) on a much longer timescale, which in turn are diagnostic of the differences in the neutral signals.

Some of these properties of the BOLD response are illustrated in the simulation of Fig. 2, for which the MRK is assumed to be the gamma function shown in Fig. 2A, right, as the basis function for the formal analysis. Gamma bases are statistical descriptors of the occurrence of discrete particles (Stacey, 1962; Farwell & Prentice, 1977) that have a simple analog implementation that is a cascade of identical lowpass filters (De Vries & Principe, 1992; Celebi &

Principe, 1995; Chen, 2006). In terms of molecular diffusion processes within neurons, the gamma function represents an optimal description of the cooperative process of the arrival of effector molecules at the channels controlling current flow through the cellular membrane (Shao, 1997). We derive the normal equation for the optimum value of the time scale parameter and decouple it from that of the basis weights. Using statistical signal processing tools, we further develop a numerical method for estimating the optimum time scale.

6. Direct forward modeling approaches

A few previous studies have made estimates of the effects of different neural models on the form of the BOLD response dynamics. For example, Mechelli et al. (2001) report a simulation study of the estimated regional cerebral blood flow (rCBF) and blood-oxygenation-dependent (BOLD) signals as a function of the duration, onset asynchrony and relative amplitudes of two brief stimuli. They included a basic model of neuronal dynamics and varied one parameter of this model – the amplitude of a slow late transient – to show its effect on the simulated BOLD responses. This exercise constitutes an unvalidated forward model of the effect of only one parameter of a simulated neural response. However, what they offer as the analysis of the effects on the BOLD waveform is described (incomprehensibly) as "the BOLD parameter estimates", which is actually a single-valued function with no specification of which parameter(s) is/are being estimated. Since no comparison is made with empirical data or their noise limitations, the fact that this study includes a proposed model for the neural dynamics does not qualify it as a validated procedure for estimating the neural population dynamics underlying the local BOLD signals (which is the goal of our study).

Buxton et al. (2004) extend their balloon model of the hemodynamic response leading to the BOLD signal by proposing a model of the neural response to account for the temporal nonlinearity in BOLD responses as a function of duration. This neural response incorporates a slow subtractive inhibitory component to the net neural signal, which has the effect of producing a neural response consisting of an initial transient followed by a sustained plateau. Model responses for three kinds of stimuli – a single short pulse, two short pulses and one long pulse, are offered as a demonstration of the properties of this model. As with Mechelli et al. (2001), no attempt is made to compare the model outputs with actual BOLD recordings, so the Buxton et al. (2004) study again does not qualify as a validated procedure for estimating the neural population dynamics underlying the local BOLD signals.

Both Mechelli et al. (2001) and Buxton et al. (2004) include parameters intended to account for the temporal nonlinearity of short duration responses (which do not fall linearly as response duration is reduced; Boynton et al., 1996; Birn, Saad & Bandettini, 2001). Both studies demonstrate the required lack of reduction in a single example of a short-duration response, but neither study provides a validation of either the waveform or the amplitude response function relative to empirical BOLD data. In principle, either model could provide a platform for such validation or the further estimation of the dynamics of the underlying neural population response, but they neither do so nor suggest procedures by which such estimation could be achieved.

7. Analytic model of the neural-BOLD coupling

To start the analysis, a specific model structure of the processes leading to the BOLD paramagnetic signal of fMRI recordings incorporates aspects of the biophysical processes that are not present in the linear convolution analyses of Friston et al. (1997, 1998, 2000), although somewhat condensed in comparison with the recent biophysical/metabolic derivations of Mechelli et al. (2001), Buxton et al., (2004) or Sotero & Trujillo-Bareto (2007, 2008).

The metabolic demand through the biophysical chain to the measured BOLD signal has two sources of nonlinearities. The major source of the BOLD waveform measured by functional Magnetic Resonance Imaging (fMRI) is the summed local field potential in the cortical region contributing to the signal for each voxel. The metabolic demand generated by the underlying neural activity is summed in parallel across the local neural sources, and is thus nonlinear with respect to the linear systems prediction for a serial system. The coupling itself also exhibits saturation nonlinearities when pushed beyond the region of small-signal linearity.

The neural responses within each voxel are treated as generated by sets of homogeneous populations with similar signal waveforms Ni(t) within each population (Fig. 3). Each neural response then generates a local metabolic demand Mi(t) that may have a nonlinear relationship to the neural signal waveform (Chatton, Pellerin & Magistretti, 2003). The MRK will be convolved with a non-linear transform of the presumed neural signal to provide an estimate of the neural metabolic demand that is being met by the combined glial and hemodynamic metabolic response. The fMRI analysis also has a finite dynamic response time, but it will be treated as incorporated in the MRK of the glial/hemodynamic response.

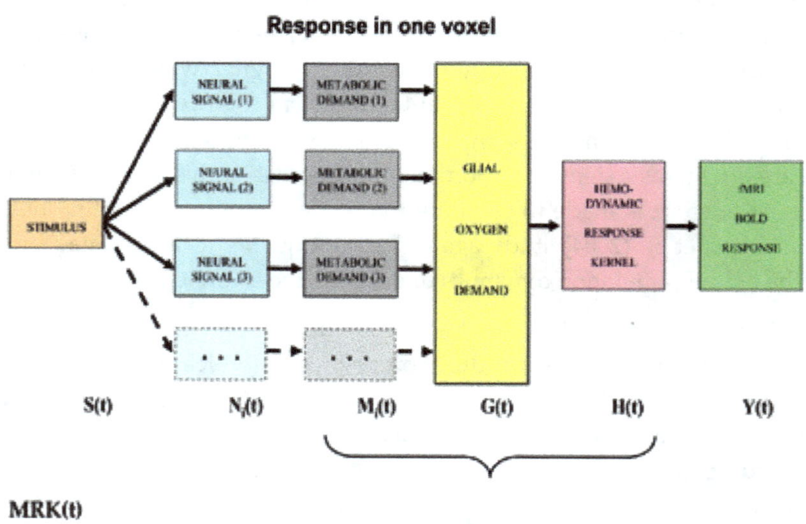

Figure 3. Block diagram of the main processing stages that lead up to the BOLD signal. The *i* subscript indicates that the stage incorporates multiple components within the voxel. See text for details.

These nonlinearities provide the opportunity to develop an analytic model of the neural signal leading to the BOLD activation. The model assumes the presence of neuronal subpopulations having response dynamics with various decay time constants in response to the stimulus. Pooling among the subpopulation responses can then explain the multiple decay characteristics of the recorded local field potentials (LFPs). Subsequent convolution with a characteristic metabolic response kernel then generates the predicted response Y(t) for the BOLD waveform for the region of cortex generating the LFP signal, accounting for concurrently recorded BOLD waveforms.

The neural responses within each voxel are modeled as sets of homogeneous populations Ni(t) with similar signal waveforms within each population. Each neural population response then generates a local metabolic demand Mi(t) that may have a nonlinear relationship to the neural signal waveform. The integrated metabolic demands are met primarily by the astrocytes, which integrate the required energy consumption over time and space and make a complementary metabolic demand G(t) on the adjacent vasculature. The hemodynamic processes H(t) replenish the energy depletion in the astrocytes, leading to the paramagnetic response that generates the BOLD signal of the differential precession rates of the oxygenated/deoxygenated hemoglobin moieties.

8. Implications for the analysis of fMRI BOLD signals

A proper understanding of the metabolic pathway underlying the fMRI BOLD signal is a necessary precursor to an analytic capability for neural signal estimation from the BOLD waveforms recorded throughout the cortex. Any such attempt must be based on a model of the known neural population dynamics underlying the BOLD metabolic signal generation, which may be progressively refined as more information becomes available about both neural response characteristics and the metabolic cascade. Given adequate signal/noise ratio, it is possible to develop approaches that overcome the temporal limitations of BOLD signal and are able to reveal relevant properties of the underlying neural signals. This analysis can provide a direct linkage between the live assessment of the functioning brain and the direct neurophysiological recordings in other species.

FMRI analysis techniques for estimating the BOLD signal typically employ Generalized Linear Model, which incorporates the convolution approach to the estimation of the underlying neural signal. Convolution is based on the assumption of a unitary BOLD waveform kernel that generates the straightforward prediction of the BOLD response waveform for any stimulus type or duration in any brain area. In fact, however, major deviations from a standard BOLD waveform may be found, even in the same cortical regions, for variations in stimulus conditions. D'Avossa, Shulman & Corbetta (2003), for example, reported strong differences in waveform when the response to the motion or color of a cue/stimulus pairing was modulated by attention. Such local waveform differences must derive from differences in the neural signals driving the BOLD activation, since the metabolic and hemodynamic processes that mediate the paramagnetic signals should be invariant within a given cortical region.

The BOLD signal measured by fMRI is often characterized as having high spatial resolution (up to a quarter of a million voxels), but low temporal resolution (0.5 – 5 s) relative to other methods for mapping human brain function (such as high-density EEG analysis). Estimation of single-parameters of the waveform, such as response delay alone, can improve the temporal resolution for the neural signal delays to 100 ms or better for narrowly targeted brain regions (Menon, Luknowsky & Gati, 1998; Henson et al., 2002) but this requires the assumption that the BOLD signal has a unitary waveform, which is often not the case (Aguirre et al., 1998; D'Avossa, Shulman & Corbetta, 2003; Handwerker, Ollinger & D'Esposito, 2004; Likova & Tyler, 2008; Tyler & Likova, 2009). Even minor deviations from a stable waveform violate the assumptions of such single-parameter analysis and invalidate the delay measure.

To evaluate the neural contribution to the differential BOLD response waveforms within the same cortical regions, Likova & Tyler (2008) developed an "instantaneous stimulus paradigm" to evoke BOLD responses to instantaneous stimulus transitions. It is typically assumed that, despite their perceptual differences, such "instantaneous" stimuli would all generate the same BOLD waveform (effectively equivalent to the MRK) for all different stimulus types. Thus, revealing any significant deviation from that prediction in the BOLD waveform elicited in one and the same cortical area can contribute to revealing the specifics of the underlying neural processing and enhance the understanding of the recurrent network of extended perceptual responses to complex stimulus configurations. Indeed, the instantaneous stimulus paradigm generated a wide variety of BOLD waveforms. Moreover, the data show dramatic differences in the BOLD waveforms properties (e.g., latency, sign, amplitude and width) even within the same brain areas as a function of the stimulus type. As there can be no vascular heterogeneity within the same area, these dramatic waveform variations must be attributed to differences in the underlying neural dynamics, not to spatial variations in the MRK. These results further imply that fMRI signals contain much more information about the neural processing than is commonly appreciated, and thus have the potential to capture them through an appropriate approach.

9. Nonlinear dynamic forward optimization

However, until recently there has been no method of transcending the BOLD temporal limitations in order to estimate the dynamics of the neural signals underlying the measured fMRI waveforms. Tyler & Likova (2009, 2011) therefore proposed a Dynamic Nonlinear Forward Optimization (NDFO) approach for the time-resolved estimation of the neural signals underlying the particular characteristics of the temporal BOLD waveforms for a particular stimulus processed by a particular cortical region. The philosophy of this approach is to utilize the information available from neurophysiological studies of the neural population dynamics and biochemical studies of the metabolic pathway coupling to the measurable blood response to provide Bayesian priors as to the likely temporal structure of the component neural signals. This method provides a compact account of the measured waveform with the minimal number of neural predictors, based on prior knowledge of the expected temporal properties of neural signals and of their consequent metabolic demand. The result is the ability to specify the prevalence of each element in the otherwise inaccessible star. In the case of the neural signals, the goal is to estimate the amplitude and time course of each of the neural components whose metabolic effects, when summed, account for the measured BOLD waveform for a particular stimulation condition and cortical region.

Rather than simply characterizing the behavior of the BOLD waveform (Birn, Saad & Bandettini, 2001; d'Avossa, Shulman & Corbetta, 2003; Fox et al., 2005; Grotz et al., 2009) or attempting to infer the potentially complex properties of the underlying neural mechanisms from the form of the BOLD response by deconvolution (Glover, 1999; Logothetis, 2002, 2003a,b; Logothetis & Wandell, 2004), the concept of forward modeling is to incorporate as much knowledge as possible about the likely neural substrate and optimize the remaining details to best fit the BOLD waveform. Here the predictors are non-linear because there is a nonlinear relationship between the neural responses and the metabolic demand that they generate, but the summative property of the paramagnetic signals throughout a voxel implies that we can assume that the component metabolic demands sum linearly together (Fig. 3). The dynamic forward modeling may incorporate a variety of possible nonlinearities into the structure of the model. The neural model that we investigate in the present version of the analysis is the sum of positive and a negative component based on delayed gamma functions convolved with the stimulus waveform

9.1. Analytic framework for the neural temporal response

The starting point for the NDFO modeling is a model of the neural signal, whose first effect in terms of the cascade of BOLD dynamics is to create a metabolic demand G(t) in the neighboring glial cells (see Fig. 3). Gamma probability density functions have the analytic form a. kt-1. e-t/τ/Γ(k), where t is the time dimension, a is a scaling parameter and k and τ are generic waveform parameters. (To equate the area to unity, the function is defined with a = 1/τk), but for the present purposes a is a free optimization parameter.) They may be termed simply "gamma functions" to emphasize their analytic rather than statistical properties. In engineering the same function is known as the n-pole filter function (with n = k), and is used to describe the dynamics of a wide range of processes. For the present application, the temporal gamma function is assumed to have integer powers of k and corresponds to the solution of differential equations with real (non-imaginary) roots. The gamma function has the analytic advantage over many other functions, such as the Gaussian, that it is by definition causal because it has the value of zero at t = 0, and is defined as zero for t < 0 (i.e., the full specification is y = kt-1. e-t/τ for t >= 0; y = 0 for t < 0). Its shape progresses from highly asymmetric around the peak for small k to approximately Gaussian and symmetric for large k (see Fig. 4). Fig. 4. Examples of delayed gamma function step responses with exponents of k = 2 (left) and 6 (right). Successive functions (colors) introduce a wide range of peak latencies for the neural signal estimates (with time constants increasing in factors of 2 and a fixed delay Δt of 40 ms).

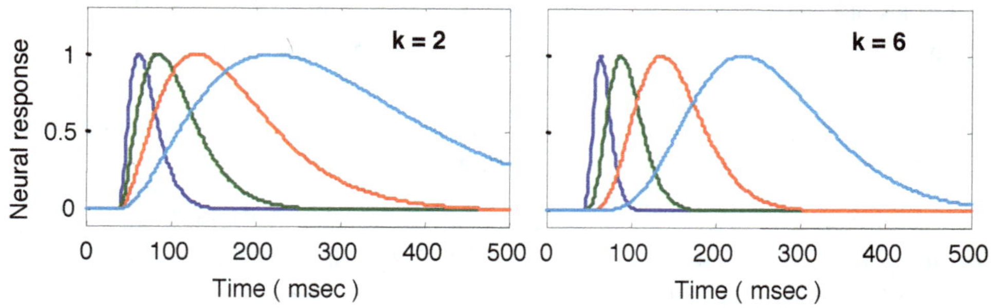

Figure 4. Examples of delayed gamma function step responses with exponents of k = 2 (left) and 6 (right). Successive functions (colors) introduce a wide range of peak latencies for the neural signal estimates (with time constants increasing in factors of 2 and a fixed delay Δt of 40 ms).

A key feature of this formalism is that the peak latency is determined by the time constant, τ, and is proportional to the width (at half height) of the response peak, which can be estimated to good accuracy by the methods described in the next section.

9.2. Neural model

A comprehensive model of the BOLD therefore requires an accurate model of the intracellular potential dynamics deriving from the sensory stimulation. Formally, we propose to use the full neural response model jointly specified in eqs 1 and 2:

$$N_p(t) = \left[|N(t)|_+ + \lambda \cdot |N(t)|_- \right] e^{-t/\eta} + \varepsilon(t) \tag{1}$$

where ε is the net source of additive noise and the function is governed by the parameter set $p = (a,\ k_\eta,\ \tau_\eta,\ b,\ \Delta t,\ \eta,\ \lambda)$

The neural signal NP(t) in eq 1 is the sum of positive and a negative component based on delayed gamma functions convolved with the stimulus waveform:

$$N(t) = a \cdot S(t) \otimes n(t - \Delta t) \tag{2}$$

where $n(t) = (1-t) \cdot t^{k_n - 1} e^{-t/\tau n} - \frac{b}{\tau_n} t^{k_n} e^{-t/\tau_n}$

(Note the convention that time series functions are capitalized, impulse response kernels are lower case, and vectors are bold-face.) The neural impulse response expression n(t) is set up so that its convolution with a step function is equivalent to the sum of a pure transient and a pure sustained component. In addition, the expression is specified with an additional transmission delay, Δt, that delays the response relative to the stimulus without affecting its waveshape with the parametrization specified in Table II, which defines the parameters in vector p of this equation. To illustrate the properties of the model, we analyze the effect of varying the inhibitory ratio implied by the negative component weight b, and the offset/ onset gain ratio λ.

a	scaling constant (a fitting parameter but not a waveshape parameter)
kn	integer exponent governing the rising phase
τn	time constant of falling phase in the neural response
Δt	transmission delay before response onset
b	sustained/transient ratio in the step response
η	time constant of nonlinear gain control in the neural response
λ	ratio of offset to onset gain in the neural response

Table 1. Nonlinear Forward Model Parameters

One issue that arises is how to measure the latency Δt of the delayed gamma functions of Fig. 4. A simple derivation can show that the peak latency tpeak of these responses is specified by the expression ($k\tau n + \Delta t$). Thus if k and Δt, both of which are well-determined from neurophysiological studies in monkey cortex, are set to means of their Bayesian priors on this basis, the peak latency tpeak is determined from the value of τ, which can be accurately derived from the model optimization.

9.3. Metabolic demand

Since little is known about the glial dynamics of transmitter recovery, we will pursue two options as to their effects. One option is that the metabolic demand driving the BOLD response derives from the transmitter recovery cycle following the activation by an axonal spike. Since axonal spikes represent only the positive aspect of the intracellular voltage and since 90% of cortical synapses are excitatory (Shank & Aprison, 1979; Wang & Floor, 1994), the signal transmitted from one cortical stage to the next may be treated as a half-wave rectified version of the dynamic neural signal. This prediction is shown as the blue curves in Fig. 5Aa (indexed in row/column notation), which is an overlay of the model estimates of the neural responses to stimulus pulses that double in duration from 8 ms to 16 s (eight doublings). For this example, the neural response has balanced excitation and inhibition, so even the prolonged pulses generate only an initial transient response, with the negative lobe at offset being thresholded out by the rectification. (Note that the local metabolic demand, Mi(t), has the same time course in this model as the transmitter recovery from which it derives. The energetic processes required for the recovery to the initial state, however, form an oxygen-based chain of glial metabolic response, G(t), that may have substantially slower time course at one or more stages.)

The other option is to consider the instantaneous metabolic demand of both excitatory and inhibitory cells, or both 'on' and 'off' cells, implying that the signal generating the metabolic demand is a full-wave rectified version of the intracellular voltage. This option is shown as the red curve in Fig. 5Aa, whose spikes represent the instantaneous metabolic demand for the offset transient for each of the pulse duration doublings (which were thresholded out in the blue curve).

9.4. Metabolic coupling

Having provided relevant variables for the linear and nonlinear components of the neural response dynamics, we may now consider the issue of the metabolic coupling of the neural signal to generate the BOLD response. This coupling has been extensively modeled over the past two decades, with the best-known example being the Buxton-Friston balloon model and the most elaborated version being by Sotero & Trujillo-Barreto (2007, 2008). However, these models are not well-validated by empirical human studies (because they contain too many interdependent variables to allow the independent assessment of each separately

10. Characteristics of the model

We may now evaluate the response to these two options for the nonlinearity of the metabolic demand through the biophysical chain of the metabolic processes to the measured BOLD signal (Table I). However, at present too little is known of the dynamics of transmitter recovery and/or the nonlinearities in the process to securely assign time constants to the astrocytic component relative to the hemodynamic component of the metabolic coupling. For the first pass, we will therefore treat the entire chain coupling the metabolic demand to the magnetic resonance signal in the traditional fashion, as a unitary linear kernel convolving the nonlinear neural signal. (As stated above, this kernel is often termed the hemodynamic response function HRF, but in view of its likely substantial astrocyte contribution, we give it the more general term of the metabolic response kernel MRK). Our main goal is to estimate the properties of the neural signal processing, and it will be seen that there is sufficient information to provide a rich analysis of these properties, and to account for the empirical nonlinearities of the BOLD signal, as long as the metabolic supply chain conforms to the linearity assumption. (As more information becomes available, nonlinear aspects of the metabolic coupling may readily be incorporated into the analysis we propose.)

The development of the peak amplitude in the BOLD temporal summation series is shown as the blue summation curve in Fig. 5Ad. The critical point of this plot is that the asymptotic corner of this summation curve occurs at 40 ms, which is the value of the time constant assumed for the neural signal in this example. Thus, the form of the BOLD amplitude summation series (Fig. 5, column d) provides a direct empirical estimate of the time constant of neural integration down to the millisecond range. There is no limit in principle to the temporal resolution that can be achieved by this methodology since it is estimated from the amplitude variation of the BOLD signal as a function of stimulus duration, not from its temporal aspects.

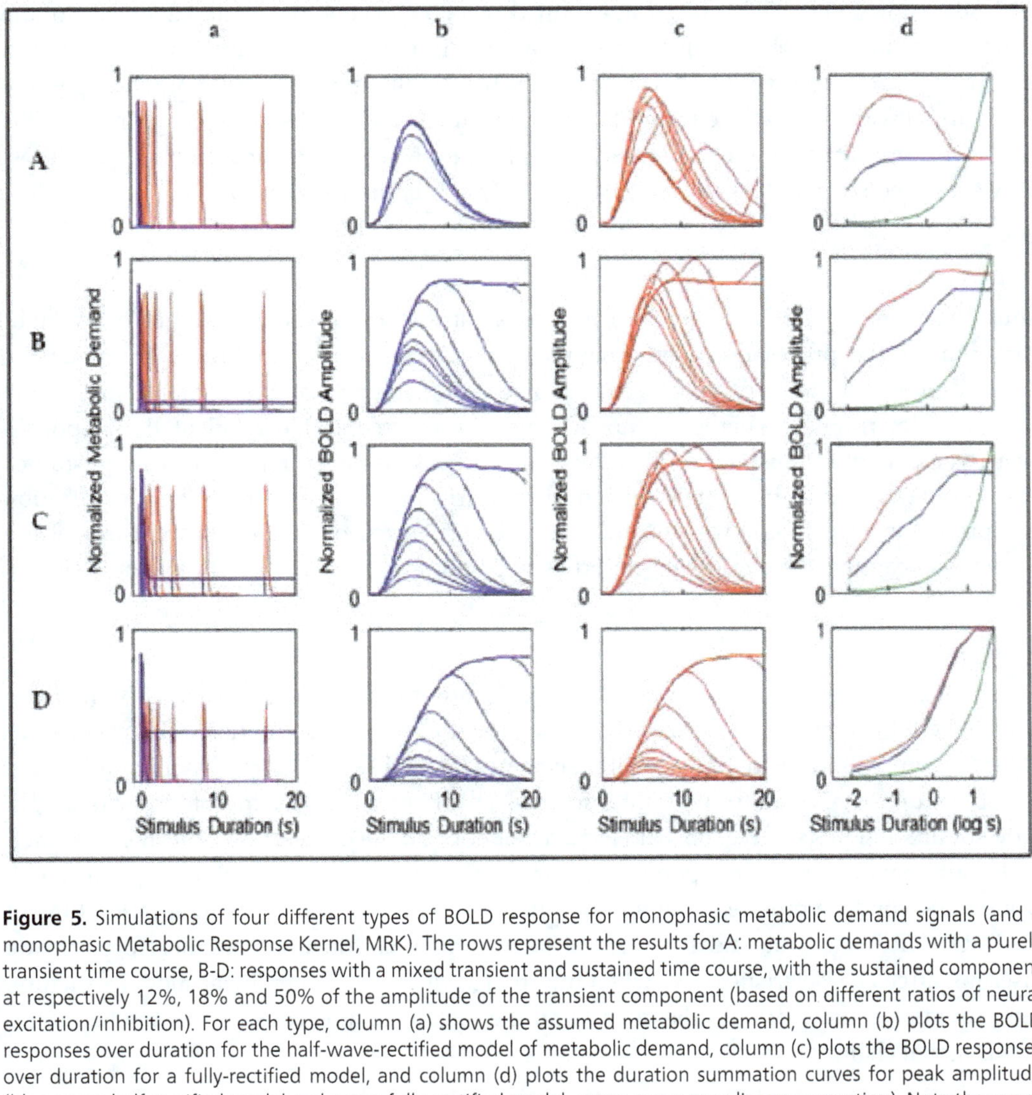

Figure 5. Simulations of four different types of BOLD response for monophasic metabolic demand signals (and a monophasic Metabolic Response Kernel, MRK). The rows represent the results for A: metabolic demands with a purely transient time course, B-D: responses with a mixed transient and sustained time course, with the sustained component at respectively 12%, 18% and 50% of the amplitude of the transient component (based on different ratios of neural excitation/inhibition). For each type, column (a) shows the assumed metabolic demand, column (b) plots the BOLD responses over duration for the half-wave-rectified model of metabolic demand, column (c) plots the BOLD responses over duration for a fully-rectified model, and column (d) plots the duration summation curves for peak amplitude (blue curve: half-rectified model, red curve: fully-rectified model, green curve: pure linear summation). Note the use of the logarithmic abscissa in column (d) to focus the analysis on the brief duration regime. The progression of the model BOLD responses with stimulus duration and the form of the summation curves are diagnostic of both the relative weighting between the sustained and transient components of the neural signal and the form of rectification feeding the metabolic demand.

The reduction in peak amplitude is captured in the red temporal summation curve of Fig. 5Ad, showing a reduction by a factor of two for long durations. (The green curve in Fig. 5Ad represents the values expected for fully proportional linear summation of the energy in the stimulus pulse; it is an accelerating curve due to the logarithmic abscissa.) The case of the full-rectification model of the metabolic demand is shown in Fig. 5Ac. Here the second neural response peak (i.e., that from the stimulus offset) plays a key role in varying the BOLD waveform, which first extends in time and then shows a two-peaked structure with reduced amplitude for long-duration stimuli.

Fig. 5Ba shows the half- and fully-rectified version of the metabolic demand to the same pulse duration series, where the neural inhibition is now assumed to be reduced in energy by 1.5% relative to the excitation. This small imbalance is magnified by the convolution with the sustained stimulus, and thus it results in a sustained component that is 12% of the am-plitude of the initial transient (blue curve in Fig. 5Ba) and then into an almost fully sustained set of BOLD response functions (Fig. 5Bb, compare to Ab).

Thus, the form of the BOLD re-sponse functions can be strongly diagnostic of even slight variations in the properties of brief neural signals. Moreover, the nature of the metabolic demand function (half- or fully-rectified) has a big impact on the form of the BOLD response, determining whether or not an offset peak occurs at the tail of the responses even when they are sustained (Fig. 5Bc). Such a peak has been reported in some studies but is not always evident. Thus it remains an empirical question to what extent rectification is representative of BOLD waveforms; inter-mediate forms of the rectification model are required to capture the empirical properties in detail.

Note that the amplitude series in Fig. 5Bb and c show bands of denser packing of the functions, where the amplitude changes were not spaced in proportion to the doublings of stimulus duration. Viewed in terms of the sequence of BOLD waveforms in Fig. 5Bb,c, the regions of dense packing form an intermediate "shelf" or partial asymptote in peak amplitude summation plots of Fig. 5Bd. It is again evident that the onset of this intermediate shelf in the summation curve corresponds to the integration time of the underlying neural signal, while the second asymptote at higher amplitude corresponds to the ~5 s integration time of the MRK (HRF). Accurate measurement of such summation functions can therefore provide discriminative characteristics that, when interpreted through the nonlinear model structure, can provide estimates of both the neural and the metabolic time constants in the neural-to-BOLD signal chain.

This point is emphasized by the response set in row C of Fig. 5, which probes the effect of varying the time constant of the neural transient. The key difference from the parameters used in row B of Fig. 5, is that the neural time constant was doubled from 50 ms to 100 ms (and the excitation/inhibition imbalance was also increased to 7% to maintain the same form of offset peak). It is evident that (i) the summation curve (Fig. 5Cd) takes a measurably different form, and that (ii) the accuracy of estimation of the neural time constant is limited not by the BOLD time constant but only by the variability of the BOLD amplitude measures. For example, this analysis shows that the neural time constant is estimable to within about 0.1 log units if the BOLD response functions can be measured to an achievable accuracy of about 10%.

log units if the BOLD response functions can be measured to an achievable accuracy of about 10%.

The final case of duration summation analyses (Fig. 5Dd) shows the NDFO predictions of increasing the excitation/inhibition imbalance of the neural response to 50%, illustrative of a system that is predominantly sustained in nature. Under these conditions, the impact of the initial transient becomes essentially negligible, and the summation curves (Fig. 5Dd) become indistinguishable from proportional summation (i.e., they run parallel to the green curve). This manipulation illustrates that the power of the NDFO analysis depends on the neural processing being predominantly transient, and that the properties of the underlying neural mechanisms would not be accessible to this form of analysis in predominantly sustained systems. Luckily, however, the well-established deviation from proportionality for short-duration stimuli implies that the neural system is, in practice, predominantly transient and is therefore amenable to this form of NDFO analysis.

11. Neural response component analysis

In a study of the fMRI components, we have recorded (Tyler et al. 2008) the sets of BOLD waveforms generated by fields of dynamic noise-patterned stimuli in differenct eccentricity bands across the visual field (Fig. 6, uppermost row). Responses were recorded in a corresponding series of retinotopic regions of interest (ROIs) defined bilaterally on V1 on the basis of serparate retinotopic mapping stimuli. An example of the variety of cortical responses obtained in retinotopic area V1 combined for both hemispheres is shown in the upper panel of Fig. 6. The responses vary not just in amplitude across stimulus types, but markedly in the waveform of the responses. Forsome stimuli, the same area may show a double-peaked on-response, a rounded on-response, a negative on-response, or a classica boxcar response. The variation in response from single cortical regions cannot be explained by variations in the hemodynamics of the blood oxygenation and strongly implies a neural origin of the differences for different stimulus type

These results support once again the important point that BOLD waveforms within particular cortical regions may vary dramatically as a function of the stimulus type, despite the fact that the metabolic/hemodynamic response kernels must remain invariant in the region (d'Avossa et al., 2003; Likova & Tyler, 2008; Tyler & Likova, 2009). The only option for a differential MRK is if the underlying neural circuitry has differential cortical layout relative to the local arterioles controlled by the astrocytes, which seems a highly unlikely structural association (and one that, if it did exist, would produce minor stastical variations in the BOLD waveform, not the radical differences among many stimulus types, as seen here). Consequently, differences in the BOLD response waveform in this ROI should be interpreted as due to differences in the *neural* response waveforms to the *different* stimuli.

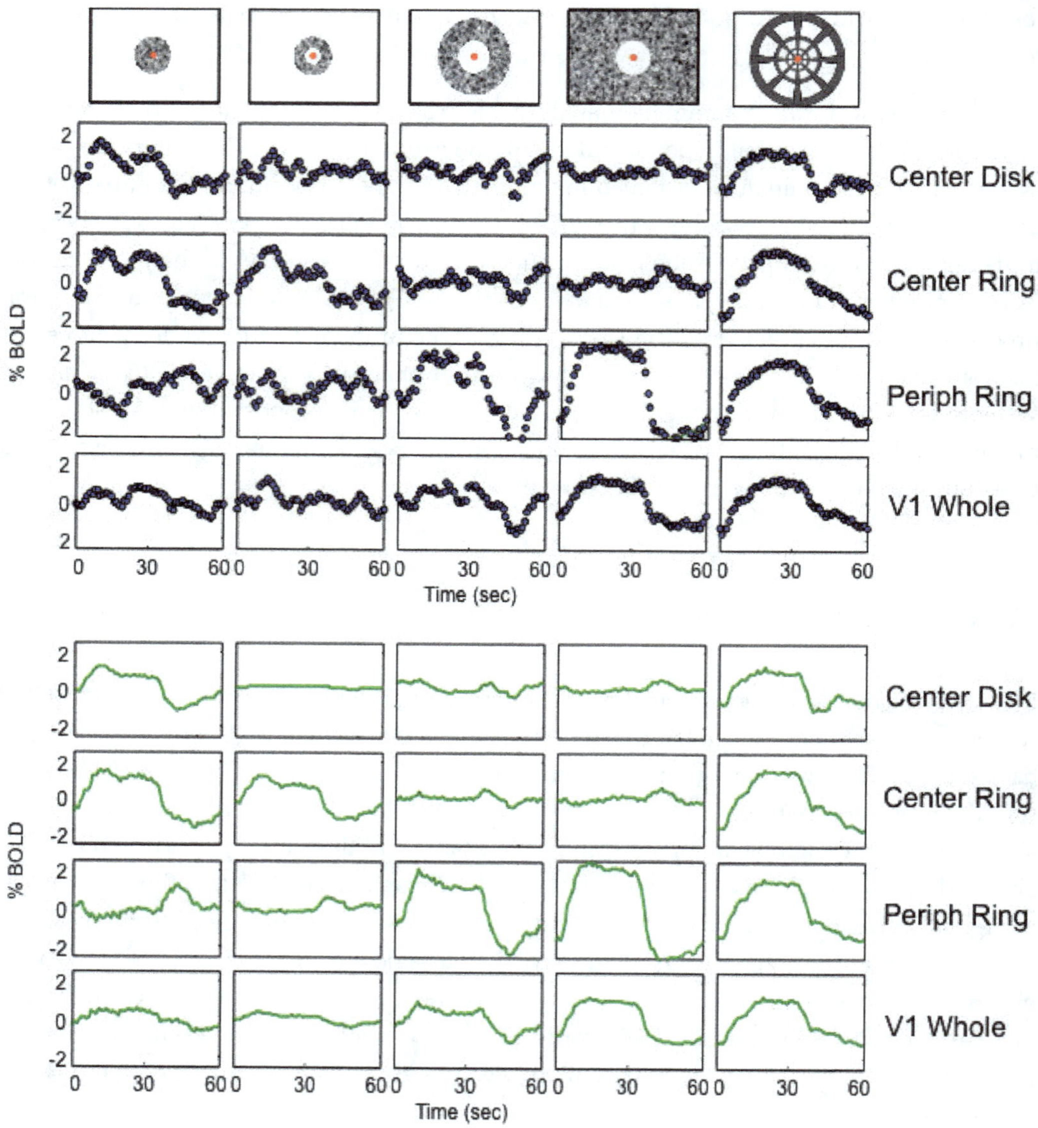

Figure 6. Upper plots: Variety of BOLD response waveforms obtained for the set of spatial noise stimuli shown along the top row in four matching ROIs deisgnated at right, in a block design of 30*s* on/ 30*s* off of fields of dynamic visual noise. Many of these responses differ substantially from the form of the typical GLM and from each other, particularly for the fine grid structure of the scaled grid in the last column. Lower plots: The independent components (IC) model does a good job of capturing this variety with the sum of the first three ICs, accounting for 92% of the variance in the empirical responses.

12. Multicomponent analysis of the neural signal contributions

Under the assumption that the neural signals in local regions of cortex consist of multiple components that are well-approximated by sets of delayed gamma-function components, they should be *dissociable* into the same vocabulary of multiple components as for the direct neural recordings through the NDFO procedure that takes into account the slow metabolic/astrocytic dynamics following the neural activation signals. The goal is to resolve the signals into the same component vocabulary, i.e., delayed gamma functions, that approximate known components of the neural dynamics.

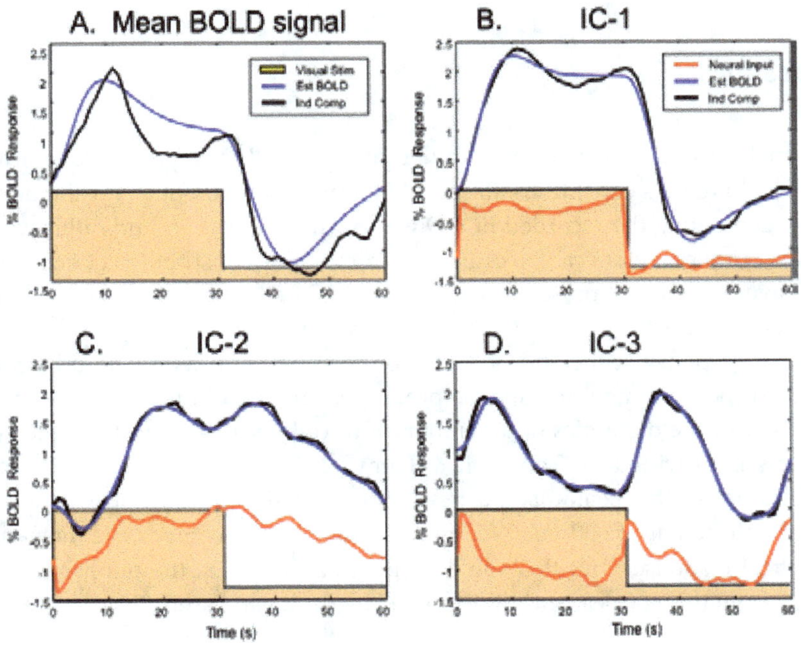

Figure 7. Dynamic forward modeling optimization of multiple neural components to the BOLD responses for cortical area V1. A. The average BOLD waveforms across the whole of V1 (black) with the fit for the Buxton-Friston balloon model. B-D. Plots of the optimized neural response estimates (red) for each of the three BOLD ICs (black curves), with the fit of the balloon model to each component (blue curves). Note the wide variety of temporal properties of the neural signals (red curves) selected by the optimization to account for the waveform differencesof the BOLD components. (from Tyler, Kontsevich & Ferree, 2008, with permission.)

The novel analysis we propose consists of (i) the simultaneous optimization of the set of neural components (ii) throught the Buxton-Friston balloon model, together with (iii) the rise and fall parameters of MRK. The results of the analysis for the V1 dataset of Fig. 6 s were sufficient to account for >95% of the BOLD variance overall (Fig. 7), which drew from the whole of the V1 ROI. Note that the mean BOLD waveform has an unusual double-peaked waveform, rising at the stimulus offset as well as the onset, and that the off-period (Fig. 7A). The IC analysis breaks this down into independent components that are differentially expressed across the individual voxels of V1 (some of this temporal waveform variety being captured in the specified ROIs within V1 shown in Fig. 6). The first IC (Fig. 7B) shows the classic form, following the predicted linear form for the balloon model (blue curve) accurately. The optimized neural signal for the fit to the actual wavform for the first IC is close to a boxcar function. The second IC has a very different form (Fig. 7B), with an early negative

BOLD peak at the stimulus onset and no corresponding rise at stimulus offset. The estimated neural signal has the same characteristic, although the negative peak has a much shorter latency. The third IC is even more non-linear, with approximately equal positive BOLD peaks at stimulus onset and offset as though responding to the stimulus events through a full-wave rectified nonlinearlity. Again, the estimated neural signal is a reflection of the same form of nonlinearity with much shorter latency.

13. Discussion

Our novel analysis of the neural signal underlying the BOLD response waveforms to a full temporal stimulus series constitutes a form of "temporal microscope" for the neural signals in the cortex generating the recorded BOLD waveforms. Thus, this study illustrates how the neural waveform parameters can be estimated from variety of stimulus effects. The estimated neural waveform for the present dataset in Fig. 5C has a strong brief transient, followed by a sustained response of about 1/10th of the peak transient response and a reduced, but rectified, offset response at the end of each stimulus. The transient should be presumed to match the corresponding neural response properties recorded in the cortex of other species. A useful survey of the dynamics of the unitary intracellular responses to single synaptic action potentials is provided by Thomson & Lamy (2007). They tabulate data from a large number of studies of the excitatory post-synaptic potential (EPSP) transient with a typical full width at half height of ~50 ms. We are not familiar with comparable meta-analyses for monkey cortical responses, but this value is clearly in line with the published examples of V1 transients from this species (such as those of Hegdé & van Essen, 2004).

The final analysis describes a search for independent response components in occipital are V1 in a relatively standard block-design stimulus paradigm incorporating a variety of spatial stimulation patterns (Tyler, Konstevich & Ferree, 2008). This analysis began with the assumptions of the balloon model of vascular hemodynamics, but the results revealed dramatic response nonlinearities, as expressed through an independent components analysis of the response variation across the cortical space of V1 and the stimulus variety (Figs. 6,7). Not shown in these figures is the way in which these nonlinear components were expressed across the cortical space, which implied that they were functional response components dependent on the relation between the stimulated and unstimulated regions, not structural differences in the vasculature. Thus, although the balloon model was an assumption of the analysis, the results raised the question of whether its assumed nonlinearities are hemodynamic in origin, given this result of profound functional nonlinearities across the space of V1, which are a fortiori of neural origin.

The neural signal components estimated to underlie the three primary ICs of Fig. 7 provide insight into the nature of the neural nonlinearities involved. Unlike the stable (linear) boxcar of Fig. 7B, the other two estimated neural waveforms have initial transients, one representing a half-wave rectification and the other a full-wave rectification. In neural signals, such nonlinearities are extremely well-known, and indeed are characteristic of neural processing in general (as "on" responses and "on-off" responses, respectively), while it is a stretch to conceptualize how they could arise from the hemodynamics per se. A more global mechanism that has such transient, rectified character is the top-down attentional mechanism, where activation may be drawn to regions of recent stimulus change in a transient fashion. These data are not sufficient to distinguish between the top-down and bottom-up hypotheses for the neural signals underlying the nonlinear BOLD responses revealed by this paradigm, but they make it clear that a rich array of neural nonlinearities should be expected to contribute to the fMRI signals recorded from the brain, which should allow the technique to answer a correspondingly abundant set of questions about the neural mechanisms involved in these response dynamics.

As knowledge evolves, more complex models of the neural/metabolic coupling and the hemodynamic response could be easily incorporated in our model. These all represent Bayesian information that, if well established, can be used to refine the model structure and enhance the fitting process when available. However, our understanding of the literature is that a) the first-order specification of the neural/BOLD coupling is well approximated by a linear response kernel, and b) that estimates of the second-order effects are contaminated by the assumption that the modeling has been purely hemodynamic, and has not taken into account potential and actual nonlinearities in the neural signals at the time scale of the BOLD signal. Thus, despite the best efforts of the proponents of elaborated hemodynamic modeling, there is no secure information about the nonlinearities of this process for the human brain in vivo.

Consequently, the present paper has tried to redress the balance by considering the effects plausible nonlinearities in the neural population responses to standard types of stimulus presentation. For clarity in this enterprise, we have assumed that the metabolic response is both linear and monophasic, illustrating a variety of BOLD response properties that could arise from such neural nonlinearities. We are not claiming to have proven that these BOLD properties are entirely determined at the neural level that, conversely, claims that they are purely properties of the vascular hemodynamics per se are suspect until they are replicated in paradigms that remove the neural component of the system. One such approach would be stimulation of the hemodynamic response by direct infusion of nitric oxide (NO) in the vicinity of the blood vessels. This experiment has apparently not been attempted, although suppression of the nitric oxide with application of the NO synthase inhibitor 7-nitroindazole completely abolishes the BOLD response while only marginally affecting the local field potentials (Burke & Bührle, 2006), establishing the role of NO in neurovascular coupling.

In particular, the nonlinearity of the transient responses at the offset of the neural response could be positive (rectifying) rather than negative (linear), and in either case show could show reduced amplitude relative to the onset response (adaptive gain control). In this example of the NDFO analysis, the offset responses are much smaller than the positive responses at stimulus onset. This analysis demonstrates that estimation of the neural response dynamics for each stimulus type is therefore not a Herculean task requiring extreme levels of signal/noise ratio, but is well within the capability of one session of normal fMRI methodology using however the appropriate combination of experimental design and theoretical analysis.

We note that a technique with a philosophy similar to the present approach has been successfully applied to the estimation of net spatial receptive field structure of small cortical regions by Dumoulin & Wandell (2008), although they used a linear rather than the full nonlinear model of the sequence of processes. Their spatial estimates were based on a model of the temporal signal to be expected as a stimulus swept across each defined point on the retina. Like us, they take the temporal stimulus waveform, convolve it with a spatiotemporal model of the response of the underlying neural population and then with a model of the hemodynamic response function to provide a basic forward model of the temporal BOLD response that is optimized to the measured BOLD response at each cortical location. Our approach takes the temporal analysis several steps further towards biological plausibility, and focuses on the temporal rather than spatial aspect of the neural population response.

14. Conclusion

The conceptualizations and techniques introduced in this paper provide an analytic capability to resolving the timing and neural signal estimation underlying the BOLD waveforms recorded throughout the cortex. Any such attempt must be based on a model of the known neural dynamics of the neural populations underlying the BOLD metabolic signal generation, which may be progressively refined as more information becomes available about both neural response characteristics and the metabolic cascade. Given adequate signal/noise ratio, the present analysis shows that it is possible to develop approaches that overcome the temporal limitations of BOLD signal and are able to reveal the relevant properties of the underlying neural signals down to their native temporal resolution. In combination, these approaches represent a notable advance in the capabilities of the fMRI technology, providing a direct linkage between the live assessment of the functioning brain and the direct neurophysiological recordings in other species.

Acknowledgements

Supported by NSF SLC grant 0846229, AFOSR grant #FA9550-09-1-0678 and CDMRP grant XWH-11-2-0066.

Author details

Christopher W. Tyler and Lora T. Likova

Smith-Kettlewell Eye Research Institute, USA

References

[1] Aguirre GK, Zarahn E, D'Esposito M (1998) The variability of human BOLD hemodynamic responses. NeuroImage, 8:360-9.

[2] Barth M, Norris DG (2007) Very high-resolution three-dimensional functional MRI of the human visual cortex with elimination of large venous vessels. NMR Biomed. 20:477-84.

[3] Bezzi P, Carmignoto G, Pasti L, Vesce S, Rossi D, Rizzini BL, Pozzan T, Volterra A (1998) Prostaglandins stimulate calcium-dependent glutamate release in astrocytes. Nature 391:281–285.

[4] Birn RM, Saad ZS, Bandettini PA (2001) Spatial heterogeneity of the nonlinear dynamics in the FMRI BOLD response. NeuroImage, 14: 817-26.

[5] Boynton GM, Engel SA, Glover GH, Heeger DJ (1996) Linear systems analysis of functional magnetic resonance imaging in human V1. J Neurosci 16: 4207-21.

[6] Buracas GT, Boynton GM (2002) Efficient design of event-related fMRI experiments using m-sequences. NeuroImage, 16: 801-13.

[7] Burke M, Bührle C (2006) BOLD response during uncoupling of neuronal activity and CBF. Neuroimage. 32:1-8.

[8] Celebi S, Principe JC (1995) Parametric least squares approximation using gamma bases. IEEE Transactions on Signal Processing, 43:781 – 784

[9] Chatton JY, Pellerin L, Magistretti PJ (2003) GABA uptake into astrocytes is not associated with significant metabolic cost: implications for brain imaging of inhibitory transmission. Proc Natl Acad Sci U S A. 100:12456-61.

[10] Chen S (2006) Signal processing. Euro. Trans. Telecomm, 17:99-110.

[11] d'Avossa G, Shulman GL, Corbetta M (2003) Identification of cerebral networks by classification of the shape of BOLD responses. J Neurophysiol, 90:360-71.

[12] De Vries B, Principe JC (1992) The Gamma Model: A new neural model for temporal processing. Neural Networks, 5:565-576.

[13] de Zwart JA, Silva AC, van Gelderen P, Kellman P, Fukunaga M, Chu R, Koretsky AP, Frank JA, Duyn JH. (2005) Temporal dynamics of the BOLD fMRI impulse response. Neuroimage 24:667-77.

[14] Dienel GA, Cruz NF (2008) Imaging brain activation: Simple pictures of complex biology. Ann NY Acad Sci 1147, 139-170.

[15] Efron B, Tibshirani RJ (1993) An Introduction to the Bootstrap. New York: Chapman and Hall.

[16] Farwell VT, Prentice RL (1977) A study of distributional shape in life testing, Technometrics 19:69–75.

[17] Filosa JA, Bonev AD, Nelson MT (2004) Calcium dynamics in cortical astrocytes and arterioles during neurovascular coupling. Circ Res. 95:73-81.

[18] Fox MD, Snyder AZ, Barch DM, Gusnard DA, Raichle ME (2005) Transient BOLD responses at block transitions. Neuroimage. 28:956-66.

[19] Friston KJ (1997) Transients, metastability, and neuronal dynamics. Neuroimage 5:164-71

[20] Friston KJ, Fletcher P, Josephs O, Holmes A, Rugg MD, Turner R (1998) Event-related fMRI: characterizing differential responses. Neuroimage. 7:30-40.

[21] Friston KJ, Mechelli A, Turner R, Price CJ (2000) Nonlinear responses in fMRI: the Balloon model, Volterra kernels, and other hemodynamics. Neuroimage. 12:466-77.

[22] Glover G (1999) Deconvolution of impulse response in event-related BOLD fMRI. Neuroimage. 9:416-29.

[23] Grotz T, Zahneisen B, Ella A, Zaitsev M, Hennig J (2009) Fast functional brain imaging using constrained reconstruction based on regularization using arbitrary projections. Magn Reson Med. 62:394-405.

[24] Handwerker DA, Ollinger JM, D'Esposito M (2004) Variation of BOLD hemodynamic responses across subjects and brain regions and their effects on statistical analyses. NeuroImage. 21:1639-51.

[25] Hakim TS, Sugimori K, Camporesi EM, Anderson G (1996) Half-life of nitric oxide in aqueous solutions with and without haemoglobin. Physiol. Meas. 17: 267

[26] Hansen KA, David SV, Gallant JL (2004) Parametric reverse correlation reveals spatial linearity of retinotopic human V1 BOLD response. NeuroImage. 23: 233-41

[27] Hegdé J, Van Essen DC (2004) Temporal dynamics of shape analysis in macaque visual area V2. J Neurophysiol. 92:3030-42.

[28] Henson RN, Price CJ, Rugg MD, Turner R, Friston KJ (2002) Detecting latency differences in event-related BOLD responses: application to words versus nonwords and initial versus repeated face presentations. NeuroImage, 15:83-97.

[29] Hoge RD, Franceschini MA, Covolan RJ, Huppert T, Mandeville JB, Boas DA (2005) Simultaneous recording of task-induced changes in blood oxygenation, volume, and flow using diffuse optical imaging and arterial spin-labeling MRI. Neuroimage. 25:701-7.

[30] Hyder F, Rothman DL, Shulman RG (2002) Total neuroenergetics support localized brain activity: implications for the interpretation of fMRI. Proc Natl Acad Sci USA 99:10771–10776.

[31] Hyder F, Patel AB, Gjedde A, Rothman DL, Behar KL, Shulman RG (2006) Neuronal-glial glucose oxidation and glutamatergic-GABAergic function. J Cereb Blood Flow Metab. 865-77.

[32] Kelly JP, Van Essen DC (1974) Cell structure and function in the visual cortex of the cat. J Physiol. 238:515-47.

[33] Koehler RC, Gebremedhin D, Harder DR (2006) Role of astrocytes in cerebrovascular regulation J Appl Physiol. 100: 307–317.

[34] Likova LT, Tyler CW (2008) Occipital network for figure/ground organization. Experimental Brain Research, 189:257-67.

[35] Lingnau A, Ashida H, Wall MB, Smith AT (2009) Speed encoding in human visual cortex revealed by fMRI adaptation. J Vis. 9:3.1-14.

[36] Logothetis NK (2002) The neural basis of the BOLD fMRI signal. Phil. Trans. R. Soc. Lond. 357:1003-1037.

[37] Logothetis NK (2003) The underpinnings of the BOLD functional magnetic resonance imaging signal. J Neurosci 23:3963-3971

[38] Logothetis NK, Wandell BA (2004) Interpreting the BOLD signal. Annual Review Physiology 66:735-769

[39] Magistretti PJ, Pellerin L (1999) Cellular mechanisms of brain energy metabolism and their relevance to functional brain imaging. Philos Trans R Soc Lond B Biol Sci. 354:1155-63.

[40] Magistretti PJ (2009) Role of glutamate in neuron-glia metabolic coupling. Am J Clin Nutr. 90:875S-880S.

[41] Margaria, R., Edwards, H.T., Dill, D.B. (1933) The possible mechanism of contracting and paying the oxygen debt and the role of lactic acid in muscular contraction. Am. J. Physiol. 106, 689–714.

[42] Martindale J, Mayhew J, Berwick J, Jones M, Martin C, Johnston D, Redgrave P, Zheng Y (2003) The hemodynamic impulse response to a single neural event. J Cereb Blood Flow Metab. 23:546–555;

[43] Menon RS, Luknowsky DC, Gati JS (1998) Mental chronometry using latency-resolved functional MRI. Proc Natl Acad Sci U S A, 95:10902-7.

[44] Metea MR, Newman EA (2006) Glial cells dilate and constrict blood vessels: a mechanism of neurovascular coupling. J Neurosci, 26:2862-70.

[45] Meyer EP, Ulmann-Schuler A, Staufenbiel M, Krucker T (2008) Altered morphology and 3D architecture of brain vasculature in a mouse model for Alzheimer's disease. Proc Natl Acad Sci U S A. 105:3587-92.

[46] Mulligan SJ, MacVicar BA (2004) Calcium transients in astrocyte endfeet cause cerebrovascular constrictions. Nature 431:195-9.

[47] Prentice RL (1974) A log-gamma model and its maximum likelihood estimation. Biometrika 61:539–544.

[48] Shank R, Aprison M (1979) Biochemical aspects of the neurotransmitter function of glutamate. In: Glutamic Acid: Advances in Biochemistry and Physiology. New York: Raven, p. 139–150.

[49] Shao XM (1997) Parametric survival analysis for gating kinetics of single potassium channels. Brain Research, 770: 96-104

[50] Shmuel A, AugathM, Oeltermann A, Logothetis NK (2006) Negative functional MRI response correlates with decreases in neuronal activity in monkey visual area V1. Nature Neurosci, 9: 569-577.

[51] Shulman RG, Rothman DL (1998) Interpreting functional imaging studies in terms of neurotransmitter cycling. Proc. Natl Acad. Sci. USA 95, 11993–11998.

[52] Sibson NR, Dhankhar A Mason GF, Rothman DL, Behar KL, Shulman RG (1998) Stoichiometric coupling of brain glucose metabolism and glutamatergic neuronal activity. Proc. Natl Acad. Sci. USA 95, 316–321.

[53] Sibson NR, Mason GF, Shen J, Cline GW, Herskovits AZ, Wall JE, Rothma DL, Shulman RG (2001) In vivo 13C NMR measurement of neurotransmitter glutamate cycling, anaplerosis, TCA cycle flux in rat brain during [2–13C]glucose infusion. J Neurochem 76:975–989.

[54] Smith AJ, Blumenfeld H, Behar KL, Rothman DL, Shulman RG, Hyder F (2002) Cerebral energetics and spiking frequency: the neurophysiological basis of fMRI. Proc Natl Acad Sci USA 99:10765–10770.

[55] Sotero RC, Trujillo-Barreto NJ (2007) Modelling the role of excitatory and inhibitory neuronal activity in the generation of the BOLD signal. Neuroimage. 35:149-65.

[56] Sotero RC, Trujillo-Barreto NJ (2008) Biophysical model for integrating neuronal activity, EEG, fMRI and metabolism. Neuroimage. 39:290-309.

[57] Stacy EW (1962) A generalization of the gamma distribution, Ann. Math. Stat. 33, 1187–1192.

[58] Tyler CW, Kontsevich LL, Ferree TC (2008) Independent components in stimulus-related BOLD signals and estimation of the underlying neural responses. Brain Research, 1229, 72-89.

[59] Tyler CW, Likova LT (2009) Neural signal estimation through time-resolved functional imaging. In: Brain Mapping Research Progress, Girard IC, Andre JS (Ed), Nova Scientific Publishers. 1-31

[60] Tyler CW, Likova LT (2011) Estimating neural signal dynamics in the human brain. Frontiers in Systems Neuroscience 5:33.

[61] Wang Y, Floor E (1994) Dynamic storage of glutamate in rat brain synaptic vesicles. Neurosci Lett, 180:175–178.

9

Phase Variations in fMRI Time Series Analysis: Friend or Foe?

Gisela E. Hagberg and Elisa Tuzzi

1. Introduction

Functional MRI studies (fMRI) are based on the blood-oxygenation-level-dependent effect (BOLD) that arises in brain areas where neuronal activity takes place (Ogawa et al., 1990, 1992; 1993). BOLD induces changes in the local magnetic susceptibility and these can be measured by Gradient Echo (GE) Echo-Planar-Imaging (EPI). The fMRI signal thus observed consists of a complex value, which is subdivided into a magnitude and a phase term. In most fMRI studies, the phase signal is discarded and only the magnitude changes are used to detect activated brain areas. In recent years, an increased interest in using both signal types has emerged, with the prospective of increasing both statistical power and spatial specificity.

This chapter describes the fMRI signal from a mathematical and biophysical view point, with emphasis on the phase signal. We will show which kind of information that the phase conveys and exemplify how it can be incorporated in the fMRI analysis pipeline. In section 2, we first describe the basics of an fMRI study, from the fundamental MR signal equations to how a whole brain image is generated in the scanner. We also describe the blood-oxygenation-level-dependent (BOLD) effect that follows neuronal activation. It alters the local magnetic susceptibility and the homogeneity of the local magnetic field and hereby alters the GE EPI signal.

Next, we discuss the phase signal in detail and we characterize the phase in comparison with the more familiar magnitude signal. We illustrate how the probability distributions of the magnitude and the phase values change as the signal-to-noise-ratio increases and how physical mechanisms, like paramagnetic and diamagnetic changes in the local field homogeneity, influence the magnitude and the phase signal in different ways. Regarding neuronal activity, we will review different biophysical models of BOLD with emphasis on the phase signal. Early models describe how the phase effect tend to cancel out for microvascular networks, while a detectable effect remains in larger vessels only (Yablonskiy and Haacke, 1994; Kiselev and Posse 1999; Menon, 2002). On the contrary, a more recent model, based on the Sphere of Lorentz effect, shows that a spatially extended, activated brain area produces a detectable change in the phase signal (Zhao et al., 2007; Feng et al., 2009).

An issue with the phase signal, addressed in the fourth section, is that the potentially valuable phase information is buried in strong phase variations that extend across the head, reflecting variations in the magnetic field homogeneity that vary both in space and in time. These noise factors are unrelated to the neuronal activity and affect the phase to a greater extent than the magnitude signal (Petridou et al., 2009; Hagberg et al., 2008).Methods that suppress or remove these unwanted effects represent a key factor fMRI analysis of phase data. We describe the sources of unwanted phase effects, how these can be modelled, and quantified. We also review several available post-processing methods that can be used to suppress or even remove these unwanted phase effects.

In the last section, we discuss emerging methods that utilize the information conveyed by the phase in the analysis of fMRI data. We will highlight a method that can be used to improve the analysis of the conventional magnitude signal. This method is derived by identifying physiological noise sources from the phase data, and by noise regression of the magnitude signal. The BOLD effect in phase images can also be usedwith the prospective of increasing statistical power and spatial specificity. For illustrative purposes, we show some phase and magnitude results obtained at the group-level in an fMRI study of a motor task performed at 3T.

2. Basics of fMRI physiology

Magnetic Resonance Imaging (MRI) is a non-invasive tomographic technique based on the principles of NMR. In virtue of being a tomographic technique it provides the reconstruction of sections of a 3D object. The capability to explore the structure of the human body non-invasively makes MRI widely employed in clinical imaging. Since the early 1990's, MRI is used not only to study brain structure but also to study brain function. Theso-called functional Magnetic Resonance Imaging (fMRI), which is based on the BOLD contrast, discovered by Ogawa et al. (1990, 1992, 1993). The great advantage of fMRI resides in its non–invasiveness and high availability, since standard equipment already existing in hospitals can be used.

Neuronal activity causes a local increase in the available oxygen due to neurovascular coupling, either due to synaptic input from other brain areas, or due to local signal processing (Logothetis, 2008). The neurovascular coupling mechanism consists of several steps, leading from an increase in the local neuronal activity to changes in blood flow. Initially, the blood oxygen concentration decreases, causing the initial dip phenomenon of the BOLD effect. As a compensatory mechanism, vasoactive substances are released by glia cells into the extracellular space. When these substances reach nearby blood vessels, the blood flow increases, and so does the relative amount of oxygenated haemoglobin, as a result of changes in the diameter of the blood vessels, the density of the red blood cells, and the amount of O_2 and CO_2. The hemodynamic BOLD response thus apparently over-compensates the oxygen use in the activated neurons, giving rise to blood oxygen levels which are higher than necessary to re-establish local tissue oxygen availability. The onset of this BOLD response is typically delayed by 1-2 seconds and peaks 4-6 seconds after onset of the neural response. Spatially, the fMRI signal spreads out due to bigger veins that drain the capillaries close to the neurons at work.

2.1. The fundamental MRI signal equations

Any atom holding a net nuclear magnetic moment, *I*, can generate an MR signal detectable by a scanner. Most MRI methods employ hydrogen atoms ^1H, owing to a high nuclear gyromagnetic moment and the high water concentrations present in the human body (ca 55M).

When hydrogen atoms are dipped into an external field, B_0, the spins tend to either align with the external field (lower energy state) or orient themselves in the opposite direction (upper energy state). At equilibrium, spins are in light excess in the former state, resulting in a non-zero net magnetic moment *M*that is aligned with the external field (Fig. 1). According to the rules of quantum mechanics, the nuclear magnetic moment cannot be exactly aligned with the external magnetic field, and are therefore oriented at an angle with respect to the field. This difference in orientation between the external field and the field of the spins causes a torque effect leading to a precession of the spins around the external field (see zoomed box, Fig. 1). The precession occurs at the Larmor frequency, ω , according to the fundamental equation of NMR, the Larmor equation:

$$\omega = \gamma B_0 \tag{1}$$

where γ is the gyromagnetic ratio (in units of radian/T/s), and $B_0$the intensity of the magnetic field.

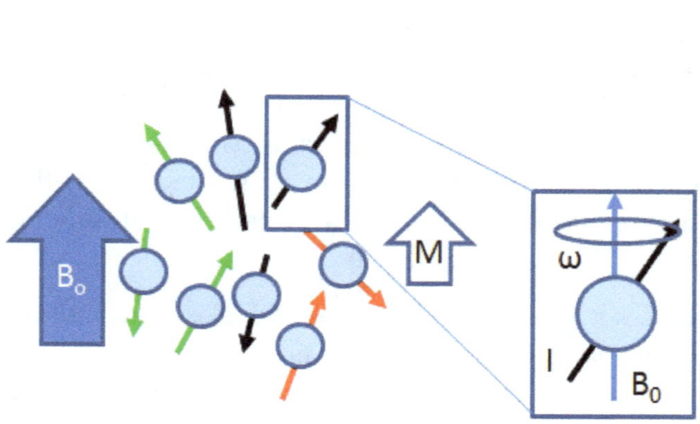

Figure 1. Net magnetic moment *M*of and ensemble of spins, each with an individual nuclear magnetic moment, *I*, placed in an external field B_0. In the zoomed inset, the precession of*I* around the B_0 axis at the Larmor frequency, ω is shown.

At equilibrium, no MR signal can be detected since the magnetization vector *M*is time independent. An MR signal can only be detected after the equilibrium condition has been perturbed, when the spin systems return to equilibrium and the spins flip from the higher to the lower energy level. The perturbation is made so that the spins can absorb the necessary energy to bridge the gap, ΔE, between the two spin states. A radiation field B_1 oscillating exactly at the Larmor frequency is used to excite the spins and induce transitions from the lower to the higher energy state. The perturbing B_1field is applied orthogonally with respect to B_0 (Fig. 2).

The induced transition to the upper energy level gives rise to a spin coherence, bringing the longitudinal equilibrium magnetization M_z into the transverse plane x-y, M_{xy}, in a fixed reference system (laboratory system) as shown in Fig. 2.

The transition from the longitudinal to the transverse direction is thus induced by a radio-frequency field B_1, or a so-called 90° pulse. When the $B_1$90° pulse is interrupted,*M* starts to precess around the B_0z-axis at the Larmor frequency, whilst re-establishing its initial equilibrium value.This causes the gradual recovery of the longitudinal component M_z and the complete extinction of M_{xy}. The temporal variation of the transverse component, M_{xy}, originates the MR signal, also known as Free Induction Decay (FID),oscillates at the Larmor frequency and is detectable as an induced voltage in the radio-frequency coil, according to Faraday's law of electromagnetic induction.

The evolution of the magnetization *M* of a spin system immersed in an external magnetic field, B_0, perturbed by an oscillating field, B_1, and the forces that rule the FID can be conjointly described by the phenomenological Bloch equations. The solutions to the Bloch equations govern the decay and recovery of the magnetization.

In the absence of local magnetic field inhomogeneities, the decay of the transverse component, M_{xy}, is described by the characteristic time constant, T_2, also known as the spin-spin relaxation time, while the characteristic time constant T_1, known as spin-lattice relaxation time, rules the recovery of the transverse component, M_z, according to:

$$M_{xy} = M_0 e^{-t/T_2} \tag{2}$$

$$M_z = M_0(1 - e^{-t/T_1}) \tag{3}$$

In the presence of local field homogeneities, that are not refocused by the imaging sequence the FID signaldecay is governed by the time constant $T_2{}^*$, or the effective transverse relaxation time:

$$M_{xy} = M_0 e^{-t/T^*{}_2} \tag{4}$$

This situation happens for gradient echo sequences used in fMRI studies. With this MR sequence, local field inhomogeneities are not refocused and in presence of a positive BOLD effect, a lengthening of $T_2{}^*$ arises due to a relative increase in the local blood concentration of oxyhemoglobin during activation. Oxyhemoglobin is less paramagnetic than deoxyhemoglobin and therefore generates a field shift which is diamagnetic relative to the baseline condition (see paragraph 4 and Fig 8). As will be discussed in greater detail further on, the presence of paramagnetic effects leads to an increase in the bulk magnetic field, with faster spin precession while the presence of diamagnetic effects causes a decreased local field, and a loss of angular precession velocity of the spins around B_0 (see Eq. 1 and Fig. 2)

A diamagnetic or a paramagnetic shift in magnetic susceptibility causes variations in the local Larmor frequency and may lead to off-resonance and dephasing effects, $\varphi(t)$ depending on whether the field is uniform or varies across the voxel. Therefore a more general signal equation for a gradient echo sequences is:

$$\begin{aligned} M_{xy} &= M_0 e^{-t/T^*_2} e^{-i\cdot\varphi(t)} \\ \varphi(t) &= \gamma \cdot \int_0^t B(\tau)d\tau \end{aligned} \qquad (5)$$

Implicitly, this equation takes into account the complex value of the MRI signal, which is described in more detail below. The decay term of [Eq. 5] is obtained from the magnitude component of the MR signal while the off-resonance dephasing effects, $\varphi(t)$are obtained from the phase.

2.2. Image generation and fMRI

The MRI signal is derived from the entire system of spins, which are excited by the RF pulse and precess at the Larmor frequency. In order to spatially distinguish between spins and to reconstruct an image, magnetic field gradients are added to the external magnetic field B_0. These gradients are applied in the three spatial directions (x,y,z), defining respectively the *slice-selection gradient*, G_z, the *phase-encode gradient*, G_y, and the*frequency-encode* (also *readout*) *gradient*, G_x. The first gradient is used to select the magnetization located inside a slice through the object, while the latter two gradients are used to encode the spatial position of this magnetization in 2D space. This information is sampled in a reciprocal space, termed k-space, and the image of the selected slice is reconstructed by a 2D Fourier Transform that maps the original magnetization distribution of the object from k-space back into object space.In an fMRI study, the signal changes caused by the BOLD response is followed by whole brain measurements that are obtained every 1-3 seconds, with typical voxel sizes between 3x3x3 and 1x1x1mm^3 in human brain studies. Due to the sluggishness of the BOLD functional brain studies generally employ gradient-echo echo-planar imaging (GE-EPI) sequences for data acquisition: a 2D image (or a slice) is acquired following a single excitation pulse, and 20-30 such slices are imaged yielding whole brain coverage within a 2-3 s long repetition time, with typical voxel sizes between 1x1x1 and 3x3x3 mm^3 (Schmitt et al., 1998). The GE-EPI sequence, in which the entire 2D k-space is filled using rapid gradient switching

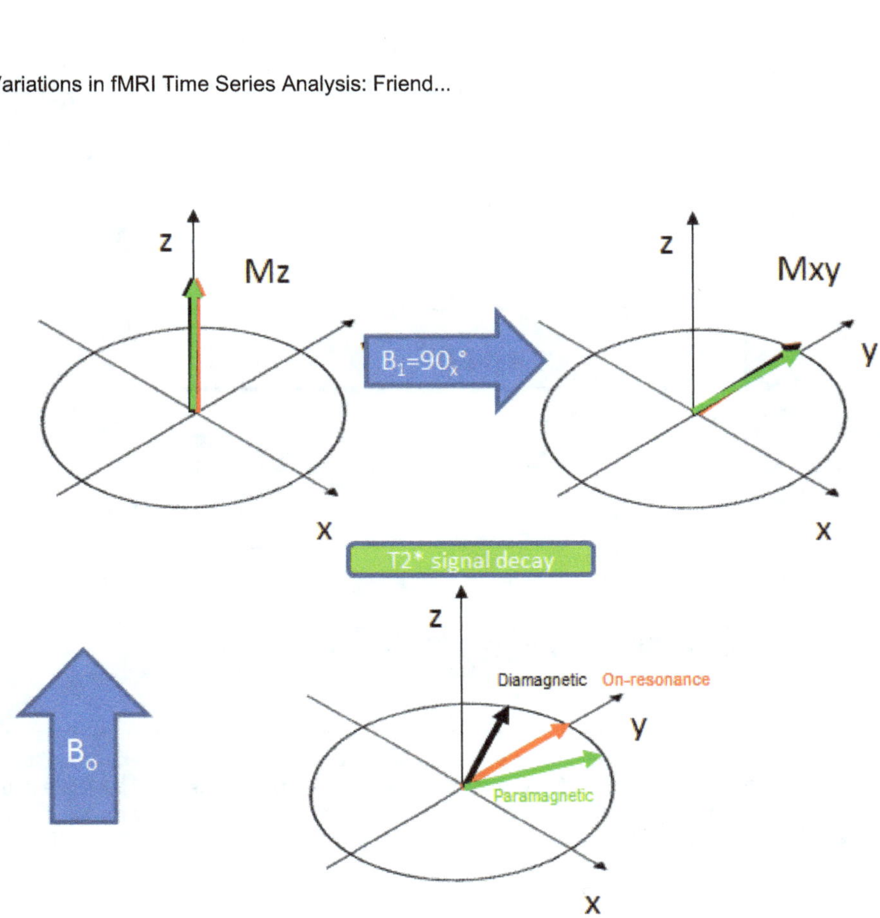

Figure 2. At equilibrium, the net magnetization is said to be longitudinal, M_z and is oriented along the direction of the external magnetic field, B_0. A radio frequency (RF) field B_1oscillating at the Larmor frequency is applied orthogonally to B_0. This so-called 90° pulse, rotates the magnetization vector into the transverse orientation M_{xy}.During the echo time, spin coherence is lost leading to a T_2* signal decay, that depends on the local magnetic susceptibility. Spins in a diamagnetic environment precesses a little slower, while spins in a paramagnetic environment precesses a little faster than the on-resonance spins. The original equilibrium condition with a longitudinal net magnetization is recovered after a time that is about five times as long as the longitudinal T_1 relaxation time.

after a single excitation pulse, begins with a slice-selective excitation pulse with a flip angle α(i.e. an RF pulse that brings the Magnetization vector at an angle $\alpha$with respect to B_0), and is followed by an EPI readout of gradient echoes (i.e. a train of gradient echoes made up of readout gradientswith alternating polarity, see G_x in Fig.3). Before each readout gradient, a brief phase-encode blip (G_y) is applied in order to quickly sample the whole k-space. Alternatively, a full 3D volume can be acquired by so-called echo-volume imaging (EVI, Mansfield, 1977). In this case no slice-selection is necessary, instead an entire volume is excited by a single RF-pulse and 3D k-space is covered by phase encoding along two spatial directions.

The advantages of using gradient-echo EPI areitsrapid image generation with minimal energy deposition, sufficient spatial resolution and ease of acquisition, yielding whole brain coverage within a short imaging time. These advantages come however at the expense of a relative low signal-to-noise ratio, which is however combined with a great BOLD contrast-to-noise ratio.

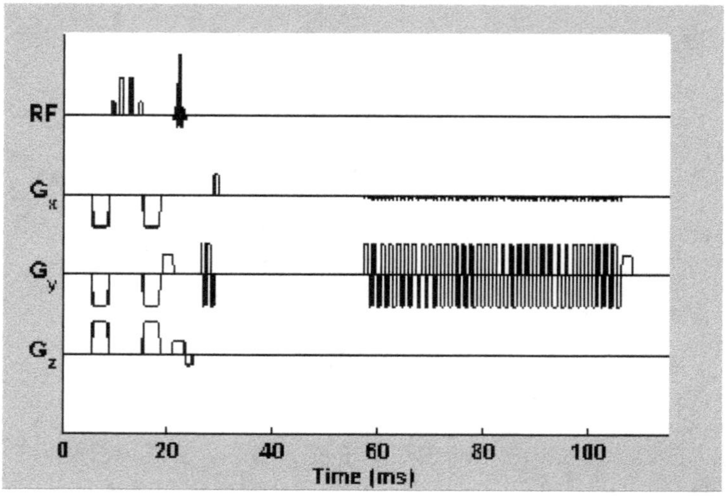

Figure 3. The gradient echo (GE) echo-planar-imaging (EPI) sequence. An RF pulse with flip angle α (first row) is applied together with a magnetic field gradient in the slice selection direction (G_z. last row). Hereby all the spins located inside the selected slice have theirmagnetization vector rotated by an angle $\alpha$with respect to B_0. k-space (the reciprocal of the image space) is sampled by a combination of brief phase-encoding blips (G_x second row) and readout gradientswith alternating polarity (G_y third row). Finally, a Fourier Transform is performed to recover the MR image of the selected slice.

To reach a sufficient BOLD contrast-to-noise ratio (CNR),several such GE-EPI images are acquired during presentation of selected stimuli, generating an fMRI time series.A typical stimulus paradigm for an fMRI experiment alternates "ON" states in which subjects are asked to perform a task, and "OFF" states (or "Control" state) in which they have to be at rest or perform a control task. Generally "ON" and "OFF" states are repeated every 20-40s, to maximize the BOLD signal, and several repetitions of such "ON"/"OFF" states are required. Typical durations of an fMRI time series is 5-10 min. An example of an fMRI experiment is shown in Fig. 4.

Besides the acquisition sequence and the stimulus paradigm, the success of an fMRI experiment depends uponthe statistical data analysis that is undertaken to individuate the cerebral regions where the variation of the magnitude MRI signal is stimulus correlated. The sensitivity of the statistical analysis depends on both the BOLD contrast and on the fMRI noise level. As we will show, the fMRI noise level can be reduced by using the information conveyed by the phase signal.

3. Characteristics of the MRI phase signal

As we will see, the MRI signal can be described by a complex number, consisting of a magnitude and a phase term. Most MRI methods only retain the magnitude term, but in some established applications, like phase-contrast angiography, Susceptibility Weighted Imaging

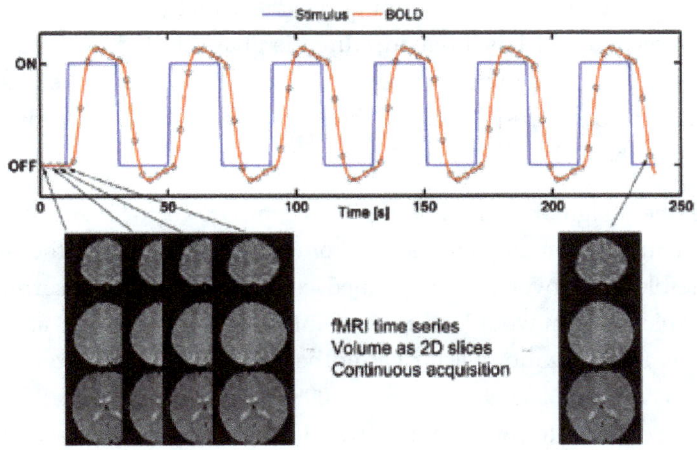

Figure 4. An fMRI experiment consisting of "OFF" and "ON" periods with a 20-40 seconds duration. Gradient-echo EPI images with whole brain coverage are acquired each 2-3 seconds, and 100 or more brain volumes make up the fMRI time series.

or anatomical phase imaging methods at high field strengths, the phase is used as a sole ingredient or in combination with the magnitude to generate image contrast.

The phase and the magnitude signals are like two sides of a coin for the MRI signal. While the magnitude signal is related to the dispersion of the underlying local magnetic field, the phase is sensitive to coherent magnetic field shifts. The reason behind this may become clear if we consider the MRI signal as a vector sum of single spin contributions located at different spatial points inside the voxel, precessing around the B_0 field according to the fundamental Larmor equation (e.g. Fig.1). In case of an ideal homogeneous magnetic field, without field dispersion or field shifts, all the vectors will precess 'on-resonance' at the same frequency generating a maximal magnitude signal at the echo time TE, and a zero phase. In the presence of a field inhomogeneity across the voxel, a field dispersion, each spin senses a slightly different field and precesses at a frequency which is slightly different from the 'on-resonance' condition. At TE, the vectors will therefore point into different directions and the vector sum generates a decreased magnitude signal, while the average phase is zero. In presence of a local deviation of the magnetic field which is uniform across the voxel, a field shift, all the vectors have the same frequency albeit different from the 'on-resonance' condition. At TE, there is a decreased magnitude signal, and an altered phase.

In the following we will discuss the different characteristics of the magnitude and phase of the MRI signal, with emphasis on some factors that are important for fMRI applications. Besides the signal and noise properties, we will describe three biophysical models for the effect of BOLD on the phase signal.

3.1. Definition of the magnitude and the phase of the fMRI signal

The MR detection systemis based on quadrature detection. The voltage induced by the oscillating net transversemagnetization$M_{xy}$is split into two channels that function with a phase difference with respect to each other. Two output signals are thus detected, the first which is 'in-phase' and the second which is 'in-quadrature' (ie phase shifted) with respect to the first. These signals can be described in mathematical terms by the real and the imaginary components of a complex vector, corresponding to the M_x and the M_y components of the detected net magnetization of the FID.

In the ideal case, the imaginary component of this complex vector is zero and all the necessary image information is contained in the real component. If this is not the case, it should in principle be possible to recover the real-valued component by'phase correcting' the data. Thereby the complex vector would be rotated into the M_x direction, and an absorption mode image of the magnetization vector would be available, as suggested bysome promising attempts (Bernstein et al., 1989, Bretthorst, 2008). However in general, due to phase imperfections that are difficult to correct, it is convenient to use the absolute (magnitude) value of the MRI signal, corresponding to the length of the complex vector. SuchMRI images are produced by taking the square root of the sum of squares of the real and imaginary components of the measured magnetization vector. The phase of the complex vector, or the argument of the complex vector, is obtained by evaluating the arc-tangent of the ratio of the imaginary and the real components (see Fig. 5):

$$S = abs(M_{xy}) = \sqrt{M_x^2 + M_y^2} \tag{6}$$

$$\varphi = \arg(M_{xy}) = \arctan(\frac{M_y}{M_x}) \tag{7}$$

In general, the phase evolves linearly with the local magnetic fieldB_{loc}in a particular voxel during the time between the excitation pulse and signal read out, i.e. the echo time, *TE*. At the time of acquisition the phase is:

$$\Delta\varphi = \gamma \cdot B_{loc} \cdot TE \tag{8}$$

where γ is the gyromagnetic ratio (in units of radian/T/s) for the observed nuclear spins (see Eq.2).

The phase evolution is defined as positive (clockwise) for increasing magnetic fields (paramagnetic shifts), and negative (counterclockwise) for decreasing magnetic fields (diamagnetic shifts). However this sign convention based on the physical torque effect on the magnetic vector is not compatible with the mathematical sign convention of complex numbers (see Fig. 2 and Hagberg, et al.,2010) and therefore often a negative sign is used in front of the expression in [Eq. 8].

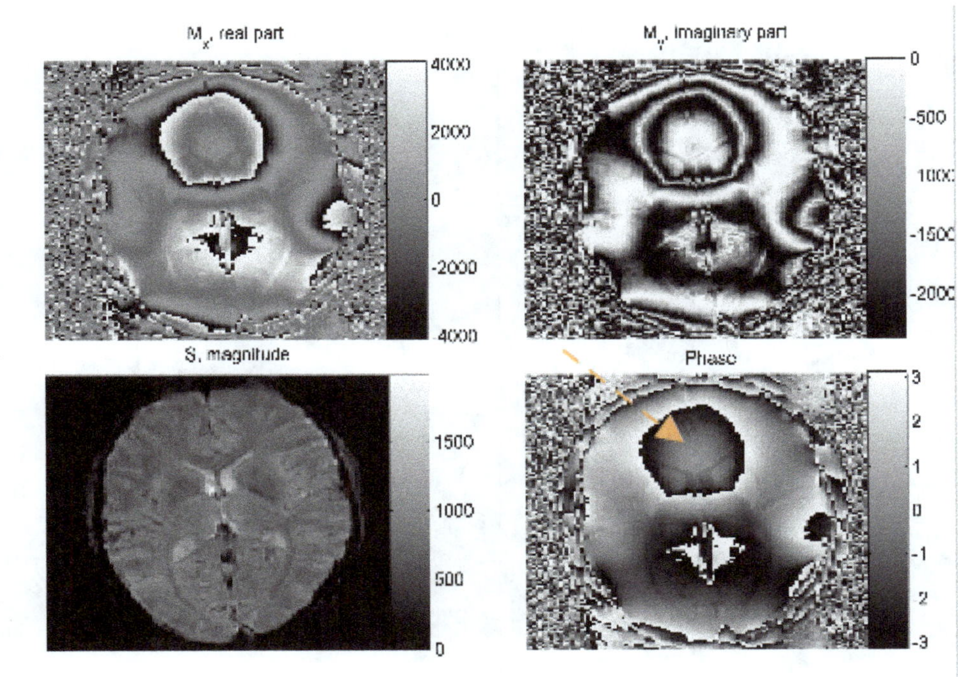

Figure 5. The MRI detection system subdivides the image information into a real and an imaginary component, corresponding to the M_x and the M_y components of the transverse magnetization. These components define a complex vector and can be rearranged to form the length [Eq. 6] and the argument [Eq.7] of the vector, corresponding to the MRI magnitude and phase signals, respectively. The red arrow indicates the area just above the frontal sinuses with strong magnetic field variations, due to the difference in susceptibility between the air in the frontal sinuses and the brain tissue.

3.2. Signal-to-noise ratio in magnitude and phase images

As we discussed above, the signal in the MRI detection system is acquired via two channels that correspond to the real and the imaginary components of a complex number. The electronic noise of each receiving channel has a Gaussian probability density function (PDF), with zero mean and variance determined by fluctuations around this mean. The PDF of the phase and magnitude noise are determined by the combined noise from both channels (Gudbjartsson and Patz 1996). The magnitude values are always greater than zero, and hence cannot have a zero mean. In presence of purely electronic noise, the noise in the magnitude image therefore follows the Rayleigh probability density function, while for SNR levels of 3 and above a Gaussian PDF is observed. The phase signal originating from pure electronic noise takes on any value in the $\pm\pi$ range with equal probability according to a uniform PDF (Eq. 9). As the SNR increases, the PDF of the phase signals evolve towards a Gaussian shape (Fig. 6). Since these the magnitude and the phase signals have a common origin in the real and imaginary components of the receiving channels, the SNR values are interrelated. For high SNR values, the PDF of the phase is obtained from the magnitude signal (Eq.9).

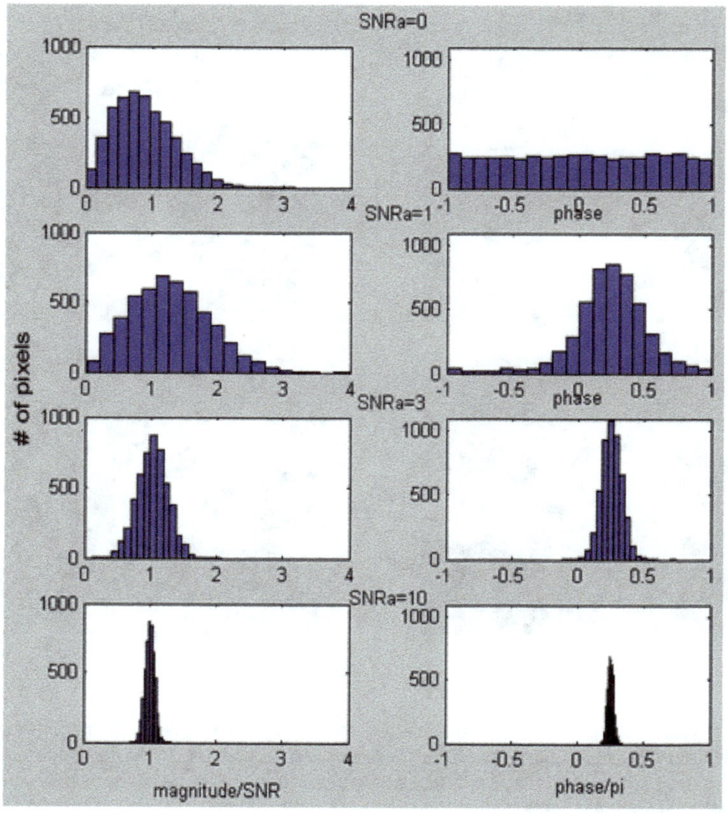

Figure 6. Histograms representing the signal-to-noise probability density functions (PDF) for the magnitude (left column) and phase (right column) signals. The following cases are shown. First row: with an SNR of zero (purely electronic noise), the magnitude values distribute according to a Rayleigh PDF, while the distribution of the phase values is uniform. In row 2-4, we show how the shape of the PDF changes as we go towards greater SNR. At low SNR levels of 1 (2nd row) a Rician PDF is observed for the magnitude data, while at an SNR of 3 (3rd row) and 10 (4th row) the shape is Gaussian. Above an SNR of 3, the phase signal also follows a Gaussian PDF, albeit with a more narrow shape, as the standard deviation of the phase signal is the inverse of the SNR observed for the magnitude signal.

$$SD_{\varphi} = \begin{cases} \dfrac{\pi}{\sqrt{3}} & \text{if SNR} = 0 \\ \\ \dfrac{1}{SNR} & \text{if SNR} >> 1 \end{cases} \tag{9}$$

These considerations evidence how the noise properties of magnitude and phase signals are interrelated at high SNR levels. Although the theory by Gudbjartsson and Patz was developed for an MRI image acquired at a single time point, their observations are also fundamental for describing the magnitude and phase fluctuations that occur during an fMRI time series, described in section 4 (see also Hagberg et al., 2008). Keeping these fluctuations as small as possible is important in fMRI, since the statistical T-values depend on them. Less fluctuations lead to higher BOLD contrast-to-noise ratios and greater statistical T-values, yielding an enhancement of the fMRI detection sensitivity.

3.3. The blood-oxygenation level dependent effect and the phase signal

The contrast in a GE-EPIsequence is generated by the signal evolution between a 90º RF excitation pulse and signal read-out (that is the echo time, TE). While the magnitude signal follows an exponential decay, the phase is linearly accrued during TE (see Eqs. 5, 8). The BOLD effect causesachange in the magnetic susceptibility difference between veins and the surrounding tissue. During the activated state, the oxygenation fraction Y is greater than during baseline states, and therefore the susceptibility difference is diminished. The effect of BOLD on the magnitude signal isdriven by a change in the dispersion (variation) of the magnetic field inside the voxel, while a change in phase is driven by a coherent shift (a net change) of the magnetic field.

The magnitude/phase evolution during TE is influenced not only by the BOLD effect per se but also by the vessel geometry and the spatial orientations of the vessels with respect to the orientation of the static magnetic field of the scanner (see Eq. 10, Fig. 7). Ideally, only the BOLD effect arising in the capillary bed close to the site of neuronal activation should be detected, however larger draining veins also contribute to the activation maps.

In order to calculate the phase variation during BOLD, let's consider the simple case of a single vessel crossinga voxel. The vessel can be modelled as an infinitely long cylinder with a different, blood-oxygenation and hematocrit dependent susceptibility than the surrounding brain tissue. In this case, the signal depends on the orientation of the vessel with respect to the static magnetic field of the scanner. Vessels oriented parallel to the field, do not 'oppose' the field as much as perpendicularly oriented vessels and hence produce a magnetic field shift that is localized inside the vessel, while in the perpendicular orientation, the vesselsproduce both extra- and intra-vascular effects. These are described by the following equations (Boxerman et al., 1995):

$$
\begin{aligned}
&\Delta B_{vessel} = iv + ev \\
&iv = 2\pi \cdot \Delta\chi_o \cdot (1-Y) \cdot Hct \cdot B_o \cdot \left(\cos^2\theta - \frac{1}{3}\right) \\
&ev = 2\pi \cdot \Delta\chi_o \cdot (1-Y) \cdot Hct \cdot B_o \cdot \left(\frac{R}{r}\right)^2 \cdot \sin^2\theta \cdot \cos(2\Psi)
\end{aligned}
\tag{10}
$$

where $\Delta\chi_0$ is the susceptibility difference between the extra (*ev*) - and intravascular (*iv*) space (in cgs units), *Y* the oxygenation level of the blood, *Hct* is the haematocrit level, $B_0$is the static magnetic field strength, *R* the vessel radius and *r* the distance from the centre of the vessel cylinder, and θ, Ψ are the angles defined in Fig 7.

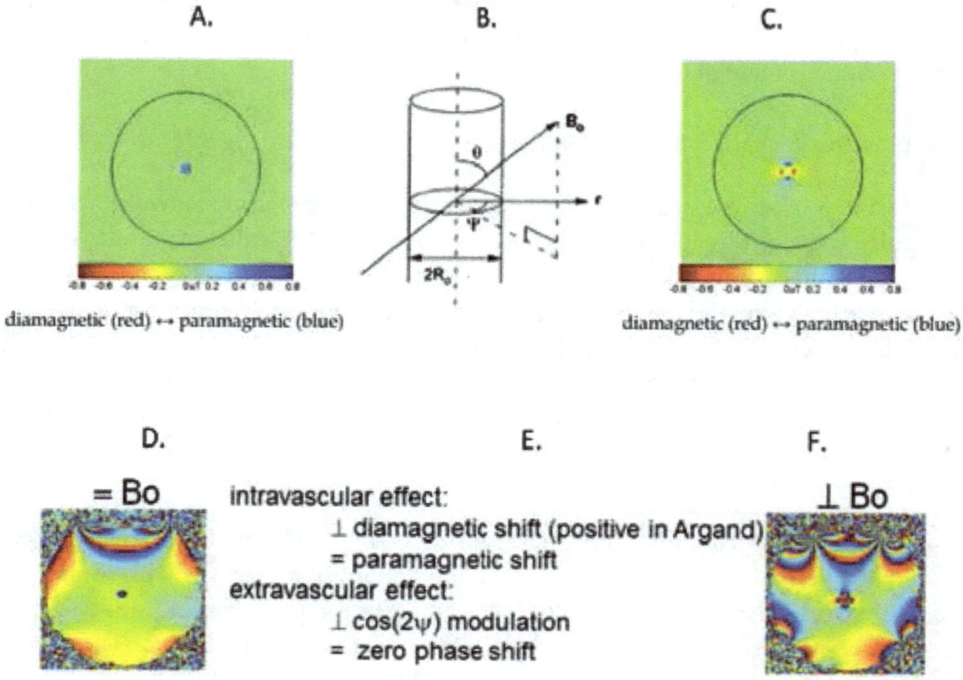

Figure 7. Biophysical cylinder model for a single vessel placed with its length axis oriented parallel (A,D, symbol: =) or perpendicular (C, F, symbol: ⊥) to the external magnetic field,B_0. B: The anglesθ, $\Psi$and the distance from the centre of the vessel, r,define the position for a point in space where a magnetic field is generated due to the blood-tissues susceptibility difference, as described in [Eq. 10]. A,C: Simulated magnetic field map for a cylinder placed in the centre of a sphere (first row: $\Delta\chi_0$=0.18ppm, hematocrit=0.4, oxygenation fraction Y=0.54). For a cylinder oriented parallel to the field, no phase modulation occur in the extravascular space (the field inside the cylinder is visible as a blue spot in the centre). For a cylinder oriented perpendicular to the external field, a cos2Ψ modulations occurs around the vessel. D,F: Measured MRI phase images (Magnetic field strength: 3T, GE-EPI, TE=20ms) for a cylinder with higher susceptibility than the surrounding water. The pattern corresponding to the dipole field is evident for the perpendicular orientation. Unwanted background variations of the field are present in the measured but not in the simulated data.E: Depending on the vessel orientation (= or ⊥) with respect to the external field, diamagnetic or paramagnetic field shifts can be observed.

In Fig. 7, phase images of a cylindrical vial containing a solution with higher magnetic susceptibility than the solution contained in the surrounding, outer area are shown for a parallel and a perpendicular orientation, with respect to the static magnetic field.The greatest extra-vascular effects are obtained for the perpendicular orientation, with a spatial cos2Ψ modulation around the vessel, and a diamagnetic phase shift inside the vessel. The size of the phase shifts will depend on the oxygenation fraction and on the geometrical factor, determined by the orientation of the vessels, as expressed by [Eq.10]. The expected phase values that occur during the resting and active conditions of an fMRI study can be obtained by straightforward calculations based on [Eq. 10]. For instance, during rest (when the oxygenation fraction is ca Y=0.54) the maximal field difference between the extra- and intravascular space amounts to ±0.62μT at 3T and appears in the tissue surrounding a perpendicular vessel (extravascular space). This value corresponds to a phase shift as high as ±4.98 radian if a

GE-EPI sequence with a TE of 30 ms is used. In presence of a BOLD response during the activated state (Y=0.68) the susceptibility difference between the blood and the tissue diminishes and therefore the maximal field difference becomes ±0.43μT (±3.45radian). In the intravascular space of a parallel vessel, the field undergoes a diamagnetic shift and is therefore reduced from 0.42 μT (3.37radian) at rest to 0.29 μT (2.33 radian) during activation. Consequently, the expected BOLD induced field change is maximal in the extravascular space for perpendicular vessels (±0.19μT, 1.52radian), while for the parallel case it is greatest in the intravascular space (-0.13μT, 1.04radian). These observations are also in line with previous work (Hoogenrad et al., 2001).

During an fMRI study the expected phase effect will be diminished due to the partial volume effects that arise when the vessel diameter is smaller than the measured voxel size (see Brainovich et al., 2010). In view of these phase shifts, Menon (2002) suggested that it should be possible to identify voxels dominated by draining vessels parallel to the field, due to the intravascular phase shift, while the contribution from perpendicular vessels should cancel out, due to signal modulation in the extravascular space that is averaged out as a consequence of partial volume effects.

The cortical region that encloses the activated neurons is characterized by a dense capillary network. Larger vessels that drain the activated region are more remotely located at the brain surface (e.g. Keller et al., 2011). The network consists of vessels with a range of different radii, and diffusion effects must also be considered to quantify the effect of the magnetic field distribution. This is not trivial to do and therefore calculations were initially done by Monte Carlo simulations (Yablonskiy and Haacke 1994) before an analytical expression was derived by Kiselev and Posse (1999, see Eqs. 5 and 25 in that paper). From these studies, it emerges that the strength of the BOLD- induced magnitude signal depends on the spatial vessel distribution, consistent with the fact that field dispersion dominates changes in the magnitude signal. On the other hand, if the single vessel model is used for the phase signal, positive and negative phase signals mutually cancel out for random vessel orientations, such as those found in the capillary network, while the phase signals add together for ordered orientations, as was recently explored in a simulation study (Chen and Calhoun, 2010).

These two models of the BOLD phase effect suggest that the interest of analyzing the phase signal resides in the possibility to exclude voxels dominated by draining veins, since predictions based on the summation of magnetic field changes in single vessels cancel out (Hoogenrad et al., 2001). A slightly different picture with regard to the BOLD effect and the variation of the phase signal emerges if the concept of the 'sphere ofLorentz effect' is taken into account (Durrant et al., 2003).Zhao et al., 2007 followed by Feng et al., 2009 showed by theory and by experiments that an extended activated brain area actually gives rise to a coherent phase shift. The sphere of Lorentz concept predicts the existence of two main effects of the BOLD response: local field changes caused by the red blood cells, and a bulk magnetic susceptibility shift which is further subdivided into a demagnetizing effect and a volume-averaged magnetization change (Durrant et al., 2003). The volume-averaged effect depends on the blood volume, the vessel geometry and the geometry of their ensuing magnetic field, as well as the size of the susceptibility effect in vessels located in the tissue surrounding the volume (Zhao et al., 2007). The spatial distribution of the phase effect that emerges from this model corresponds to a magnetic dipole and, similarly to the single vessel case, it depends on the geometry and orientation of the activated brain region with respect to the external field (Fig. 8).

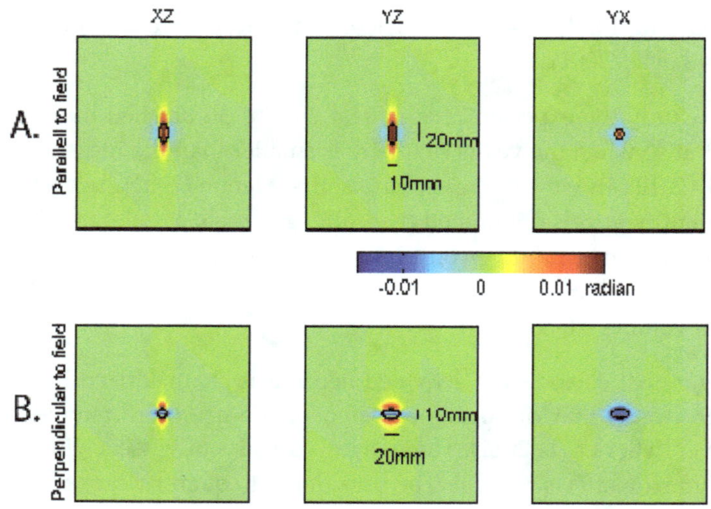

Figure 8. Simulation of the spatial pattern of the phase effect generated by the BOLD response in a brain area with an elliptic Gaussian shape (contours of the region are overlaid on the phase images). The external, static, magnetic field, B_0 is applied along the Z-direction, and the phase effect is shown in three planes: XZ, YZ, and YX. Similarly to the case of a single vessel, the phase effect depends on the orientation of the cortical regions with respect to B_0. A. When the longest axis of the region is oriented parallel to B_0, a paramagnetic shift that increases the local field occurs. B. When the longest axis of the region is oriented perpendicular to B_0, a diamagnetic effect that tends to decrease the field is generated.

In Fig. 7, phase images of a cylindrical vial containing a solution with higher magnetic susceptibility than the solution contained in the surrounding, outer area are shown for a parallel and a perpendicular orientation, with respect to the static magnetic field.The greatest extra-vascular effects are obtained for the perpendicular orientation, with a spatial $\cos 2\Psi$ modulation around the vessel, and a diamagnetic phase shift inside the vessel. The size of the phase shifts will depend on the oxygenation fraction and on the geometrical factor, determined by the orientation of the vessels, as expressed by [Eq.10]. The expected phase values that occur during the resting and active conditions of an fMRI study can be obtained by straightforward calculations based on [Eq. 10]. For instance, during rest (when the oxygenation fraction is ca Y=0.54) the maximal field difference between the extra- and intravascular space amounts to ±0.62μT at 3T and appears in the tissue surrounding a perpendicular vessel (extravascular space). This value corresponds to a phase shift as high as ±4.98 radian if a GE-EPI sequence with a TE of 30 ms is used. In presence of a BOLD response during the activated state (Y=0.68) the susceptibility difference between the blood and the tissue diminishes and therefore the maximal field difference becomes ±0.43μT (±3.45radian). In the intravascular space of a parallel vessel, the field undergoes a diamagnetic shift and is therefore reduced from 0.42 μT (3.37radian) at rest to 0.29 μT (2.33 radian) during activation. Consequently, the expected BOLD induced field change is maximal in the extravascular space for perpendicular vessels (±0.19μT, 1.52radian), while for the parallel case it is greatest in the intravascular space (-0.13μT, 1.04radian). These observations are also in line with previous work (Hoogenrad et al., 2001).

During an fMRI study the expected phase effect will be diminished due to the partial volume effects that arise when the vessel diameter is smaller than the measured voxel size (see Brainovich et al., 2010). In view of these phase shifts, Menon (2002) suggested that it should be possible to identify voxels dominated by draining vessels parallel to the field, due to the intravascular phase shift, while the contribution from perpendicular vessels should cancel out, due to signal modulation in the extravascular space that is averaged out as a consequence of partial volume effects.

The cortical region that encloses the activated neurons is characterized by a dense capillary network. Larger vessels that drain the activated region are more remotely located at the brain surface (e.g. Keller et al., 2011). The network consists of vessels with a range of different radii, and diffusion effects must also be considered to quantify the effect of the magnetic field distribution. This is not trivial to do and therefore calculations were initially done by Monte Carlo simulations (Yablonskiy and Haacke 1994) before an analytical expression was derived by Kiselev and Posse (1999, see Eqs. 5 and 25 in that paper). From these studies, it emerges that the strength of the BOLD- induced magnitude signal depends on the spatial vessel distribution, consistent with the fact that field dispersion dominates changes in the magnitude signal. On the other hand, if the single vessel model is used for the phase signal, positive and negative phase signals mutually cancel out for random vessel orientations, such as those found in the capillary network, while the phase signals add together for ordered orientations, as was recently explored in a simulation study (Chen and Calhoun, 2010).

These two models of the BOLD phase effect suggest that the interest of analyzing the phase signal resides in the possibility to exclude voxels dominated by draining veins, since predictions based on the summation of magnetic field changes in single vessels cancel out (Hoogenrad et al., 2001). A slightly different picture with regard to the BOLD effect and the variation of the phase signal emerges if the concept of the 'sphere ofLorentz effect' is taken into account (Durrant et al., 2003).Zhao et al., 2007 followed by Feng et al., 2009 showed by theory and by experiments that an extended activated brain area actually gives rise to a coherent phase shift. The sphere of Lorentz concept predicts the existence of two main effects of the BOLD response: local field changes caused by the red blood cells, and a bulk magnetic susceptibility shift which is further subdivided into a demagnetizing effect and a volume-averaged magnetization change (Durrant et al., 2003). The volume-averaged effect depends on the blood volume, the vessel geometry and the geometry of their ensuing magnetic field, as well as the size of the susceptibility effect in vessels located in the tissue surrounding the volume (Zhao et al., 2007). The spatial distribution of the phase effect that emerges from this model corresponds to a magnetic dipole and, similarly to the single vessel case, it depends on the geometry and orientation of the activated brain region with respect to the external field (Fig. 8).

Simulations of the BOLD effect thatincludes the sphere of Lorentz effect can be performed by a three-dimensional Fourier transform of the magnetic field distribution (Marques and Bowtell, 2005). Similar to the approach used by Feng et al. (2009), we performed such calculations for the BOLD response in a cortical region with an elliptic Gaussian field distribution described by:

$$\Delta B = -2\pi \cdot \Delta\chi_o \cdot \Delta Y_{cap} \cdot Hct \cdot B_o \cdot \left(\exp(-\frac{X^2}{2\cdot\sigma_x^{\,2}} - \frac{Y^2}{2\cdot\sigma_y^{\,2}} - \frac{Z^2}{2\cdot\sigma_z^{\,2}} \right)$$
$$\sigma_i = \frac{FWHM_i}{2\cdot\sqrt{2\cdot\ln(2)}} \qquad (11)$$

where ΔY_{cap} is the change in oxygenation in the capillaries (0.08) due to BOLD, *X*, *Y* and *Z* are the Cartesian coordinates in 3D space, $FWHM_i$ expresses the spatial extent of the area in terms of the full width half maximum value for the coordinates in the *i*-direction, where *i=X,Y,Z;* and the other parameters are the same as in [Eq.10] and in Fig. 7. We varied the size of the activated region between 5-40mm (FWHM of the shortest length axis) and the strength of the BOLD response. Values for the BOLD induced magnetic field change were close to those observed above for the single vessel model (± 0.05-0.25 μT). The results from these simulations are shown in Figs. 8 and 9. We found that both the spatial extent of the activated area and the strength of the BOLD response influence the size of phase change. For instance, magnetic field shifts of ±0.1 μT lead to phase shifts in the range of 0.01-0.04 radian, depending on the spatial extent of the region. As shown in Fig. 9, the greatest phase effect was found in small areas with a strong BOLD response. The size of these expected phase changes are thus about two orders of magnitude lower than those found for fully sampled large draining vessels, despite similar size of the BOLD induced magnetic field change. This fact highlights the difference between biophysical models.

With regard to the time evolution of the phase effect, studies have shown that it closely follows that of the magnitude signal (Zhao et al., 2007). This observation is in agreement with a common BOLD origin for both the phase and magnitude signals.

As we have seen, three differentbiophysical models for describing the phase signal changes caused by the BOLD effect are available in the literature. The first modelis based onthe signal behaviour in large draining veins, the second in capillary networks, while the third model describes the BOLD phase effect caused by a spatially extendedcortical region. The spatial pattern of the BOLD effect is different for the phase than for the magnitude images, but from the literature we know that their temporal evolution is similar (Zhao et al., 2007; Feng et al., 2009).

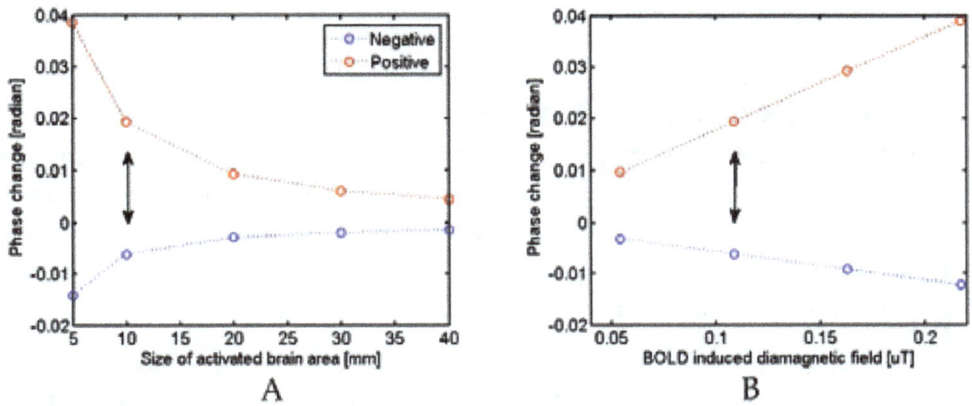

Figure 9. Simulations of the phase effect with positive (red) and negative (blue) sign generated by the BOLD response in a brain area, with an ellipsoid Gaussian shape. As in Fig. 9, the longest axis is oriented along B_0.A: Variation of the phase effect with the spatial extent of the activated area (indicated as the FWHM of the shortest length axes, see Eq. 11 and Fig.8). The BOLD response is fixed (±0.10 μT). The phase effect is greatest when the size of the region is small, but diminishes as the size of the activated region increases. B: Variation of the phase effect with the strength of the BOLD responses. The spatial extent of the activated brain area is fixed (FWHM=10mm). The positive (negative) phase increases (decreases) with increasing BOLD field changes. The arrow indicates equivalent points in Fig. 9 A and 9B where the FWHM is 10mm and the BOLD response has a field change of ±0.10 μT.

4. Unwanted phase effects and their removal

The phase value can be considered a fingerprint of the voxel averaged magnetic field. Therefore any effect that causes local or global dishomogeneities of the field leads to phase variations in space. Furthermore, during breathing and motion, the phase will vary from scan to scan in an EPI time series (Hagberg et al., 2008; Petridou et al., 2009). Since the expected BOLD-related phase changes are weak, correcting all unwanted phase fluctuations is of utmost importance.

MRI phase images are characterized by phase wrapping effects dueto an inherent limit of the MRI detection system: the range of phases that can be detected is limited to ±π and therefore phase wraps occur if this limit is exceeded. The true underlying phase value is thus equal to the observed phase ± an integer number of revolutions on the unit circle:

$$\varphi_{\text{true}} = \varphi_{\text{obs}} \pm 2\pi \cdot k \tag{12}$$

where k can take on any integer value. Such phase wraps occurin space and in time (Hagberg et al., 2008). For instance, close to air-tissue borders where the magnetic susceptibility difference is important, and therefore the phase value also varies greatly, especially if long TE times are used for the measurements, leading to phase jumps in the vicinity of such air-tissue borders (see [Eq.8], and Fig. 5). Temporal phase wraps may also occur in fMRI time series, as the magnetic field may vary with time due to physiological and scanner fluctuations.

4.1. Physiological and scanner noise in phase fMRI images

Unwanted field non-uniformities can be subdivided into static and dynamic magnetic susceptibility differences considering the duration of a 2D image acquisition and they are caused both by the subject and by the scanner (see Hagberg et al., 2008). Static effects are caused by factors that are considered to remain unchanged during the acquisition of a single image, while dynamic effects are caused by factors with a varying influence from slice to slice. Examples of static effects are imperfect shimming and slowly evolving field drifts, examples of dynamic effects are breathing, motion and system vibrations.

The magnetic susceptibility varies greatly across the brain, due to air-tissue bordersas well as due to more local susceptibility differences between the vessels,the sub-cortical structures, the grey and the white matter (Collins et al., 2002, see also the strong phase variations in brain regions just above the frontal sinuses in Fig. 5). When the brain is placed in an external magnetic field, these variations in magnetic susceptibility lead to field dishomogeneties. The scanner hardware compensates for some dishomogeneities by a procedure known as 'shimming', i.e. we try to make the field more uniform by activating the shim-coils. How good the shim can get depends on the hardware, and on some clinical scanners only linear correction terms are available, while other commercial systems are capable of performing corrections up to the 2nd order, therefore higher order field imperfections remain, despite the shimming procedure. Since the shim-values are generally set at the beginning of the fMRI experiment they do not compensate for field variations during scanning caused by respiration, that modifies the susceptibility difference between the lungs and the brain, see Ray et al., 2000, and by small micromovements of the brain during the respiratory and cardiac cycles (Le and Hu 1996; van Gelderen et al., 2007). These effects can be noticeable also in the fMRI magnitude signal (see Fig. 10), and must therefore be regressed out if more subtle effects are to be studied, like for instance in resting state studies. New hardware developments may in the future make such corrections unnecessary. One possibility is to change the shim-currents on-the-fly during the fMRI experiment, so that the effects caused by respiration are compensated (van Gelderen et al., 2007). Another possibility is to use magnetic field monitoring during image acquisition (Barmet et al., 2009). This information can either be used for image post-processing or for re-calibration of the shim-currents (Vannesjo et al., 2012).

Not only the subject, but also the scanner contributes to static effects, linked with the aforementioned imperfect shimming issue and slow magnetic field drifts. Time-dependent dynamic effects are caused by helium-pump related system vibrations, and concomitant field gradients arisingfrom Maxwell effects, eddy-current fields, and gradient non-linearities (Hagberg et al., 2008). In a typical fMRI time-series, the scan-to-scan variability of most of these factors can be neglected, except for system vibration, magnetic field drift and heating of the gradient system (Foerster et al., 2005).

4.2. Removal of unwanted phase effects

The unwanted phase effects that originate from different sources can be removed by different post-processing approaches that will be briefly described. We exemplify the effects of these methods on some data sets we acquired (Hagberg et al., 2008; 2012).

Phase wraps, defined in [Eq. 12], can be efficiently removed by performing phase unwrapping. Unwrapping is a straightforward process if it is applied across the time dimension, independently for each voxel in the fMRI time series (Hagberg et al., 2008). Alternatively, spatial phase unwrapping can be applied (e.g. Cusack and Papadakis, 2002; Jenkinson, 2003). Finally, the reference phase method has been proposed, that effectively removes phase wraps by referencing subsequent phase images to the first phase image acquired in the fMRI time series (Tomasi and Caparelli, 2007).

Logically, sources of unwanted phase effects must be unambiguously identified and characterized before removal. Recent studies have shown, that the dominating source of phase variations during fMRI time courses are induced by respiration and the cardiac beat (Petridou et al., 2009; Hagberg et al., 2008; 2012). The importance of respiratory and cardiac effects on the phase data becomes clear from Fourier analysis of the fMRI time series data (Fig.10). After spatio-temporal phase unwrapping, the physiological noise components are slightly less pronounced than after temporal unwrapping alone, while the reference phase method seems more efficient for removal of the respiratory component. The magnitude data is also affected by respiration and the heartbeat, and a very popular method for removal of physiological noise from magnitude data is RETROICOR (Glover et al, 2000). It uses the respiratory and cardiac traces to create regressors for noise removal. The benefit of this approach for phase fMRI time series acquired at 7T has been demonstrated (Petridou et al., 2009).

For long it has been known that information regarding respiration and heartbeat can be extracted from the phase value of the central k-space point (Hu et al., 1995; Le and Hu 1996). One possibility is thus toperform noise regression based on the phase of the central k-space point, instead or in combination with RETROICOR (Hagberg et al., 2012).

Other techniques specifically aim to compensate the scan-to-scan off-resonance effects in k-space. Available techniques are the DORK (acronym for dynamic off-resonance in k-space) and TOAST (temporal off-resonance alignment of single-echo time series technique) methods. In DORK, the global field-changes are estimated by the phase evolution of the central k-space point between subsequent TRs and then each read-out line is corrected in k-space assuming a linear phase accrual in time (Pfeuffer et al., 2002). In TOAST, phase rewinding is performed based on a voxel wise estimate of the B_0 changes from the smoothed difference between the phase at each single time point and the average phase in the entire fMRI time series (Hahn et al., 2009). In the next paragraph, we will show how these methods compare in terms of eliminating physiological noise.

Finally, an alternative method that we have explored is based on spatial high-pass filtering. In the human brain at 3T, we observed that the unwanted phase effects were characterized by a low spatial frequency (Hagberg et al., 2012). This characteristic is present also for phantom measurements as can be seen in Fig. 7. We found that the phase fluctuations became similar to the ones observed in magnitude data in healthy human subjects,after application of Gaussian filters that removed all components extending 20mm or more (Hagberg et al., 2012). Fourier analysis also shows that the scanner Helium pump artefact at 2Hz and the respiratory artifact are completely removed by spatial filters, while some cardiac pulsation effects remained (Fig. 10, Hagberg et al., 2012).

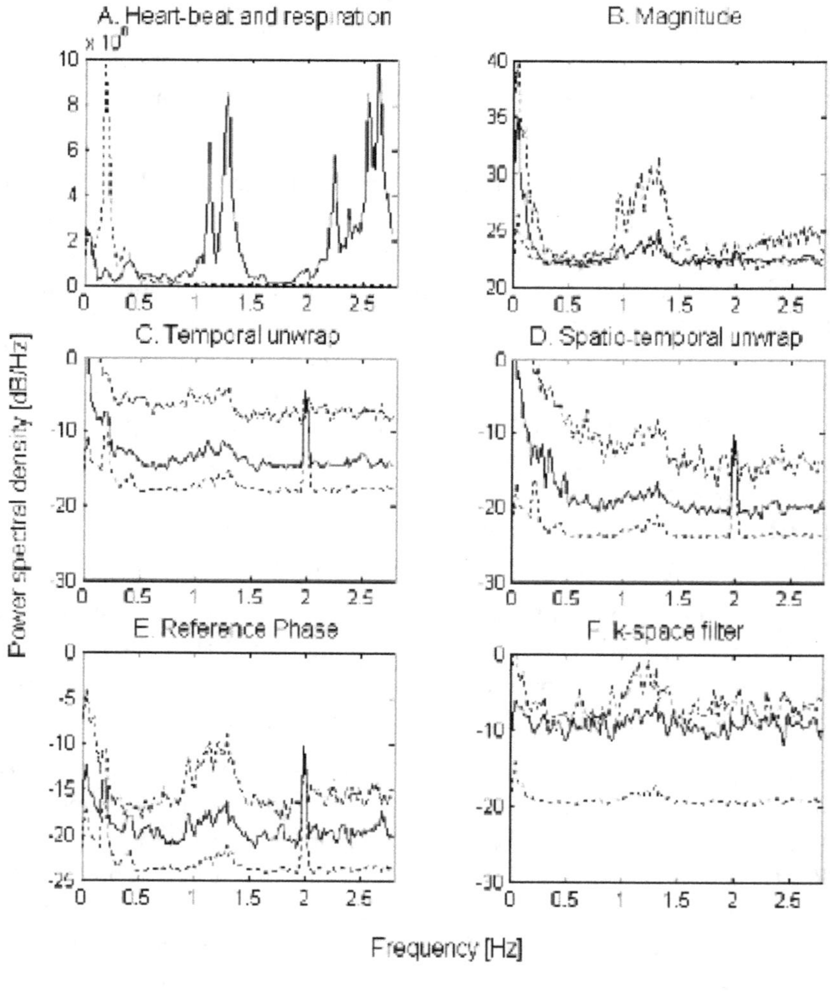

Figure 10. Fourier analysis of the heart beat and the respiratory cycle (A) and their relation to the MRI signal in magnitude (B) and phase (C-F) images. A: Respiration occurs between 0.12 and 0.25 Hz, and the first and second harmonics of the heart-beat around 1.2 and 2.4 Hz, respectively. B: In magnitude images, respiration induced fluctuationscause the typical 1/f decrement at low frequencies, but instabilities are also prominent around the first cardiac harmonic. Note the relative absence of disturbances around 2Hz, caused by the scanner Helium pump and visible in most of the phase time-series. Results are shown for gray matter (solid line), white matter (dotted line), and CSF (dashed line). C: temporal unwrap and detrending of the phase time-series (Hagberg et al., 2008); D: spatial unwrapping followed by temporal unwrapping and detrending, (Hagberg et al., 2008); E: Reference phase method (Tomasi and Caparelli, 2007); F: k-space filtering (Hagberg et al., 2012).

The efficiency of each technique for removal of phase instabilities can be evaluated and compared with results from the magnitude data. Krueger and Glover (2001) proposed a model that quantifies the available temporal stability of magnitude data, *tSNR* based on the factor λ_M that expresses the proportionality between the magnitude signal and the physiological noise. Basically this model implies that the available temporal signal-to-noise level reaches a maximum limiting value for high signal-to-noise-ratios at a single time point, SNR_0, calculated from the average signal in each voxel across the GE-EPI timecourse, *S*, divided by the Rayleigh corrected noise level, *N*:

$$SNR_o = \frac{S}{1.53 \cdot N}$$
$$tSNR = \frac{SNR_o}{\sqrt{1 + \lambda_M^2 \cdot SNR_o^2}} \tag{13}$$

In accordance with the Gudbjartsson and Patz relationship between the noise in magnitude and phase images (Eq. 9), we can derive three models for the temporal fluctuations in phase images. In the first model, the noise components induce greater fluctuations in the phase than in the magnitude images, in the second model the contributions are similar in both image types and in the last model the noise is less pronounced in phase than in magnitude images, following the relationship (Hagberg et al., 2008):

$$tSD_\varphi = \frac{1}{tSNR} = \frac{\sqrt{1 + \lambda_\varphi^2 \cdot SNR_0^2}}{SNR_0} \tag{14}$$

where $\lambda_M < \lambda_\varphi$; $\lambda_M = \lambda_\varphi$; or $\lambda_M > \lambda_\varphi$, respectively for the three noise models.

The *tSNR* obtained for the magnitude signal and $1/tSD_\varphi$ images obtained after different phase processing methods are shown in Fig. 11 and illustrates that the phase noise is generally greater than the magnitude noise, but can be efficiently reduced by adequate post-processing methods. (Fig. 11, see also Hagberg et al., 2012). Spatial high-pass filtering currently represents the best approach for removal of unwanted phase fluctuations. If adequately adapted, similar or even reduced λ_φ values are obtained for the phase compared to magnitude data. In general, the amount of filtering must be adapted to the field strength of the scanner, the echo time and voxel size of the GE-EPI sequence. For instance, at 3T, a TE of 30ms, and a voxel size of 3x3x3mm^3 we found that a Gaussian filter with a 20mm FWHM suffices to reach the a similar stability in both phase and magnitude time series (Hagberg et al., 2012). Filters with a FWHM close to the voxel size, reduces the phase noise to less than half the magnitude noise. For most other post-processing methods, including spatio-temporal unwrapping, regression based on the phase evolution central k-space point (NVR), RETROICOR, and TOAST, the phase noise was always greater than the magnitude noise.

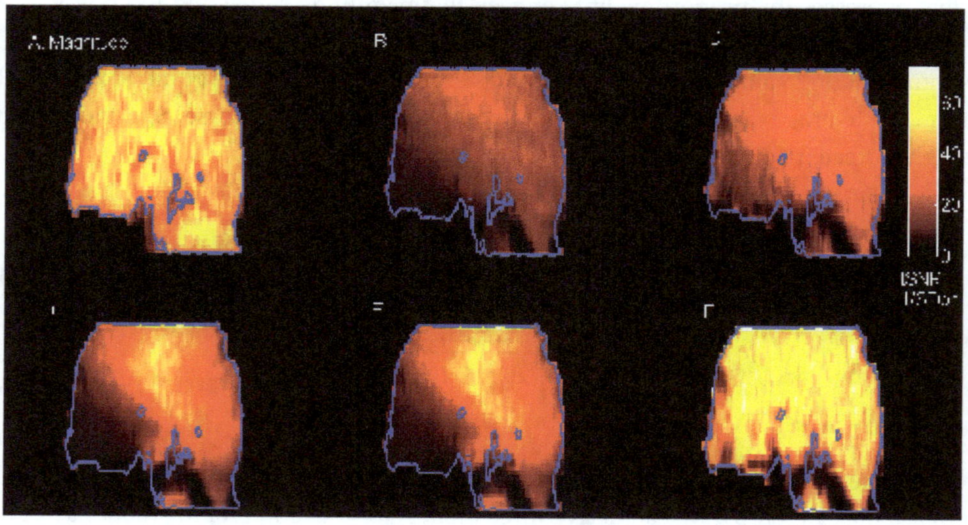

Figure 11. Temporal stability in magnitude (A) and phase (B-F) images. The phase images were post-processed by different methods prior to calculation of the inverse of the standard deviation of the phase across the time series (see Eq. 14). (B) RETROICOR; (C) TOAST; (D) noise regression based on the phase of the central k-space point; (E) combined approach based on both thecentral k-space point and RETROICOR; (F) : k-space High pass filtering of the phase data by a Homodyne filter based on a Gaussian kernel in k-space (Hagberg et al., 2012).

5. On the use of phase information in fMRI studies

The phase signal possesses many interesting features that may be used to extract valuable information without the need for additional scanning time. The question that remains is howthe phase information best is used in order to improve currently available standard fMRI methods. At the time being, no clear-cut answer emerges in the literature. Ongoing work will probably give us an answer in the near future. What follows is a brief overview of some possible approaches that are currently being explored. In the last paragraph, we will also show an example of the outcome of an fMRI analysis performed for both the magnitude and the phase signals within the framework of the standard General Linear Model, using different phase post-processing methods.

We have seen how unwanted phase fluctuations due to respiration or heartbeat are well visible in the phase data. The phase can thus be used to identify and characterize the temporal evolution of different noise sources. This information can be used to remove contributions from common noise sources from the magnitude data sets.

We have seen how the BOLD response influences the phase signal as described by different biophysical models. The dipole of the ensuing magnetic field effect is manifest at different length-scales, depending on whether draining veins or microvascular networks drive the response. Indeed, a phase effect arises both at the level ofsingledraining vessels with diameters of 100-500μm and inextended cortical regionswith BOLD activation. Therefore, the phase signal may be used to exclude single voxels dominated by draining veins (Menon, 2002) or to potentiate the statistical fMRI analysis based on magnitude data (Rowe and Logan, 2004).

5.1. Improving the magnitude signal: noise reduction

Physiological noise is a known limiting factor in fMRI studies (Krüger and Glover, 2001). Improving temporal stability is desirable, as it directly influences the statistical T-values. As pointed out above, studies show that the phase evolution at the centre of k-space in fMRI time series closely reflects field variations due to respiration and the cardiac beat (Hu et al, 1995, Le et al., 1996). Therefore the phase signal can be used as a proxy for physiological (and scanner) fluctuations. The magnitude signal could then be de-noised by simply regressing out unwanted fluctuations (Hagberg et al., 2012). This kind of use of the phase data may thus improve the outcome of fMRI analysis based on magnitude data.

The improvement in temporal stability of the magnitude signal was evaluated for different post-processing strategies (Hagberg et al., 2012). The standard RETROICOR method is based on signal regression (Glover, 2000). The onset of respiration and heart beat is obtained from measurements with a respiration belt and a pulse oxymeter synchronized to the acquisition of the fMRI time series. A set of 8 or more regressors are then created and used for signal regression and de-noising of the magnitude signal. In our approach, that we termed phase based nuisance variable regression (NVR, Hagberg et al., 2012), we used the phase evolution in the centre of the k-space as the only noise regressor. We also evaluated the possibility to combine the RETROICOR noise regressors with the regressor based on the phase evolution in central k-space (Table 1 and Fig. 12). We found that the temporal stability of the magnitude fMRI time course improved by 5% after NVR, which was slightly less than RETROICOR (Hagberg et al., 2012). It should be noted that RETROICOR is based on the cardiac and respiratory traces that must be acquired in synchrony with the fMRI time course, while NVR can be applied without this information. In addition, we found that a combination of RETROICOR and phase-based magnitude correction could improve the overall signal stability more than RETROICOR alone.

Tissue	Raw magnitude data	RETROICOR	NVR	RETROICOR and NVR combined
Gray matter voxels	0.0102±0.0042	0.0083±0.0041	0.0093±0.0041	0.0079±0.0039
White matter voxels	0.0056±0.0022	0.0040±0.0024	0.0050±0.0022	0.0035±0.0026
CSF voxels	0.0199±0.0076	0.0159±0.0066	0.0176±0.0065	0.0150±0.0058

Table 1 Stability in magnitude images in terms of the physiological noise parameter λ_M (see Eq. 13) for raw images and after noise-regression.

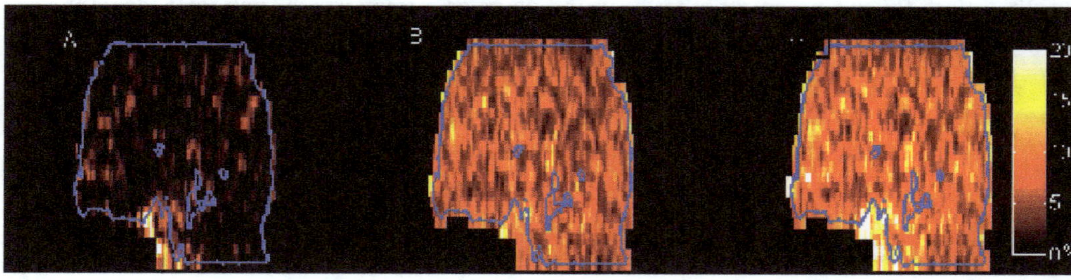

Figure 12. Increase in temporal stability of the magnitude signal for different magnitude post-processing methods. The data shown is the percent increase in temporal signal-to-noise ratio with respect to no post-processing for (A)after NVR; noise regression based on the evolution at the centre of k-space; (B) after RETROICOR; and (C) after a combined approach based on both NVR and RETROICOR methods. Data were obtained during a 5min acquisition of resting-state fMRI data. A sagittal plane showing the results for all acquired transverse slices is shown.

5.2. Statistical analysis methods incorporating the phase effect

Basically, two methods that incorporate phase signals in the fMRI analysis have been suggested. The first method aims at excluding those voxels from the analysis where the phase changes are great. These voxels are most probably related to draining veins (Menon 2002). The second method is the constant phase model of Rowe and Logan (2004) that extends the General Linear Model GLM to complex values. This model was further refined by Rowe (2005) who combined the real and the imaginary terms of the MRI signal into a single matrix expression. The General Linear Model which is used to evaluate magnitude images is:

$$abs(y_t) = X \cdot \beta + \eta \tag{15}$$

For complex numbers, GLM can be rewritten as (Rowe, 2005):

$$\begin{bmatrix} \mathrm{Re}(y_t) \\ \mathrm{Im}(y_t) \end{bmatrix} = \begin{bmatrix} \cos\varphi_t & 0 \\ 0 & \sin\varphi_t \end{bmatrix} \cdot \begin{bmatrix} x & 0 \\ 0 & x \end{bmatrix} \cdot \begin{bmatrix} \beta^{re} \\ \beta^{im} \end{bmatrix} + \begin{bmatrix} \eta^{re}{}_t \\ \eta^{im}{}_t \end{bmatrix} \tag{16}$$

where y_t is the complex valued fMRI time course, φ_t is the phase at each time point, x, $X$are the design matrices for the complex vector and the magnitude signals, respectively;$\beta_t{}^{re}$, $\beta_t{}^{im}$, β the parameter estimates obtained after model fitting; and$\eta_t{}^{re}$, $\eta_t{}^{im}$, η the noise of the real, imaginary and magnitude signals.

Examples of using this model indicate the difficulties that may arise when assessing fMRI results (Rowe 2005). Indeed at least three sets of maps showing activated voxels can be identified, dependent on which signals show significant activations: magnitude only (MO), phase only (PO), or activations in both magnitude and phase images (M&P). Considering the dipolar pattern that the BOLD response has (see Fig. 8), both positive and negative phase changes occur. Therefore we actually end up with as much as 5 sets of activation maps: MO; PO_positive; PO_negative, M&P_negative; M&P_positive (Rowe, 2005; Arja et al., 2010). At the time being, no method is available that brings the analysis of these maps one step further, so that a single activation map showing where in the brain activation takes place with a high sensitivity and specificity, is available. For instance, it is not clear what a PO activation which is visible in the phase but not in the magnitude images actually means. As we have seen in the earlier paragraphs, such an effect could be generated by a draining vessel, or by the sphere of Lorentz effect of the activated cortical patch, or perhaps by an unwanted phase effect that was not completely removed prior to analysis. It is desirable that methods that allow us to combine the activation maps are developedin the future. Such an approach could be based on the available biophysical models for the BOLD effect in phase images, perhaps even by performing quantitative susceptibility mapping (Balla et al., 2012), and may in the future bring us closer to the goal of correctly assigning the cerebral networks where the neuronal activity has its origin at the highest specificity and sensitivity.

5.3. On the use of phase images in an fMRI study

In the following, we will show an example of an fMRI study that incorporates both phase and magnitude images. The goal of the analysis was to investigate possible global phase effects according to the models that describe the phase signal changes caused by the BOLD effect. In order to make sure that we adequately handle unwanted phase effects, different approaches for removal of these were explored and their impact on the final activation maps were investigated.

Five healthy right handed subjects (three females and two males, 24-27 years) volunteered to participate in the fMRI study (approved by the local IRB). They performed index finger tapping in synchrony with a visual stimulus flashing at 1.7 Hz, in a block design paradigm: left hand tapping for 18s, 9s rest; right hand tapping for 18s, 9s rest; repeated 4 times. Complex valued BOLD fMRI time series were collected (Gradient echo EPI, 75 volumes, TR=3s, TE=39 ms, slice thickness: 3 mm and a 50% gap between 24 slices, bandwidth: 3396 Hz/px, voxel size: 3 x 3 x 4 mm3). Phase wraps and unwanted phase effects related to spatial static magnetic field gradients were removed by three different methods: a) spatio-temporal phase unwrapping, b) pixel wise noise regression based on the phase of the central k-space point and c) spatial high-pass filtering. For the spatial filtering method, a homodyne k-space approach was used based on the following three window functions: Hanning window, Gaussian window (with three different window widths: 5, 10 and 20mm) and a spline window, that was adapted to the magnitude k-space data of each image slice and each timepoint in the fMRI time series (Hagberg et al., 2012). Normalization to the MNI brain space was based on the magnitude image and subsequently applied to the phase images, and conventional spatial smoothing of the pre-processed images was applied to both phase and magnitude images, prior to statistical analysis using SPM5. Statistical analysis was first performed at the single-subject level, then the contrast images were included in a second-level group analysis to reveal the common activation pattern. We thus did not specifically use the Rowe and Logan model in [Eq. 16], but could rely on standard statistical analysis within the framework of the General Linear Model, using standard statistical methods.

Activation patterns for magnitude and phase images achieved after post-processing and statistical analysis are shown in Fig. 13. No significant activations were found in the phase data after a) spatio-temporal unwrapping or b) phase-regression. Only after post-processing by c) spatial homodyne high-pass filtering, significant activation patterns were obtained. Voxels with significant magnitude changes were located in the primary motor cortex. Some of these voxels also showed significant positive changes of the phase, however most voxels with a significant phase effect were located outside M1. In general, the parameter estimates for the phase signal were smaller than for the activations revealed in the magnitude data, leading to lower statistical Z and T-values (Table 2). The T-values for the magnitude images reached levels of 15, while the T-values for the phase data depended on which spatial homodyne window function that had been used. Satisfactory values of the statistical T-value (≥ 8) were obtained with the Homodyne approach using a Hamming window and a Gaussian function with FWHM=20mm, which most probably removes all unwanted phase effects at this field strength and for this echo time (Hagberg et al., 2012). The statistical parametric maps (SPMs) achieved with three of the five filters could be thresholded with $p<0.001$ (uncorrected for multiple comparison). The other two sets of data were thresholded with $p<0.1$ uncorrected, in order to reveal the significant activations (Fig. 13).

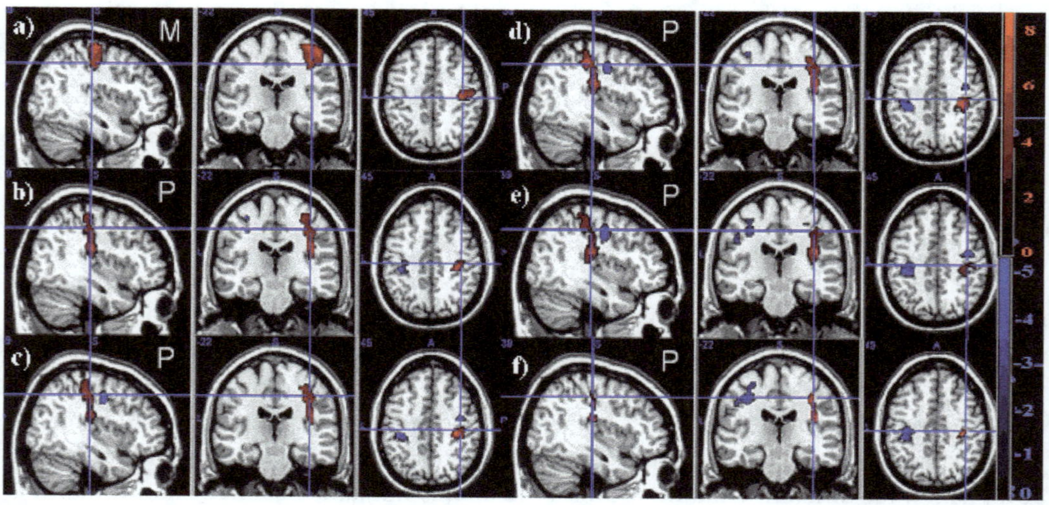

Figure 13. Activation patterns for a motor task obtained from a) magnitude (M) and b-f) phase (P) images. Unwanted phase effects were removed by five different homodyne (spatial high-pass) filters: b) Hamming window; c) Gaussian 20mm; d) Gaussian 10mm; e) Gaussian 5mm and f) k-space spline window. The statistical maps have been thresholded at a statistical significance level of $p<0.001$(uncorrected for multiple comparisons). Color bars indicate statistical T-value ranges.

	Cont	# voxels in cluster	Tvalue	Zvalue	p-value	MNI coordinates
Phase						
Hamming n=32	Pos	Clmax 659	8.57	5.08	$p_u<0.001$	34, -26, 46
	Neg	85	5.84	4.16	$p_u<0.001$	38, -6, 42
Gauss FWHM 20mm	Pos	Clmax 792	8.04	4.93	$p_u<0.001$	32, -26, 48
	Neg	92	5.74	4.11	$p_u<0.001$	38, -6, 40
Gauss FWHM 10mm	Pos	Clmax 841	7.80	4.86	$p_u<0.01$	42, -20 22
	Neg	Clmax 238	5.38	3.96	$p_u<0.01$	38, -6, 44
Gauss FWHM 5mm	Pos	Clmax 1064	6.61	4.46	$p_u<0.01$	34, -26, 44
	Neg	Clmax 381	5.02	3.79	$p_u<0.01$	-40, -30, 52
k-spline filter	Pos	Clmax 606	8.62	5.10	$p_u<0.001$	42, -20, 18
	Neg	Clmax 213	5.28	3.90	$p_u<0.001$	-40, -30, 42
Magnitude						
Raw data	Pos	Clmax 950	15.06	6.37	FWE=0.5	52, -14, 54

Table 2 Results obtained in a second level analysis. T and Z statistical values and size of the activated clusters (agglomerate of activated voxels) for magnitude and phase images are reported. Corresponding p-values and Montreal Neurological Institute (MNI) coordinates of their centre are shown for positive (Pos) and negative (Neg) phase changes, and for the positive magnitude activation.

After identification of voxels with significant signal changes in the second-level group analysis, the timeseries were extracted from these voxels for each subject. In Fig. 13, the extracted phase and magnitude timeseries, in brain regions with significant, stimulus correlated signal changes, are shown. In agreement with the work by Zhao et al. (2007), the time evolution of the phase and magnitude signals closely follow each other. The maximal change of the magnitude signal is 1-2% while the maximal phase change is 0.005-0.010 radians. The contrast-to-noise ratio was smaller for the phase than the magnitude data, both for the negative and for the positive phase changes. With respect to the size of the observed phase changes these were in agreement with those found for the simulated data (Figs. 8 and 9). The size of the activated clusters was 1000 voxels or less, corresponding to a region with an extension (FWHM) of 12mm. For this size, the observed phase changes of 0.005-0.01 radian would correspond to a diamagnetic field shift of ca 0.05-0.10 μT or less, which in turns corresponds to a change in the oxygenation fraction of ca 0.04-0.08 in a capillary network.

This preliminary study suggests how the phase information can be incorporated into the fMRI analysis. In a previous study, (Hagberg et al., 2008) we showed that it is possible to identify voxels with large phase changes in draining veins, by strong positive and negative phase changes close to the brain surface, where the largest vessels are found (Menon 2002). In the present study we used the same set of data but with a different post-processing approach, that included phase post-processing by Homodyne high pass filtering followed by normalization to a standard brain space and spatial smoothing of the final images. This approach allowed to remove contributions from strong positive and negative phase changes in draining vessels and enabled the detection of quite subtle phase changes. These results are consistent with a BOLD response in an extended brain area that generates a magnetic dipole effect (Durrant et al., 2003; Zhao et al., 2007).

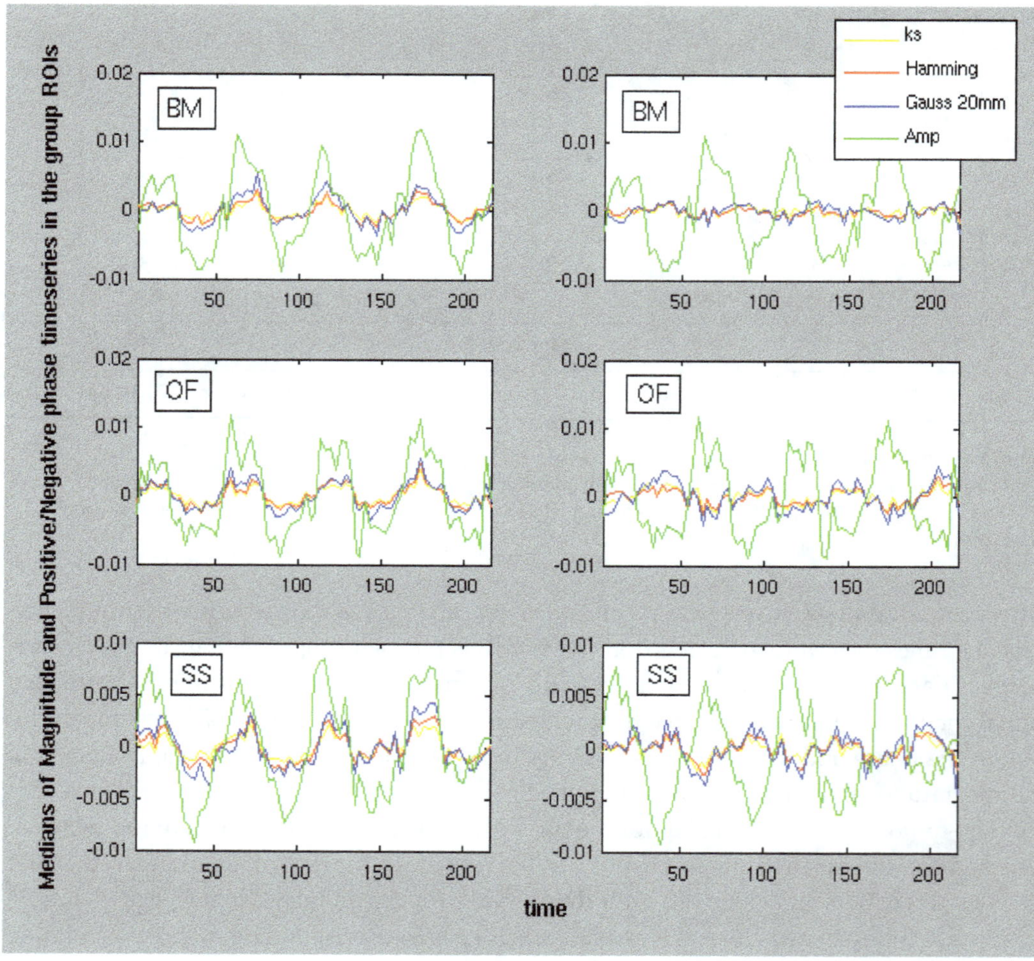

Figure 14. Timeseries extracted from brain regions with significant, stimulus correlated signal changes in three different subjects (SS, BM, and OF). Positive (left) and negative (right) phase signals are shown, overlaid on the magnitude signal (Amp, green). The phase signal clearly has a lower contrast-to-noise ratio than the magnitude signal. The temporal evolution of the phase and magnitude timeseries are similar.

6. Conclusion

Functional MRI methods based on the evaluation of magnitude image data may benefit from the inclusion of the information conveyed by the phase images. For instance, it is possible to directly improve the quality of the magnitude data by noise regression derived from the phase signal. In order to reveal subtle BOLD related activations in phase images, the many unwanted phase effects must first be accounted for. Spatial high-pass filtering that removes the spatially slowly evolving B_0 signal components currently represent the best approach for achieving this goal. We show that phase changes consistent with a dipolar activation pattern caused by an extended cortical region can be detected. Future work must address the question of how the BOLD related phase activation patterns can be incorporated in the statistical analysis pipeline, in order to improve the specificity and the sensitivity of fMRI.

Acknowledgements

The authors would like to thank Valentina Brainovich, who helped us with the fMRI study, and a grant from the Italian Ministry of Health (RF05.103).

Author details

Gisela E. Hagberg[1,2] and Elisa Tuzzi[1]

1 Fondazione Santa Lucia IRCCS, Rome, Italy

2 Max Planck Institute for Biological Cybernetics, Tübingen, Germany

References

[1] Arja, S. K., Feng, Z., Chen, Z., Caprihan, A., Kiehl, K. A., Adali, T., & Calhoun, V. D. (2010). Changes in fMRI magnitude data and phase data observed in block-design and event-related tasks. *Neuroimage*, 49(4), 3149-3160.

[2] Balla, D., Sanchez-panchuelo, R. M., Wharton, S., Hagberg, G. E., Scheffler, K., Francis, S. T., & Bowtell, R. (2012). Functional quantitative susceptibility mapping (fQSM). Proc Intl Soc Mag Reson Med. 20 :325.

[3] Barmet, C., De Zanche, N., & Pruessmann, K. P. (2008). Spatiotemporal magnetic field monitoring for MR. Magn Reson Med. , 60(1), 187-97.

[4] Bernstein, M. A., Thomasson, D. M., & Perman, W. H. (1989). Improved detectability in low signal-to-noise ratio magnetic resonance images by means of a phase-corrected real reconstruction. Med Phys. , 16(5), 813-817.

[5] Boxerman, J. L., Hamberg, L. M., Rosen, B. R., & Weisskoff, R. M. (1995). MR contrast due to intravascular magnetic susceptibility perturbations Magn Reson Med.; , 34(4), 555-566.

[6] Brainovich, V., Sabatini, U., & Hagberg, G. E. (2009). Advantages of using multiple-echo image combination and asymmetric triangular phase masking in magnetic resonance venography at 3 T. Magn Reson Imaging 27(1) , 23 EOF-37 EOF.

[7] Bretthorst, G. L. (2008). Automatic phasing of MR images. Part II: Voxel-wise phase estim. ationJournal of Magnetic Resonance , 191-193.

[8] Chen, Z., & Calhoun, V. D. Magnitude and Phase Behavior of Multiresolution BOLD Signal. (2010). Conc Magn Reson B 37B(3) , 129 EOF-145 EOF.

[9] Cusack, R., & Papadikis, N. (2002). New robust 3-D phase unwrapping algorithms: application to magnetic field mapping and undistorting echoplanar images. *Neuroimage*, 16, 754-764.

[10] Durrant, C. J., Hertzberg, M. P., & Kuchel, P. W. (2003). Magnetic susceptibility: further insights into macroscopic and microscopic fields and the sphere of Lorentz. ConcMagn. Reson. 18A(1): 72- 95.

[11] Feng, Z., Caprihan, A., Blagoev, K. B., & Calhoun, V. D. (2009). Biophysical modeling of phase changes in BOLD fMRI. *Neuroimage*, 47(2), 540-548.

[12] Foerster, B. U., Tomasi, D., & Caparelli, E. C. (2005). Magnetic field shift due to mechanical vibration in functional magnetic resonance imaging. Magn Reson Med 54(5) , 1261 EOF-7 EOF.

[13] Glover, G. H. (1999). Deconvolution of Impulse Response in Event-Related BOLD fMRI. *NeuroImage*, 9, 416-429.

[14] Glover, G. H., Li, T. Q., & Ress, D. (2000). Image-based method for retrospective correction of physiological motion effects in fMRI: RETROICOR. Magn Reson Med 44(1), , 162 EOF-7 EOF.

[15] Gudbjartsson, H., & Patz, S. (1995). The Rician distribution of noisy MRI data. Magn Reson Med 34(6) , 910 EOF-4 EOF.

[16] Hagberg, G. E., Bianciardi, M., Brainovich, V., Cassarà, A. M., & Maraviglia, B. (2008). The effect of physiological noise in phase functional *magnetic resonance imaging*from blood oxygen level-dependent effects to direct detection of neuronal currents. Magn Reson Imaging 26(7), , 1026 EOF-1040 EOF.

[17] Hagberg, G. E., Welch, E. B., & Greiser, A. (2010). The sign convention for phase values on different vendor systems: definition and implications for susceptibility-weighted imaging. Magn Reson Imaging. , 28(2), 297-300.

[18] Hagberg, G. E., Bianciardi, M., Brainovich, V., Cassarà, A. M., & Maraviglia, B. (2012). Phase stability in fMRI time series: effect of noise regression, off-resonance correction and spatial filtering techniques. *Neuroimage*, 59(4), 3748-3761.

[19] Hahn, A. D., Nencka, A. S., & Rowe, D. B. (2009). Improving robustness and reliability of phase-sensitive fMRI analysis using temporal off-resonance alignment of single-echo timeseries (TOAST). *Neuroimage*, 44(3), 742-52.

[20] Hoogenraad, F. G., Pouwels, P. J., Hofman, M. B., Reichenbach, J. R., Sprenger, M., & Haacke, E. M. (2001). Quantitative differentiation between BOLD models in fMRI. Magn Reson Med. , 45(2), 233-246.

[21] Hu, X., Le, T. H., Parrish, T., & Erhard, P. (1995). Retrospective estimation and correction of physiological fluctuation in functional MRI. Magn Reson Med 34(2) , 201 EOF-12 EOF.

[22] Jenkinson, M. (2003). Fast, automated N-dimensional phase-unwrapping algorithm. Magn Reson Med. 49(1), 193-197.

[23] Kiselev, V. G., & Posse, S. (1999). Analytical model of susceptibility-induced MR signal dephasing: effect of diffusion in a microvascular network. Magn Reson Med. , 41(3), 499-509.

[24] Krüger, G., & Glover, G. H. (2001). Physiological Noise in Oxygenation-Sensitive Magnetic Resonance Imaging. Magn Reson Med 46(4) , 631 EOF-7 EOF.

[25] Le, T. H., & Hu, X. (1996). Retrospective estimation and correction of physiological artifacts in fMRI by direct extraction of physiological activity from MR data. Magn Reson Med 35(3) , 290 EOF-8 EOF.

[26] Logothetis, N. K. (2008). What we can do and what we cannot do with fMRI. *Nature*, 453(7197), 869-78.

[27] Mansfield, P. (1977). Multi-planar image formation using NMR spinechoes. 1. Phys. C. 10:LL58., 55.

[28] Marques, J. P., & Bowtell, R. (2005). Application of a Fourier-based method for rapid calculation of field inhomogeneity due to spatial variation of magnetic susceptibility. Concepts Magn Reson Part B 25B , 65-78.

[29] Menon, R. (2002). Postacquisition Suppression of Large-Vessel BOLD Signals in High-Resolution fMRI Magn Reson Med 47(1), 1-9.

[30] Ogawa, S., Lee, T. M., Nayak, A. S., & Glynn, P. (1990). Oxygenation-sensitive contrast in magnetic resonance image of rodent brain at high magnetic fields. Magn Reson Med. , 14(1), 68-78.

[31] Ogawa, S., Tank, D. W., Menon, R., Ellermann, J. M., Kim, S. G., Merkle, H., & Ugurbil, K. (1992). Intrinsic signal changes accompanying sensory stimulation: functional

brain mapping with magnetic resonance imaging. Proc Natl Acad Sci U S A. , 89(13), 5951-5955.

[32] Ogawa, S., Menon, R. S., Tank, D. W., Kim, S. G., Merkle, H., Ellermann, J. M., & Ugurbil, K. (1993). Functional brain mapping by blood oxygenation level-dependent contrast magnetic resonance imaging. A comparison of signal characteristics with a biophysical model. Biophys J , 64(3), 803-812.

[33] Pfeuffer, J. Van de Moortele P.-F, Ugurbil K, Hu X, Glover GH, (2002). Correction of Physiologically Induced Global Off-Resonance Effects in Dynamic Echo-Planar and Spiral Functional Imaging. Magn Reson Med. , 10, 344-353.

[34] Petridou, N., Schäfer, A., Gowland, P., & Bowtell, R. (2009). Phase vs. magnitude information in functional *magnetic resonance imaging*time series: toward understanding the noise. Magn Reson Imaging 27(8) , 1046 EOF-57 EOF.

[35] Raj, D., Paley, D. P., Anderson, A. W., Kennan, R. P., & Gore, J. C. (2000). A model for susceptibility artefacts from respiration in functional echo-planar magnetic resonance imaging. Phys Med Biol 45(12) , 3809 EOF-20 EOF.

[36] Rowe, D. B., & Logan, B. R. (2004). A complex way to compute fMRI activation. *Neuroimage,* 1078 EOF-1092 EOF.

[37] Rowe, D. B. (2005). Modeling both the magnitude and phase of complex-valued fMRI data. *Neuroimage,* 25, 1310-1324.

[38] Schmitt, F., Stehling, M. K., & Turner, R. (1998). Echo-Planar Imaging: Theory, Technique and Application. Springer Verlag

[39] Van Gelderen, P., De Zwart, J. A., Starewicz, P., Hinks, R. S., & Duyn, J. H. (2007). Real-time shimmingto compensate for respiration induced Bo fluctuations. Magn Reson Med , 57, 362-368.

[40] Tomasi, D. G., & Caparelli, E. G. (2007). Macrovascular cobtribution in activation patterns of working memory. J Cereb Blood Flow Metab , 27, 33-42.

[41] Vannesjo, SJ, Haeberlin, M, Kasper, L, Pavan, M, Wilm, BJ, Barmet, C, & Pruessmann, KP. (2012). . Gradient system characterization by impulse response measurements with a dynamic field camera. Magn Reson Med. doi: 10.1002/mrm.24263.

[42] Yablonskiy, D. A., & Haacke, E. M. (1994). Theory of NMR signal behaviour in magnetically inhomogeneous tissues: the static dephasing regime. Magn Reson Med , 32(6), 749-763.

[43] Zhao, F., Jin, T., Wang, P., Hu, X., & Kim, S. G. (2007). Sources of phase changes in BOLD and CBV-weighted fMRI. Magn Reson Med , 57, 520-527.

Permissions

All chapters in this book were first published by InTech Open; hereby published with permission under the Creative Commons Attribution License or equivalent. Every chapter published in this book has been scrutinized by our experts. Their significance has been extensively debated. The topics covered herein carry significant findings which will fuel the growth of the discipline. They may even be implemented as practical applications or may be referred to as a beginning point for another development.

The contributors of this book come from diverse backgrounds, making this book a truly international effort. This book will bring forth new frontiers with its revolutionizing research information and detailed analysis of the nascent developments around the world.

We would like to thank all the contributing authors for lending their expertise to make the book truly unique. They have played a crucial role in the development of this book. Without their invaluable contributions this book wouldn't have been possible. They have made vital efforts to compile up to date information on the varied aspects of this subject to make this book a valuable addition to the collection of many professionals and students.

This book was conceptualized with the vision of imparting up-to-date information and advanced data in this field. To ensure the same, a matchless editorial board was set up. Every individual on the board went through rigorous rounds of assessment to prove their worth. After which they invested a large part of their time researching and compiling the most relevant data for our readers.

The editorial board has been involved in producing this book since its inception. They have spent rigorous hours researching and exploring the diverse topics which have resulted in the successful publishing of this book. They have passed on their knowledge of decades through this book. To expedite this challenging task, the publisher supported the team at every step. A small team of assistant editors was also appointed to further simplify the editing procedure and attain best results for the readers.

Apart from the editorial board, the designing team has also invested a significant amount of their time in understanding the subject and creating the most relevant covers. They scrutinized every image to scout for the most suitable representation of the subject and create an appropriate cover for the book.

The publishing team has been an ardent support to the editorial, designing and production team. Their endless efforts to recruit the best for this project, has resulted in the accomplishment of this book. They are a veteran in the field of academics and their pool of knowledge is as vast as their experience in printing. Their expertise and guidance has proved useful at every step. Their uncompromising quality standards have made this book an exceptional effort. Their encouragement from time to time has been an inspiration for everyone.

The publisher and the editorial board hope that this book will prove to be a valuable piece of knowledge for researchers, students, practitioners and scholars across the globe.

List of Contributors

Reza Farivar
Massachusetts General Hospital and Harvard Medical School, USA
McGill Vision Research Unit, McGill University, Canada

Wim Vanduffel
Massachusetts General Hospital and Harvard Medical School, USA
Katholieke Universiteit Leuven, Belgium

Yeji Han, Sung Suk Oh and HyunWook Park
Korea Advanced Institute of Science and Technology, Republic of Korea

Joong Koo Kang
Asan Medical Center, Republic of Korea

Wei Gao, Weili Lin and Dinggang Shen
Department of Radiology and Biomedical Research Imaging Center, UNC-Chapel Hill, USA

Hongtu Zhu
Department of Biostatistics and Biomedical Research Imaging Center, UNC-Chapel Hill, USA

Kelly S. Giovanello
Department of Psychology and Biomedical Research Imaging Center, UNC-Chapel Hill, USA

J. Keith Smith
Department of Radiology, UNC-Chapel Hill, USA

John H. Gilmore
Department of Psychiatry, UNC-Chapel Hill, USA

John Schlerf
Johns Hopkins University, USA

Timothy Verstynen
Carnegie Mellon University, USA

Tobias Wiestler and Jörn Diedrichsen
University College London, UK

Nasser H Kashou
The Children's Radiological Institute, Nationwide Children's Hospital, USA

Hiroki Yamamoto
Graduate School of Human and Environmental Studies, Kyoto University, Japan

Luis Hernandez-Garcia and Hesamoddin Jahanian
University of Michigan, FMRI Laboratory, USA

Christopher W. Tyler and Lora T. Likova
Smith-Kettlewell Eye Research Institute, USA

Gisela E. Hagberg
Fondazione Santa Lucia IRCCS, Rome, Italy
Max Planck Institute for Biological Cybernetics, Tübingen, Germany

Elisa Tuzzi
Fondazione Santa Lucia IRCCS, Rome, Italy

Index

www.ingramcontent.com/pod-product-compliance
Lightning Source LLC
LaVergne TN
LVHW080625210926
848485LV00003B/213